Psychological Insights for Understanding COVID-19 and Families, Parents, and Children

With specially commissioned introductions from international experts, the *Psychological Insights for Understanding COVID-19* series draws together previously published chapters on key themes in psychological science that engage with people's unprecedented experience of the pandemic.

This volume collects chapters that address prominent issues and challenges presented by the SARS-CoV-2 pandemic to families, parents, and children. A new introduction from Marc H. Bornstein reviews how disasters are known to impact families, parents, and children and explores traditional and novel responsibilities of parents and their effects on child growth and development. It examines parenting at this time, detailing consequences for home life and economies that the pandemic has triggered; considers child discipline and abuse during the pandemic; and makes recommendations that will support families in terms of multilevel interventions at family, community, and national and international levels. The selected chapters elucidate key themes including children's worry, stress and parenting, positive parenting programs, barriers which constrain population-level impact of prevention programs, and the importance of culturally adapting evidence-based family intervention programs.

Featuring theory and research on key topics germane to the global pandemic, the *Psychological Insights for Understanding COVID-19* series offers thought-provoking reading for professionals, students, academics, policy makers, and parents concerned with the psychological consequences of COVID-19 for individuals, families, and society.

Marc H. Bornstein holds positions at the *Eunice Kennedy Shriver* National Institute of Child Health and Human Development, the Institute for Fiscal Studies, and UNICEF. He is President Emeritus of the Society for Research in Child Development, Editor Emeritus of *Child Development*, and founding Editor of *Parenting: Science and Practice*. Bornstein has written and edited several books, including the five-volume *Handbook of Parenting* for Routledge.

Psychological Insights for Understanding COVID-19

The *Psychological Insights for Understanding COVID-19* series aims to highlight important themes in psychological science that engage with people's unprecedented experience of the COVID-19 pandemic. These short, accessible volumes draw together chapters as they originally appeared before COVID-19 descended on the world but demonstrate how researchers and professionals in psychological science had developed theory and research on key topics germane to the global pandemic. Each volume includes a specially commissioned, expert introduction that contextualises the chapters in relation to the crisis, reflects on the relevance of psychological research during this significant global event, and proposes future research and vital interventions that elucidate understanding and coping with COVID-19. With individual volumes exploring society, health, family, work and media, the *Psychological Insights for Understanding COVID-19* series offers thought-provoking reading for professionals, students, academics and policy makers concerned with psychological consequences of the pandemic for individuals, families and society.

Titles in the series:

Psychological Insights for Understanding COVID-19 and Families, Parents, and Children
Edited by Marc H. Bornstein

Psychological Insights for Understanding COVID-19 and Media and Technology
Edited by Ciarán Mc Mahon

Psychological Insights for Understanding COVID-19 and Society
Edited by S. Alexander Haslam

Psychological Insights for Understanding COVID-19 and Work
Edited by Cary L. Cooper

Psychological Insights for Understanding COVID-19 and Health
Edited by Dominika Kwasnicka and Robbert Sanderman

For more information about this series, please visit: www.routledge.com/Psychological-Insights-for-Understanding-COVID-19/book-series/COVID

Psychological Insights for Understanding COVID-19 and Families, Parents, and Children

Edited by Marc H. Bornstein

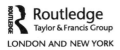
Routledge
Taylor & Francis Group

LONDON AND NEW YORK

First published 2021
by Routledge
2 Park Square, Milton Park, Abingdon, Oxon OX14 4RN

and by Routledge
52 Vanderbilt Avenue, New York, NY 10017

Routledge is an imprint of the Taylor & Francis Group, an informa business

British Library Cataloguing-in-Publication Data
A catalogue record for this book is available from the British Library

Library of Congress Cataloging-in-Publication Data
A catalog record for this book has been requested

ISBN: 978-0-367-68300-9 (hbk)
ISBN: 978-0-367-68298-9 (pbk)
ISBN: 978-1-003-13681-1 (ebk)

Typeset in Times New Roman
by Apex CoVantage, LLC

Selected chapters are taken from the following original Routledge publications

Emotional Development from Infancy to Adolescence: Pathways to Emotional Competence and Emotional Problems
Dale F. Hay
ISBN: 978-1-84872-014-5 (pbk) ISBN: 978-1-31584-945-4 (ebk)

Family Based Prevention Programs for Children and Adolescents: Theory, Research, and Large-Scale Dissemination
Edited By Mark J. Van Ryzin, Karol L. Kumpfer, Gregory M. Fosco and Mark T. Greenberg
ISBN: 978-1-84872-485-3 (pbk) ISBN: 978-1-315-76491-7 (ebk)

Handbook of Parenting: Volume 4: Social Conditions and Applied Parenting, Third Edition
Edited By Marc H. Bornstein
ISBN: 978-1-138-67081-5 (pbk) ISBN: 978-0-429-39899-5 (ebk)

Positive Youth Development in Global Contexts of Social and Economic Change
Edited by Anne C. Petersen, Sílvia H. Koller, Frosso Motti-Stefanidi, and Suman Verma
ISBN: 978-1-138-67081-5 (pbk) ISBN: 978-1-315-30727-5 (ebk)

Understanding Children's Worry: Clinical, Developmental and Cognitive Psychological Perspectives
Charlotte Wilson
ISBN: 978-0-8153-7888-4 (pbk) ISBN: 978-1-351-22766-7 (ebk)

Contents

Contributors

Katharine T. Bamberger, Department of Human Development and Family Studies, Pennsylvania State University, USA.

Bernadine Brady, School of Political Science & Sociology, National University of Ireland, Galway, Galway, Ireland.

Jeanne Brooks-Gunn, Columbia University's Teachers College and College of Physicians and Surgeons, USA.

Brian Bumbarger, Evidence-based Prevention and Intervention Support Center, Pennsylvania State University, USA.

Shayna S. Coburn, George Washington University School of Medicine and Health Sciences, USA.

Keith A. Crnic, Department of Psychology, Arizona State University, USA.

Patricio Cumsille, Pontificia Universidad Católica de Chile, Chile.

Pat Dolan, National University of Ireland, Galway, Ireland.

David L. DuBois, School of Public Health, University of Illinois at Chicago, USA.

Gregory M. Fosco, Department of Human Development and Family Studies, Pennsylvania State University, USA.

Mary Agnes Hamilton, Cornell University, USA.

Stephen F. Hamilton, Bronfenbrenner Center for Translational Research, Cornell University, USA.

Wen-Jui Han, School of Social Work, New York University, USA.

Nina Philipsen Hetzner, Office of Planning, Research, and Evaluation, Administration for Children and Families in Health and Human Services, USA.

Sheetal Kanse, Continuing Education and Community Engagement, University of Utah, USA.

Karol L. Kumpfer, Department of Health Promotion and Education, University of Utah, USA.

Catia Magalhães, Department of Psychology and Education Sciences, Polytechnic Institute of Viseu, Portugal.

M. Loreto Martínez, Pontificia Universidad Católica de Chile, Chile.

Jenna McWilliam, School of Psychology, The University of Queensland, Australia.

Susana Núñez Rodriguez, University Salgado de Oliveira, Brazil.

Matthew R. Sanders, Parenting and Family Support Centre, University of Queensland, Australia.

Deborah E. Sellers, Bronfenbrenner Center for Translational Research, Cornell University, USA.

Karen M. T. Turner, Parenting and Family Support Centre, University of Queensland, Australia.

Charlotte Wilson, University of Dublin, Trinity College, Ireland.

Jing Xie, Cultural and Health Research Center, University of Houston, USA.

Introduction: The SARS-CoV-2 pandemic

Issues for families, parents, and children

Marc H. Bornstein

> *Chuck Woolery, for three decades the host of wildly popular game shows on U.S. television, such as 'Love Connection,' 'Wheel of Fortune,' and 'Scrabble,' tweeted to his 691,000 followers that 'Masks are nothing more than a symbol of capitulation,' and that 'Everyone is lying' about the virus – 'the CDC, Media, Democrats, our Doctors.'*
>
> *Woolery soon after deleted his Twitter account announcing that his son had tested positive for the coronavirus.*

The 2020 SARS-CoV-2 pandemic triggered an unprecedented series of events that upended the lives of families, parents, and children around the globe. The pandemic constitutes the worst public health crisis in a century and cratered economies, skyrocketed unemployment, and disrupted most aspects of everyday life. It shuttered businesses, schools, daycares, camps, libraries, and parks and isolated families in their homes with little outside support. The pandemic also fomented continuing and deep uncertainties about how families, parents, and children should conduct their lives during the spread of the disease and into the future.

At this writing in the fall of 2020, the novel coronavirus has taken a grim and tragic toll on the world's population, exceeding 50,000,000 confirmed infected people and 1,250,000 total deaths across 190 countries and regions worldwide (coronavirus.jhu.edu). These numbers certainly represent undercounts of true values (on account of limitations on testing) and are equally certain to continue mounting. As the world awaits a vaccine against SARS-CoV-2, families, parents, and children must rely on their own and their communities' informed and considerate behaviors. During the pandemic, vulnerabilities of families, parents, and children were exposed or exacerbated by community lockdowns, business failures, protective and other service suspensions, and childcare and school closures that were deemed necessary to slow the spread of the disease – "flatten the curve" (Mervosh, Lu, & Swales, 2020).

Where do families, parents, and children fit in the unfolding drama of the global SARS-CoV-2 pandemic? Everywhere, as it turns out. Family life and effective parenting are central to children's well-being and to their achieving their potential (Bornstein, 2019). Families and parents are responsible for children's physical well-being and mental health, their growth and development, their safety and protection; families and parents organize children's environments, experiences, and opportunities for learning and in life. With unexpected suddenness, the SARS-CoV-2 pandemic cast parents as children's and families' "first responders," and parents across the globe have been challenged to care for their families and children in novel and numerous ways in the face of unprecedented circumstances.

This timely volume collects chapters (as they were originally published) that felicitously address several prominent issues and challenges presented by the SARS-CoV-2 pandemic to families, parents, and children. This introduction first provides a short history (to date) of the SARS-CoV-2 pandemic and reviews some general information on how disasters like the pandemic are known to impact families, parents, and children. The novel coronavirus which gave rise to the pandemic has proved to follow a highly idiosyncratic, variable, unpredictable, and kaleidoscopically changing course, so even by the time of publication or reading this collection, some information in this volume may have fallen out of date. However, the material presented in this chapter constitutes a faithful representation of the state of affairs for families, parents, and children at this juncture in the SARS-CoV-2 pandemic in the fall of 2020, and the general information in the chapters reprinted here is relevant now as it will be into the foreseeable future.

This introductory chapter next discusses where families, parents, and children fit into developmental and parenting sciences that focus on responsibilities of parents and their meaningfulness for child growth and development. The introduction then turns specifically to consider parenting in the time of SARS-CoV-2 detailing consequences for home life and economies that the pandemic has triggered. Childcare privation and school closures have tasked parents with significantly greater caregiving, didactic, disciplinary, and managerial responsibilities than they normally shoulder. The introduction concludes with a brief case study application to the fraught issue of child discipline and abuse during the pandemic and recommendations that will support families, parents, and children in terms of multilevel interventions at family, community, and national and international levels.

The SARS-CoV-2 pandemic

A brief history of the COVID-19 disease and pandemic

Coronavirus and COVID-19. A coronavirus is a type of infectious agent. Strains of coronaviridae have circulated among human beings as well as many species of mammals historically and are known to cause predominately respiratory tract illnesses. Coronavirus is one of the most common etiologies of the common cold as well as lower respiratory tract infections, behind only rhinovirus (Mäkelä et al., 1998). In December 2019, a novel coronavirus (because it was not previously identified) emerged in Wuhan, China, and on 11 February 2020 was named by the World Health Organization (WHO, 2020a) "coronavirus disease 2019" (initially 2019-nCoV, eventually COVID-19; Gorbalenya et al., 2020). This coronavirus causes a severe acute respiratory syndrome (the second of its kind, hence SARS-CoV-2) and is the virus responsible for the pandemic that engulfed the globe in

2020. The virus that causes COVID-19 may have originated in the horseshoe bat, however exactly how SARS-CoV-2 entered the human population is (at this writing) unknown. Indeed, as will become clear, numerous facets and features of this disease – from genetic and biological to behavioral and epidemiological – continue to be shrouded in mystery, and as will also become abundantly clear the unquestionable watchword of the COVID-19 pandemic is *uncertainty*. The WHO (2020b) declared the COVID-19 outbreak a Public Health Emergency of International Concern on 30 January 2020 and a "pandemic" on 11 March 2020. COVID-19 arrived in our homes early in 2020 and in blazingly short order altered daily life for families, parents, and children. An updated chronology of SARS-CoV-2 can be found at https://en.wikipedia.org/wiki/Timeline_of_the_COVID-19_pandemic.

When it emerged, the coronavirus was (as indicated) novel to the world. In consequence, all key characteristics of the disease were shrouded in uncertainty, and germane to this volume each of the following characteristics of the virus has presented troubling to dire implications for the adjustment and well-being of families, parents, and children.

Diagnosis and symptomatology. COVID-19 has proved to be a highly unpredictable and potentially deadly infectious disease. Considerable uncertainty surrounded early diagnosis of COVID-19 in large measure because of vast individual differences in symptomatology, in severity of disease, in organ involvement, and in testing. First, COVID-19 patients run the full gamut from asymptomatic to those who easily sustain a transient headache or low-grade fever or temporarily lose smell and taste to those with more symptoms severe enough to warrant hospitalization or confinement to Intensive Care Units (ICU) with ventilation-assisted breathing for extended periods to "long-haulers" who partially recover but endure symptoms for months to the now million who have tragically succumbed to the disease. About 40 percent of COVID-19 cases are asymptomatic, 40 percent experience only mild or passing symptoms, 15 percent have more severe infections (perhaps requiring oxygen), and 5 percent have critical infections requiring ICU care and ventilation (Beigel et al., 2020; Cha, 2020). COVID-19 carries a mortality rate that exceeds those of flus (Layne, Hyman, Morens, & Taubenberger, 2020; Schuchat, 2020).

COVID-19 is primarily a respiratory disease, with the coronavirus embedding itself into the lungs and compromising breathing. Early symptoms of infection expectedly include cough and shortness of breath (in 73 percent of patients younger than 18 years of age and in 93 percent of patients 18 to 64 years of age) and (in line with its association with colds) headache, sore throat, runny nose, and fever and chills, which appear as soon as two days or as long as two weeks after exposure to the virus (American College of Emergency Physicians, 2020).

However, this coronavirus was also revealed to affect other body organs, including the brain, heart and blood vessels, liver and kidneys, and the gastrointestinal tract (nausea and diarrhea are additional symptoms; Fifield, 2020). One-quarter to one-third of patients experience neurological dysfunction, and a small percentage suffer "impaired consciousness" (Koralnik & Tyler, 2020). Cardiovascular complications, including stroke, are also common; a study in Germany reported that nearly 80 percent of COVID-19 patients had heart abnormalities several months after infection (Puntmann et al., 2020). *In extremis*, COVID-19 triggers an intense inflammatory response in the immune system ("cytokine storm") which sometimes proved fatal by itself (Ragab, Eldin, Taeimah, Khattab, & Salem, 2020).

A particularly worrisome condition that came to be recognized only as the pandemic persisted is a diversity of lingering symptoms in patients months after clearing viral infection. These "long-haulers" (at least 23,000 of whom formed a Facebook group: Long Covid Support Group) complain of brain fog, trouble breathing, elevated heart rate, leg pain, hair loss, depression, and severe fatigue (Cleveland Clinic, 2020). In accord with the multisystem syndrome that is COVID-19, one long-hauler reportedly consults a pulmonologist, a cardiologist, a neurologist, a respiratory therapist, a physical therapist, and a social worker (Bernstein, 2020). So far, there appears to be no clear determination when or if long-hauler symptoms subside. As reported in one British study, an estimated 10 percent of COVID-19 patients suffer such prolonged symptoms (Greenhalgh, Knight, A'Court, Buxton, & Husain, 2020). In March 2020 soon after the outbreak in China, coronavirus emerged for an unprepared population in Bergamo, Italy. Now in the fall of 2020 half a year later, among the first 750 survivors screened, approximately 30 percent have lung scarring and breathing trouble, and an additional 30 percent have problems associated with inflammation and clotting, such as heart abnormalities and artery blockages (Harlan & Pitrelli, 2020). A confirming study of 100 patients who had recovered from COVID-19 documented some form of heart abnormality in 78 percent of these cases, despite the lack of a relevant preexisting condition (Puntmann et al., 2020).

Testing for COVID-19 has presented a raft of challenges. Tests for coronavirus come in two general lots. Tests that diagnose the presence of coronavirus through analysis of viral genetic material in fluid samples from the nose and throat (e.g., polymerase chain reaction or antigen) and tests that determine whether one had coronavirus through serological analysis of antibodies (U.S. Centers for Disease Control and Prevention [CDC], 2020a).

Antibodies are proteins in the blood produced by the immune system made in response to infections. Antibodies show the body's efforts to fight off an infection and are present after recovery. The presence of antibodies indicates likely past infection and may also indicate some immunity, but not how much or for how long. Tests return results in minutes, while others take several days. All tests are in some degree inaccurate and unreliable. Test quality is a first-order factor: A good test has 95 percent sensitivity and 95 percent specificity, meaning that even a good test is wrong 5 percent of the time. If 1,000,000 people are tested (a big number but a fraction of any nation's population), that's 50,000 built-in errors . . . for a *good* test.

A "false positive" incorrectly identifies an infection when there is none; a "false negative" fails to identify an infection when there is one. Problematically, a negative test is not dispositive proof of no viral infection. A test might return negative when a person is actually infected for any number of reasons: Timing is one factor (if tested too early in the illness, the amount of virus in the airway may be too little to detect; also, a test is only "valid" for a single point in time as between the time of a test and a negative result a person could become infected); how a test is done may have different levels of accuracy (swab collection may retrieve samples from the back of the nose, the throat, or outer nose and so give different evidence); handling or transport of the swab and laboratory error are additional factors. The U.S. Food and Drug Administration (2020) advised that because test results are not always accurate, symptoms should be a factor in a diagnosis.

Our understanding of the extent of infection – in the family, parent, child, or nation – depends on testing and accuracy of reporting. The number of actual coronavirus infections is likely 2 to 13 times greater than the number of reported cases based on studies of antibodies (Havers et al., 2020). Clearly, less is known than is desirable about the diagnosis and symptomatology of COVID-19. Understanding disease transmission, equally important to families, parents, and children, is growing but still woefully incomplete.

Infection transmission. It quickly became known that the virus spread easily person-to-person. However, critical information was missed early on, compounded by initial uncertainties that surrounded the routes of transmission. On the one hand, as early as February 2020 the disease was spreading throughout Japan, but epidemiological data had already documented that people with no or few symptoms could disseminate the disease and that certain conditions promoted its dissemination (now known as "super-spreader events"; Oshitani, 2020). On the other hand, the virus was first thought to linger on surfaces, according to a March 2020 report (National Institutes of Health, 2020), so frequent hand washing, avoiding touching the face, nose, and eyes, and disinfecting countertops, door handles, food packaging, and other frequently touched places became public health preventative measures. In May 2020 the CDC (2020b) updated its guidelines to state that, although surface transmission is possible, it was no longer thought to be the main route by which the virus transmits. By July 2020 scientific opinion in some quarters had changed (radically) to view deep cleaning services in restaurants, on airplanes, and at other public places as merely "an expensive distraction" (Thompson, 2020).

After several notable false starts as late as March 2020 (CDC, 2020c; WHO, 2020c), the coronavirus was eventually recognized to transmit primarily as an airborne disease between individuals in close contact (Morawska & Milton, 2020). When people cough or sneeze, breathe or talk, sing or shout, they ballistically expel the virus in respiratory droplets of different amounts and sizes. Large droplets usually fall to the ground within 15 minutes and within a range of only approximately 6 feet/2 meters (CDC, 2020d), so physical distancing helps to mitigate spread of the virus. After some time and investigation, it became recognized that the virus is also "aerosolized," that is transmitted in small particles that can travel as far as 45 feet and float in the air for hours, thereby potentially transmitting infection at great distances and for long times (Hamner et al., 2020). (One scientist described a theoretical exhalation of coronavirus as akin to the plume of smoke from a cigarette. "Once you get beyond that plume, anything that small enough to stay floating in the air can travel . . . quite far all the way across the room." When inhaled, even aerosols can infect anew. In regard to the essentially airborne transmissibility of the virus, it was eventually recognized that face masks or coverings would offer the most effective approach in preventing droplets of the coronavirus from being exhaled or inhaled (Guarino, Janes, & Cha, 2020; WHO, 2020d).

Before mitigation (e.g., masking), the coronavirus reproduction number was estimated at about 2.5, meaning that each infected person infected an average of two to three other people, similar to a more common influenza. Also, when the pandemic was just beginning, a modeling study revealed that different outcomes would depend on the relative restrictiveness of steps taken to limit transmission of the virus (Ferguson et al., 2020). The study recommended restrictive suppression efforts. Different people and different nations followed nearly the full gamut of possibilities from widespread lockdowns to total disregard. The virus itself also contributed to variation as genetic sequencing revealed continual accumulation of mutations, at least one of which was deemed to have increased contagiousness (Long et al., 2020; Volz et al., 2020): Patients infected with that strain had higher loads of virus in their upper respiratory tracts. We now know that coronavirus transmission is fostered by the "3Vs": voice, venue, and ventilation (in Japanese, *san mitsu*, the 3Cs: closed locations with poor ventilation, crowded places, and close-contact settings where conversations are taking place).

With time and experience, a series of factors that aggregate into "super-spreading" events was identified that relate back to the 3Vs. Poor ventilation in an enclosed venue with people vocalizing, especially for any long duration, greatly increases the probability of infectious spread. Early well-documented cases in which the coronavirus spread rapidly and widely in an enclosed or indoor environment included a restaurant in Guangzhou, China, a bus traveling in China's Zhejiang province, and a call center in Seoul, South Korea (Birnir, 2020). Adults with positive SARS-CoV-2 test results are approximately twice as likely to have reported dining at a restaurant than were those with negative SARS-CoV-2 test results (K. A. Fisher et al., 2020). Widely publicized (and confirming) examples of super-spreading events were then identified as choir practices (Hamner et al., 2020), weddings (Zdanowicz, Jackson, & Orjoux, 2020), summer camps (Szablewski et al., 2020), cruise ships (Moriarty et al., 2020), a motorcycle rally (COVID Alliance, 2020), and even White House gatherings (Mandavilli & Tully, 2020). By the summer and fall of 2020, holiday making and packed bars and nightclubs resulted in mini-epidemics: Foot traffic to bars one week after they reopened is associated with an increase in COVID-19 cases three weeks later (Weiner, Alcantara, & Ba Tran, 2020). However, it has also become clear that people tend to let their mitigation guards (masking, physical distancing, etc.) down in small and informal social gatherings (barbecues, retirement parties, and birth celebrations) that set the stage for viral spread.

To learn the risk in different situations, consult the calculator at https://www.microcovid.org/. Likewise, as a primary route for novel coronavirus spread is through the air, schools, offices, airplanes, and other venues need to gauge the risk of coronavirus transmission: Air changes per hour is a metric (Ossola, 2020).

Distribution of infections. An especially insidious characteristic of the novel coronavirus, identified early in Japan but eventually confirmed through pervasive testing, is that asymptomatic individuals can spread infection (Dong et al., 2020; Götzinger et al., 2020; Huang et al., 2020). Indeed, people with the coronavirus are maximally infectious in the 48 hours just before they develop symptoms (Harvard Medical School, 2020). Likewise, people with certain characteristics, notably underlying health issues, such as cancer, chronic kidney disease, chronic obstructive pulmonary disease, heart conditions, immunocompromised states, obesity, diabetes, and others, proved to be especially vulnerable to the disease (CDC, 2020e) – hence the devastation to nursing homes (which account for 35-40 percent of all COVID-19 deaths in the United States; Burki, 2020; Chidambaram, 2020; Szczerbińska, 2020) and especially high rates of illness and mortality among the elderly and minorities (Mallapatty, 2020). Furthermore, social disparities place certain categories of people (the poor, ethnic minorities) at higher risk: crowded living conditions, food and housing insecurity, being or being related to an essential worker, wealth and education gaps, and difficulty accessing health care because of a lack of family resources or insurance (Hubler, Fuller, Singhvi, & Love, 2020).

COVID-19 proved to be an equal opportunity disease, infecting babies as well as presidents. Once sufficient public health data had aggregated, however, illness and mortality from the novel coronavirus that gave rise to the COVID-19 pandemic were found to be cruelly biased in the sense that the pandemic struck different "social addresses" with unequal ferocity. Consider the following U.S. national and international statistics:

• Age. The pandemic follows a steep age gradient such that older and older individuals have proved to be at increasing risk of the most severe symptoms, hospitalizations, and death rates (CDC, 2020f). Eight out of every 10 deaths attributed to COVID-19 in the United States have stricken adults 65 and older (CDC, 2020g; Mallapatty, 2020). This is not to say that young people are immune (bald assertions from the highest government officials to the contrary notwithstanding). As mentioned, young people tend to suffer few or mild or brief symptoms, require hospitalization less often, and succumb to the disease at much lower rates than adults (Kim et al., 2020; Lu et al., 2020; Smith, 2020), even if exceptional and worrisome cases regularly arose in both symptom severity and mortality among the young. By September 2020, there were more than 500,000 child COVID-19 cases in the United States, with children representing 10 percent of the cumulative number of reported cases, 1.7 percent of total hospitalizations, and 0.07 percent of total deaths (0.01 percent of child cases result in death; American Academy of Pediatrics, 2020a; Leeb et al., 2020; Sisk, Cull, Harris, Rothenburger, & Olson, 2020). There is even a steep mortality age gradient among children: Only 10 percent of deaths occurred in infants age 1 or younger, 20 percent between ages 1 and 9, and 70 percent between ages 10 and 20 (Bixler et al., 2020).

At a political rally in Swanton, Ohio, on 21 September 2020, President of the United States Donald J. Trump incorrectly claimed that COVID-19 affects "nobody young. Below the age of 18, like, nobody. They have a strong immune system, who knows? . . . But it affects virtually nobody. It's an amazing thing" (https://www.washingtonpost.com/nation/2020/09/22/trump-coronavirus-young-people/). However, as reported by Bob Woodward (2020) in his book *Rage*, in an interview on 19 March 2020 Trump told the *Washington Post* associate editor that the coronavirus affected "plenty of young people. . . . Now it's turning out it's not just old people, Bob. . . . Young people too, plenty of young people" (https://ix.cnn.io/projects/2020/trump-woodward-audio-embeds/index.html?src=./data/audio-transcript-05.json).

The novel coronavirus behaves differently from other viruses, such as seasonal influenza. Most viruses pose dangers for the very young and very old. Why, then, most children have no symptoms or only mild disease remains another mystery. Likely, valuable treatment information could be gleaned from answering why.

- Gender. Men and women catch the virus at similar rates, but men disproportionately die from the disease (57 percent of U.S. deaths; Griffiths et al., 2020; Mallapatty, 2020).
- Ethnicity. Across a number of indicators – financial to mortality – Latin, African, and Native Americans have been more adversely affected by COVID-19 than European Americans (NPR, Robert Johnson Wood Foundation, & Harvard T. H. Chan School of Public Health, 2020). Latin (72 percent), African (60 percent), and Native American (55 percent) households report facing serious COVID-19 induced financial problems, while fewer European American (36 percent) households so report. As to infection rates, one U.S. study examined leftover blood plasma samples from a randomly selected group of 28,500 kidney dialysis patients at one of 1,300 centers in 46 states in July 2020 (Anand et al., 2020). Testing revealed about 8 percent of patients had coronavirus antibodies, unequally distributed among ethnicities: 16 percent for patients who lived in majority African American communities and 11 percent in majority Latin American communities against 4 percent in European American communities. The coronavirus also hospitalizes and kills Latin, African, and Native American children and adults in much higher numbers than their European American peers (Bixler et al., 2020; Rodriguez-Diaz et al., 2020; Thebault, Ba Tran, & Williams, 2020; Thebault & Fowers, 2020). For example, adjusted for population the Navajo Nation reported more virus deaths than any U.S. state (Navajo Nation Department of Health, 2020). Latin American children are approximately 8 times more likely, and African American children 5 times more likely, to be hospitalized with COVID-19 than their European American peers (Kim et al., 2020). Of children who perished because of COVID-19, more than 75 percent have been Latin (45 percent), African (29 percent), or Native American (4 percent), even though these minorities represent only 41 percent of the U.S. population (Bixler et al., 2020).

- Income. Of households with annual incomes below $100,000, 54 percent reported facing serious financial problems during the coronavirus outbreak, compared with 20 percent of households with annual incomes of $100,000 or more (NPR et al., 2020). In England before the lockdown, learning time among primary school children was fairly homogeneous; during the lockdown, the richest third of primary school children spent about 4.5 hours per week more on distance learning than the poorest third of primary school children (Andrew et al., 2020a).
- Region. The U.S. plasma dialysis study referred to earlier revealed a stark variation in infections by zip code, with a 10-fold higher risk for patients living in urban compared to rural settings (Anand et al., 2020). When it appeared, the coronavirus tended first to strike more densely populated urban areas across nations. The dialysis study was conducted in July 2020. By October 2020, the virus had spread to rural U.S. communities, far from the coastal cities stricken early in the pandemic (Achenbach & Dupree, 2020).
- Political party affiliation. A July 2020 survey found that Democrats ranked the coronavirus pandemic as first of the top five leading threats to U.S. vital interests (followed by climate change, racial inequality, foreign interference in U.S. elections, and economic inequality); the coronavirus pandemic did not even rank in the top five for Republicans (Smeltz, Daalder, Friedhoff, Kafura, & Helm, 2020). Mask wearing became a politicized statement in the United States, with Democrats more likely than Republicans to wear a mask all or most of the time (Igielnik, 2020). Little wonder that by October 2020, U.S. counties with the most intense leanings toward Republicans witnessed the largest increases in COVID-19 cases, whereas counties that lean Democratic tended to be flat (Achenbach & Dupree, 2020).
- Nation. It has been observed that no one factor determines so much about a person's lifecourse as the country where the person is born. The United States has approximately 4 percent of the world's population but more than 25 percent of global COVID-19 cases (Williams & Sedgwick, 2020). COVID-19 kills 103 and 89 Peruvians and Belgians per 100,000 population, respectively, whereas Vietnamese and Taiwanese suffer rates of 0.04 and 0.03, respectively (Johns Hopkins University of Medicine, 2020). COVID-19 kills 65 people per 100,000 population in the United States and 64 in the United Kingdom.

As was observed relatively early in its spread, the "COVID-19 pandemic is a fundamentally disequalizing event. Its effects are expected to be most damaging for children in the poorest countries [and] on the poorest households within countries" (United Nations Foundation, 2020).

Treatment. At this writing, there is still no cure for COVID-19. Since the descent of the coronavirus on the world, treatment has significantly improved and medical management of patients is becoming routine if still challenged by lack of supporting equipment even in high-income countries (Harris, 2020). Simpler courses of therapy have been learned (supplemental oxygen, expecting and treating complications like blood clots with blood thinners, lying patients prone rather than supine all the time). False starts with some drugs (hydroxychloroquine) were superseded by still experimental steroids (Dexamethasone; RECOVERY Collaborative Group, 2020), antivirals (Remdesivir; Palca, 2020), monoclonal antibodies (REGN-COV2; PR Newswire, 2020), and other medications (convalescent plasma; Harris, 2020; Palca, 2020) to treat sick patients and improve survival around the world (Armstrong, Kane, & Cook, 2020).

Lingering questions. Accurate scientific information is widely acknowledged as critical to guide fundamental everyday choices families, parents, and children face. With all that came to be understood about the COVID-19 infection in a remarkably rapid amount of time, more than three-quarters of a year into the pandemic many basic questions still defy definitive answers. Can just breathing the air where an infected person has passed infect another person with the novel coronavirus? Where and how long does the virus linger in the air and remain infectious? What quantity ("inoculum") or amount of virus exposure infects? Are masks and physical distancing effective against aerosol particles of virus? Are groceries (where most people obtain necessary foodstuffs) safe? How is it safest to patronize a restaurant or store, attend a conference or a concert, or travel by train or plane? Can you contract coronavirus twice? If exposed, for how long should one quarantine; if infected, for how long should one isolate? Where do those incredible individual differences in infectability and symptomatology come from? Which promotes resistance: the "inoculum," family genetics, or a residue of childhood viral exposure? For families, parents, and children, more specific questions abound. Are children and adolescents equally susceptible to catching or avoiding the virus and equally responsible for spreading the virus? Should daycares, schools, and camps open and under what precautions? Do children suffer greater harm from risking disease at school or from lack of in-person schooling? This chapter raises many other still unanswered questions. Six feet/2 meters was a guideline, not a magic number; screening and diagnostic testing proved problematic; language was faulty and misleading with people using "social distancing" when they really meant to use "physical distancing," and using "isolation" (to separate sick people with a contagious disease from people who are not sick) versus "quarantine" (to separate and restrict the movement of people who were exposed to a contagious disease to see if they become sick) interchangeably. Uncertainty is a powerful toxin that begets anxiety, and anxiety erodes physical, mental, and emotional health.

As the first human cases of the infection were identified in China, much early biobehavioral research emanated from there. A preliminary study reported the presence of fear, clinging, inattention, and irritability in Chinese children associated with the COVID-19 pandemic (Jiao et al., 2020). A study of 8,079 junior and senior high school students in China found that approximately 37 percent experienced anxiety and 44 percent experienced depressive symptoms during the epidemic (Zhou et al., 2020). Another survey reported as many as 14 percent of Chinese children experienced more severe symptoms of PTSD (Liang et al., 2020). These sorts of untoward population-level sequelae are not uncommon in the face of disasters and crises of various kinds.

Disasters, families, parents, and children

Natural and manmade disasters are well recognized to cause extensive and damaging physical and mental health to families, parents, and children (Masten, Narayan, Silverman, & Osofsky, 2015; Masten & Palmer, 2019; North, 2016). Posttraumatic stress disorder (PTSD), anxiety, and depression (Bolt, Helming, & Tintle, 2018; Jose, Holman, & Silver, 2019) have been documented in the wake of natural disasters – typhoons (Labarda, Jopson, Hui, & Chan, 2020), earthquakes (Seto, Imamura, & Suppasri, 2019), hurricanes (Fussell & Lowe, 2014), and wildfires (Sprague et al., 2015) – manmade disasters – nuclear catastrophes (Bolt et al., 2018), acts of terror (Calderoni, Alderman, Silver, & Bauman, 2006; Hendricks & Bornstein, 2007; Jose et al., 2019), and political violence (Cárdenas Castro, Arnoso Martínez, & Faúndez Abarca, 2019; Gelkopf, Berger, Bleich, & Silver, 2012) – as well as, of course, earlier public health crises, such as the SARS and H1N1 outbreaks (Hawryluck et al., 2004; Rubin, Amlôt, Page, & Wessely, 2009). Like other disasters, the novel coronavirus propagated traumatic stress, likely aggravated existing mental health difficulties, and led to the emergence of diverse other disorders (Horesh & Brown, 2020). The world has learned that knowledge of anticipated health effects is critical to obviate or respond effectively to disasters to protect families, parents, and children. Hence, the dearth of accurate knowledge about the coronavirus and its course has compounded the physical and medical consequences of COVID-19.

One major public health recommendation to emanate at the onset of the pandemic, and to be reinforced as other public health measures (e.g., face covering, physical distancing, hand washing) failed to take hold, was to quarantine or isolate. (Quarantine derives from the Italian *quarantena*, meaning "forty days," originating in 14th–15th-century Venice to designate the period before passengers and crew on arriving ships could disembark during the Black Death plague epidemic.) By themselves, quarantine and isolation are stressful experiences (Carleton, 2016; Sweeny, 2018) that have known deleterious psychological effects (Brooks et al., 2020; Hawryluck et al., 2004; Sprang & Silman, 2013), including anger, confusion, and PTSD which are compounded by infection-related fears, frustration, boredom, deprivation, misinformation, financial loss, and stigma. To date, however, relevant studies of quarantine and isolation outcomes have been limited to small numbers of diseased and symptomatic people for short and defined periods of time. The impact of quarantine and isolation on millions of people for an indefinite period, as is the case during the worldwide COVID-19 pandemic, is therefore unknown.

Effects of the COVID-19 pandemic are likely especially detrimental for families, parents, and children (Sprang & Silman, 2013). Children are by definition developing organisms, their brain architecture is rapidly maturing, and they are especially sensitive to "adverse childhood experiences" (Roubinov, Bush, & Boyce, 2020). Children's daily activity routines, which normally contribute to stability and predictability in their lives, have been severely disrupted by the COVID-19 epidemic (Wisner et al., 2018). For example, as many as 220 million

Chinese children and adolescents were quarantined on account of COVID-19. They experienced disruptions to their daily routines, and prolonged school closure and home confinement during the disease outbreak was thought to put at risk their physical health (activity, screen time, sleep patterns, diets, weight gain, and cardiorespiratory fitness) and mental health (stress, fears of infection, frustration and boredom, inadequate information, lack of in-person peer contacts; Wang, Zhang, Zhao, Zhang, & Jiang, 2020). A population survey of 1,099 residents of the United Kingdom revealed that the community pandemic increased respondents' anxiety and harmed family relationships, possibly mediated by lockdowns, social isolation, physical distancing, and lack of access to mental health resources (Academy of Medical Sciences, 2020).

Parents normally buffer their children's stress, and so play a critical role in responding maturely and constructively to a disaster for themselves and for their children. However, the COVID-19 pandemic increased parents' own distress as they (mothers especially) suddenly had to shoulder increased responsibilities for childcare, distance learning, and homemaking. Many also faced income loss and unemployment and manifold threats associated with both (elaborated later in this chapter) that commonly "spill over" to undermine family relationships in the home (Masarik & Conger, 2017). Developmental scientists have advanced a Family Investment Model that spells out how economic hardships first undermine families' ability to meet housing, food, clothing, and medical care needs and then in turn become detrimental to the mental health and development of all individuals in the family (Conger, Conger, & Martin, 2010; Duncan, Magnuson, & Votruba-Drzal, 2017). Harsh parenting and interparental conflict are also likely to emerge in economically insecure families (Conrad, Paschall, & Johnson, 2019; Schofield, Conger, Gonzales, & Merrick, 2016), both of which create a risk for child physical health and mental well-being (elaborated later in this chapter).

SARS-COV-2, families, parents, and children: where families, parents, and children fit into parenting and developmental science

The prevailing theory in developmental science is a contextual bioecological one which places the family, parent, and child at the center of a system of interconnected nested distal to proximal forces . . . from culture and social class to mass media and extended family to peers and daycare (Bronfenbrenner & Morris, 2006). In this scheme, parenting is the final common pathway to early childhood oversight and caregiving and, in turn, child development and stature, adjustment and success. Parents have the special and continuing task to prepare their children for the physical, economic, and psychosocial situations that are characteristic of the environments and cultures in which their children must survive and thrive (Bornstein, 2015). Moreover, the amount of interaction between parent and offspring is greatest in early childhood, and early childhood is the time when human beings are especially susceptible to influences of experiences they will carry with them for the balance of the life course . . . in essence, long after leaving their family of origin.

Indeed, what is special about human beings, and one of the most significant characteristics of our species, is the long period of developmental plasticity during which physical and neural as well as mental and socioemotional structures emerge in close attunement with the effective environment (Gould, 1977; Hoynes, Schanzenbach, & Almond, 2016). Human infants and young children are "altricial" and do not and cannot grow up as solitary individuals; infants and young children are totally dependent on parents for survival and development. Childhood is the time when we first make sense of the physical world, first learn to express and read basic emotions, and forge our first social bonds. Parents escort children through all these dramatic firsts. In the enigmatic words of one notable British psychoanalyst, "There is no such thing as an infant" (Winnicott, 1965, p. 39). Human children only exist as part of reciprocal systems with their caregivers (Lerner, 2018).

Parents are therefore tasked with many responsibilities in rearing their children to become competent, well-functioning mature adult members of their social group. Parents influence children via their genetic endowment (but there is precious little that can be done about that after assortative mating) and via the environments they create for children and the experiences they provide children. Developmental science shows that environments and experiences influence children's growth at all levels . . . from cells to cradle to culture. Effective parenting parses into two lots: parents' cognitions (their thoughts, attitudes, knowledge, etc. about parenthood and childhood, children and child development) and parents' practices (the actual environments and experiences parents create for children). In the realm of early child development, parents engage children in diverse overlapping, but individually identifiable, caregiving practices. Box 1.1 outlines the several caregiving responsibilities of parents and their intersections with the COVID-19 pandemic.

BOX 1.1   The several caregiving responsibilities of parents and their possible intersection with the COVID-19 pandemic

Nurturant Caregiving . . . meets the biological, physical, and health requirements of offspring. Parents are responsible for promoting children's wellness and preventing their illness. Parents nurture offspring, meeting needs and maintaining homeostatic balance by providing sustenance, routine care, protection, supervision, grooming, comfort, and the like. With respect to the COVID-19 pandemic, for example, parents have the responsibility to keep themselves virus free, to safeguard their children and adolescents from the virus, and to ensure that their children and adolescents do not spread the coronavirus infection to others.

Physical Caregiving . . . promotes gross and fine psychomotor development in offspring. The child is beginning to reach out and grasp the world, and later locomotes within it. With respect to the COVID-19 pandemic, for example, parents have the responsibility to promote their children's and adolescents' face covering, hand washing, and physical distancing.

Social Caregiving . . . includes visual, verbal, and affective behaviors that engage offspring emotionally and manage their interpersonal exchanges. Social caregiving focuses on the dyad; through sensitivity and responsiveness, positive feedback, and emotional closeness, parents make children feel valued, accepted, and approved of. Social caregiving helps children regulate their own affect and emotions. With respect to the COVID-19 pandemic, for example, parents have the responsibility to reassure their children and adolescents that they are safe, to allay their children's and adolescents' worries, anxieties, and fears (Wilson, 2021, in this volume), and to comfort their children and adolescents in the event of family tragedy.

Didactic Caregiving . . . includes strategies that stimulate offspring to engage and understand the environment outside the dyad and to enter the world of learning. Didactics means introducing, mediating, and interpreting the external world to the child; teaching, describing, and demonstrating; as well as provoking or providing opportunities to observe, to imitate, and to learn. With respect to the COVID-19 pandemic, for example, parents have the responsibility to communicate to their children and adolescents coherent evidence-based explanations of the coronavirus situation that are clear, simple, and concrete (Stein et al., 2019) and that take into account the child's age, emotional and mental intelligence, as well as the child's level of understanding illness and death (Dalton, Rapa, & Stein, 2020). *A Family Guide to Covid*, a free, downloadable e-book, answers questions about COVID-19 from "Why has my life changed?" to "What are the long-term effects?" (Haseltine, 2020). It would seem especially important to school adolescents, who are in the natural developmental stage of striving for autonomy from parents, about the risks of flocking to bars or hanging out with friends or attending so-called COVID parties (events where people congregate in close proximity in attempts to infect themselves and develop immunity to the virus). Widespread infections and secondary surges have been attributed to just such super-spreader events.

Material Caregiving . . . includes parents' provision and organization of their offspring's environments as in responsibility for the number, character, and variety of toys, books, and household objects available to the child, the level of ambient stimulation, limits on physical freedom, and overall safety and physical dimensions of children's experiences. With respect to the COVID-19 pandemic, for example, parents have the responsibility to keep their children's and adolescents' physical environments well ventilated, to provision children's and adolescents' learning and entertainments, and to keep their children and adolescents physically distant from others who may be unwittingly infectious themselves.

Language Caregiving . . . is vital to offspring's mental and social development. Early language skills merge into higher-order verbal and mental functioning and so have predictive validity for the development of speech, grammar, reading, academic achievement, and intelligence. Language skills also predict behavioral adjustment in children. Children's and adolescents' achievements in language and literacy open doors to education, occupation, income, and health. With respect to the COVID-19 pandemic, for example, parents have the responsibilities, specifically, to engage their children and adolescents in meaningful discussions about all facets of the disease and, generally, to foster their children's and adolescents' language abilities so that they become responsible educated citizens.

It should be noted in this connection that the effects of parenting cognitions and practices on children are not global, but specific (Bornstein, 2017). Specific parent cognitions and practices tend to influence specific child outcomes. Providing a rich verbal environment may foster a child's verbal competence, but will not necessarily speak to the child's development of empathy or social competence. Rather, *specific experiences specific parents provide specific children at specific times exert effects in specific ways over specific aspects of child growth.* This specificity view matches UNICEF's (United Nations Foundation, 2018) orientation away from averages to honor variation in what, how, for whom, where, and when parenting and parent intervention programs are effective.

Parenting in the time of SARS-COV-2

At the time of this writing in the fall of 2020, parents' multivocal responsibilities have been complicated and compounded by the global coronavirus pandemic. As childcare, schools, and other support systems for parents collapsed, parents have been tasked with many responsibilities over and above caregiving. At this time, it seems that they are likely to be so encumberd for an indefinite period. (With more than one-third of U.S. parents admitting to serious problems keeping their children's education going [NPR et al., 2020], never have parents appreciated teachers so much!)

Lockdowns or quarantines at home may have salutary effects on some families, parents, and children who have not been impacted by the disease, financial distress, or other associated privations. They have provided opportunities for families to engage in activities together, with fathers and mothers at home to share cooking and meals, chores and game nights, and for parents and children to come to know one another more intimately than the centrifugal humdrum of pre-COVID normal daily routines ever allowed. Some parents and children may benefit from new realizations about each other and deeper appreciations of one another. Some extended families have "sheltered-in-place" so that grandparents, parents, and children occupy family "pods" or "bubbles" deepening intergenerational family ties.

These grandparents praise the joy of constantly watching a girl or boy as they grow and change. Together, families have shared the experience of the pandemic which may be critical to negotiating it successfully (Hafstad, Haavind, & Jensen, 2012). Furthermore, the pandemic can be fearful and paralyzing, even for those not directly affected (Liu, Bao, Huang, Shi, & Lu, 2020), but as the Yerkes–Dodson law teaches anxiety and fear in small amounts can be motivating to behave sanely and appropriately. Indeed, adversity can be a springboard to the development of new strengths and skills.

As daycares and schools closed, children have had to adapt to (sometimes cope with) distance learning and parents have been thrust into the role of ersatz teachers. Propitiously, the pandemic offers parents so inclined with unique occasions to discuss news-drenched medical, social, and behavioral science with their children as well as model resilience and character virtues to their children, as examples of how "good works" can spread as rapidly as the virus (#GivingTuesday, 2020; Masten & Palmer, 2019; White-Cummings, 2020). Of course, some children and parents decry the "frustration and boredom" born of distance learning and constrained computer-based social interaction; the upside fact is, however, that through online schooling the pandemic has offered children a realistic glimpse into and, importantly, preparation to operate more effectively in a future post-pandemic world of daily life and professional work more and more likely constructed of virtual meetings and collaborations. Indeed, the miscues associated with having the teacher and peers at school be able to peer into one's home, and overhear a family conversation, set the perfect occasion for a conversation about how to think about privacy, risks to privacy, and how to reduce them. Moreover, remote learning may be a struggle or misadventure for many students, but other anxious, withdrawn, conflict averse, embarrassed, or intimidated children have found a safe haven and thrived. Boys tend to dominate classroom participation, and online learning removes social barriers that can keep girls from excelling. Online, children are able to ask questions of their teachers privately, enter digital "break-out rooms" with staff, and get one-on-one instruction apart from other students. Still other special education children with disabilities of diverse kinds (ADHD, language disorders) have found it helpful to see their teacher directly in front of them on a computer screen, improved concentration with removal from the sometime chaos of a school classroom, and profited from working at their own pace and when they want.

Even if more work and challenge, for their part teachers ("DJs of Zoom") have touted some advantages of remote instruction such as the ease of handling some discipline issues with the "mute all" button. Some educators now ponder how the experiences of students who have improved under distance learning can be applied to benefit in-person learning in the future.

Moreover, not all of the pandemic's social, economic, or environmental consequences have been adverse. Some sufferers of mental illness have reported relenting symptoms, a well-known by-product of a more measured pace of life, more routine, more time spent with loved ones, and reprioritizing life's "to-dos." For some individuals now working at home, common stresses of the work-a-day world have been relieved, as they escape commuting, performance anxiety, and competitive coworkers. Other positive adjustments have accompanied the pandemic and embedded themselves in our lives to degrees that the world is unlikely to abandon. People have adapted to new modes of working and learning, different ways of relating, conversing, and meeting, and novel venues of seeking entertainment and medical care. Concomitantly, some attitudes have changed; for example, walks of life heretofore taken for granted – grocery store employees, nurses, teachers – are now thought of as "essential workers." For families, not currently shopping, dining out, or travelling, overall household debt has relented (Federal Reserve Bank of New York, 2020), and some items (disinfectant wipes, toilet paper) and businesses (Amazon, Netflix, Zoom) clearly emerged as pandemic economic "winners" (Lynch, 2020). Diverse enterprises have altered everyday operations and policies, restaurants and cafes have appropriated sidewalks, and towns and cities have transformed streets into pedestrian walkways. Global carbon-dioxide emissions are estimated to fall by as much as 10 percent in 2020 compared to 2019 due to the "COVID crash" cutting automobile and air travel and generally boosting a green economy (Evans, 2020). On a macroeconomic level, it was originally thought that, as large numbers of migrants languished in unemployment, remittances (payments that migrants send back to their low- and middle-income countries of origin) would decline (World Bank, 2020a), virtually assuring that more of the world's poorest families would have less access to housing, food, and medicine; instead of folding, however, remittances from the United States to Central and Latin America increased year-over-year in five of the first six months of 2020 (Slef, 2020).

Those positive and valuable effects aside, for most families, especially those of essential workers and those without extensive resources, lockdowns and quarantines introduced new and momentous stresses. Some consequences of the pandemic directly affect parents, children, and parent-child relationships in the family. We can gather them together generically under an aegis of "home life" consequences. Other consequences exert indirect effects on parents, children, and parent-child relationships in the family through changes in community, economy, and nation state. We can organize them generically under a rubric of "economic" consequences.

Home life consequences

. . . for parents

The abrupt emergence and ubiquity of the COVID-19 pandemic disoriented adults. Housebound lockdowns and the "zoomification" of life and work led to misplaced time on account of shapeless days, structureless weeks, and months that passed like hours. Working adults lost the quotidian rhythms and routines of normal existence of being out the door, getting into a car, going to an office, and engaging with adult workmates in person . . . even as workdays around the globe grew longer (DeFilippis, Impink, Singell, Polzer, & Sadun, 2020). The mind normally segments reality based on changes in the environment, a phenomenon called "event boundaries" (Swallow, Zacks, & Abrams, 2009). Spatial location is an essential human mnemonic, and things all happening in the same place unmoored from regularity become distorted, and they interfere with and erode memory.

Parents *qua* adults have experienced increased challenges related to mental health, personal adversities, professional trials, and economic losses (Abgrall, Deloche-Gaudez, Neff, & Akhounak, 2020), which in documented cases eventuated in strains on leisure time, interpersonal communication, problem solving, management, and critical thinking. The COVID-19 pandemic was new to the world in the new year, but by February 2020 the threat had successfully insinuated itself and had a significant impact on mental health. The numbers of prescriptions filled per week for anti-depressant (18.6 percent), anti-anxiety (34.1 percent), and anti-insomnia (14.8 percent) medications increased between mid-February and mid-March, when COVID-19 was declared a pandemic. More than three quarters (78 percent) of all three types of prescriptions filled during the week ending 15 March were for new prescriptions; the number of new prescriptions between February and March for all three categories was 25.4 percent (Express Scripts, 2020). An April–June 2020 survey of 5,500 UK mothers and fathers found that, during the lockdown, both were doing some childcare during an extra four hours each day: In 2014, some 70 percent of parents reported having leisure time at around 7 p.m., whereas during lockdown only 40 percent did (Andrew et al., 2020a). The National Opinion Research Center at the University of Chicago has conducted an annual survey of the U.S. national mood since 1972; it found that the proportion of people describing themselves as "very happy" plummeted to 14 percent in the summer of 2020 (NORC, 2020). More telling and disturbing data arrived at the same time from converging sources. The prevalence of symptoms of an anxiety disorder was three times as high, and symptoms of depression were four times as high, in June 2020 than in the second quarter of 2019 (Czeisler, Lane, et al., 2020). According to a July 2020 Kaiser Family Foundation Tracking Poll, 53 percent of adults in the United States reported that their mental health had been negatively impacted due to worry and stress over the coronavirus, an increase from 32 percent reported in March (Panchal et al., 2020). Negative impacts on mental health and well-being included difficulty sleeping (36 percent) or eating (32 percent), increases in alcohol consumption or substance use (12 percent), and worsening chronic conditions (12 percent). Pandemic-related anxiety has been documented to erode adult mental health in a diversity of ways, from COVID-induced nightmares (Weaver, 2020) and "coronasomnia" (Morin & Carrier, 2020) to "doomsurfing" (Roose, 2020) to "coronaphobia" (Coronavirus Anxiety Project, 2020, has developed a *Coronavirus Anxiety Scale*). A survey of 6,514 adults in the United States found that those with higher daily hours of COVID-19-related media exposure, and exposure to conflicting COVID-19 information in the media, were at greater risk for pandemic-related acute stress and depressive symptoms (Holman, Thompson, Garfin, & Silver, 2020). Recognizing this kind of rapidly deteriorating circumstance, the WHO (2020e) urgently called for substantial measures aimed at averting a massive increase in mental health risks as a result of the pandemic.

Three examples illustrate implications of these developments for adult adjustment, one concerned with physical health, the second with work-life balance, and the third with spiritual well-being. First, because of concerns about COVID-19 an estimated 41 percent of U.S. adults delayed or avoided medical care including urgent or emergency care and routine care (Czeisler, Marynak, et al., 2020). Second, adults suddenly at home with children are still wage-earners who must balance their professional commitments with attentive childcare; this now commonplace conundrum was brought home vividly (and hilariously) during a September 2020 zoomed CNN interview with a research director at a science nonprofit (Schwedel, 2020). Third, many people are spiritual or devout (Mahoney & Boyatzis, 2019): An estimated 25 percent of U.S. Americans attend a house of worship every week, and almost 40 percent more consider themselves to be very religious (Duffin, 2020). The COVID-19 pandemic unsettled religious life. By anecdotal report, 35 million Americans who seldom pray or darken the door of a house of worship started praying during the coronavirus epidemic (ROTW, 2020). At the same time, however, houses of worship closed; for example, North Point Ministries in Georgia with a congregation of 30,000 spread across six ministries suspended in-person adult worship until 2021 (Gjelten, 2020). These and other compromised features of adulthood likely spill over into family life.

For parents *qua* parents, particularly mothers who traditionally bear the larger burden of family management and child caregiving (Bornstein, 2015), the pandemic has had multiple serious aftermaths, including augmented responsibilities for childcare, supervising full-time schooling, and disruptions of work life, self-care, and own pursuits, to name a few. As indicated earlier, adults suffer anxiety and stress in disasters (Abgrall, Akhounak, & Neff, 2020; Abgrall, Neff, Deloche-Gaudez, & Akhounak, 2020; Fussell & Lowe, 2014; Maeda & Oe, 2017) – mothers and fathers especially so – which are almost always accompanied by escalations in depression, PTSD, substance use, a broad range of mental and behavioral disorders, domestic violence, and child abuse (Cluver et al., 2020; Galea, Merchant, & Lurie, 2020; Park, Russell et al., 2020b).

Parenting can be joyous, uplifting, and fulfilling in ways few other human experiences ever match (Nelson-Coffey & Stewart, 2019), but it can also be demanding, stressful, and frustrating as parents sometimes struggle with the developmental and behavioral twists and turns that accompany the many exigencies of childrearing. Whether under conditions of high risk or facilitative developmental contexts, fault-line stresses of parenting are readily apparent (Crnic & Coburn, 2019, in this volume). The COVID-19 pandemic exposes and amplifies those stresses by saddling mothers with additional housekeeping duties and childtending all day long while the whole family remains housebound. Particularly heavy responsibilities fall on the shoulders of mothers who still cannot escape popular indictments of "mom shaming" (Kitchener, 2020). Additionally, COVID-19 incites specific and urgent fears of infection and hospitalization for family members (children, spouses, self, and own parents), and the absence of clear, reliable, and consistent information still challenges adherence to guidelines for preventing COVID-19. Mothers make approximately 80 percent of health care decisions for their children and are more likely to be the caregivers when a child falls ill (Bornstein, Cote, Haynes, Hahn, & Park, 2010; U.S. Department of Labor, 2020a). Witte and Allen (2000) reported a direct association between disease-related fear/worry and preventative health behaviors.

So, expectedly, parents' mental health difficulties as well as child behavior problems increased from the onset of the pandemic (Fisher, Lombardi, & Kendall-Taylor, 2020). The impact of the coronavirus reached beyond physical health and safety, as people suffer adverse mental health effects of spending more time confined indoors, deprived of the company of loved ones, and threatened with unemployment (Huckins et al., 2020) on top of known adverse effects of stress (including substance abuse, alcohol consumption, excessive work or exercise, binge eating, or other distractions through the Internet or social media) or physical escape (including suicidal ideation; Mikolajczak, Brianda, Avalosse, & Roskam, 2018; Mikolajczak, Gross, & Roskam, 2019). After China, Italy was the first country to experience the rapid spread and sustain the devastating effects of COVID-19 (de Best, 2020). The Italian government swiftly imposed stringent containment procedures, including school closures and a stay-at-home order (*#IoRestoaCasa*; Government, 2020). A study that explored parents' and their 2- and 14-year-old children's individual and dyadic adjustment one month into the quarantine revealed that parents' perception of the difficulty of quarantine undermined their own and their children's well-being and that parents' depression, anxiety, stress, and parenting stress each mediated the impact of the quarantine on children's behavioral and emotional problems: Parents who reported more difficulties in coping with quarantine, in terms of taking care of their children's learning, finding space and time for themselves, their partner, and their children, and for activities they routinely did before the lockdown, showed more stresses which, in turn, amplified their children's emotional symptoms, hyperactivity-inattention, and conduct problems (Spinelli, Lionetti, Pastore, & Fasolo, 2020).

As a concrete example, parental "burnout" materialized as a home hazard. Parental burnout is a context-specific syndrome that can arise as a result of chronic stress that depletes personal resources and the ability to manage stress effectively (Hallsten, 2005). The COVID-19 pandemic lockdown constituted just the kind of stressful contingency likely to increase the risk of parental burnout. Emotional regulation skills, self-efficacy beliefs, family organization, positive parenting attitudes, coparenting with respect to educational practices, and marital satisfaction play protective roles against parental exhaustion and can enhance parents' ability to cope with such adverse situations (Mikolajczak et al., 2018). During the COVID-19 pandemic, many parents have become deprived of support from relatives and childcare and hence susceptible to potentially harmful consequences of disrupted extended family relationships (grandparents) and absence of help from alloparents (caregivers). Others, the lucky ones who enjoy willing partners, formed pods with extended family and sometimes even with neighbors to share parenting responsibilities.

. . . for children

As indicated earlier, coronavirus infection symptoms, hospitalizations, and mortality are mitigated, but *not* absent, in infants, young children, and even adolescents. In the United States, children younger than 18 years of age represent fewer than

10 percent of all cases and constitute fewer than 4 percent of hospitalizations and less than 1 percent of deaths (Michaud & Kates, 2020). Especially worrisome, however infrequent, was the emergence in May 2020, approximately two to four weeks after infection with COVID-19, of nearly 1,000 confirmed cases of children and adolescents manifesting a rare multisystem inflammatory syndrome (MIS-C; CDC, 2020h), marked by severe complications including cardiac dysfunction (40.6 percent), shock (35.4 percent), coronary artery dilatation or aneurysm (18.6 percent), and acute kidney injury (18.4 percent; CDC, 2020h; Godfred-Cato et al., 2020; Ludvigsson, 2020); 19 deaths were attributed to MIS-C (American Academy of Pediatrics, 2020b).

Despite the overall innocuous infection statistics, the COVID-19 pandemic eventuated in an unanticipated yet pervasive raft of unhappy consequences for children. Generally, children caught up in disasters report lower direct exposures than their parents, but still experience the same overall levels of distress as their parents (Juth, Silver, Seyle, Widyatmoko, & Tan, 2015). Children are of course developing organisms, and the maturing brain for instance is highly sensitive to environmental adversity. Long-term follow-up studies of individuals conceived and *in utero* during environmental disasters (pandemics and famines) – documented examples include the 1918–1919 worldwide flu pandemic, the 1944 Dutch hunger winter, the 1998 Canadian ice storm, and the 2010 Chilean earthquake – have revealed that such shocks cast a long negative shadow across the life course (Almond, 2006; King & Laplante, 2015; Lumey et al., 2007). Research from the CDC and WHO has shown strong correlations between such adverse childhood experiences (ACEs) and increased lifetime rates of depression, suicide, alcohol and drug use, obesity, HIV infection, chronic obstructive pulmonary disease, and heart disease (Anda et al., 2006). More immediate examples of childhood risks proliferated during the 2020 pandemic as parents of children under 6 years of age reported delaying health care (Fisher et al., 2020), including well-care pediatric visits (American Academy of Pediatrics, 2020c) and children's normal vaccination schedules (Santoli et al., 2020), potentially rendering them more vulnerable to vaccine-preventable childhood diseases (WHO, 2020f). More than one-half (55 percent) of U.S. parents surveyed reported that their child "acted out" more since the start of the pandemic (American Psychological Association, 2020; NPR et al., 2020). As lockdowns at home persisted, children have lost out on normative peer relationships and play interactions as well as enriching experiences with grandparents and relatives, non-parental caregivers, and teachers (Honig, 2019). During the pandemic, a large majority of U.S. parents (71 percent) surveyed reported being worried about its impact on their child's social development (American Psychological Association, 2020; NPR et al., 2020). Cross-cultural data extend the pervasiveness of this reaction: In 484 families in five countries (Italy, the Philippines, Sweden, Thailand, and the United States), notably diverse with respect to the timing and spread of the COVID-19 outbreak and governmental response, higher levels of reported disruption after the onset of the COVID-19 pandemic related to increases in internalizing (depression, anxiety) and externalizing (anger, argumentativeness) behaviors in mothers, fathers, and their 20-year-olds (Skinner et al., 2020).

The further stunning consequence of the COVID-19 pandemic for infants and toddlers, and children and adolescents, struck in the rushed and then lasting closures of daycares and schools (see Box 1.2, daycare, school, and work, where steps parents can take to help their children cope with these stressors are detailed).

BOX 1.2   Daycare, school, and work

Almost one-third of U.S. workers have children under 18 years of age at home (Long, 2020). About 56.6 million students enroll in elementary, middle, and high schools across the United States attended to by 3.2 million public school teachers and 500,000 private school teachers plus staff (NCES, 2020).

Early reports from China advised that quarantined children experience disruptions to their daily routines, with potential negative impacts on their physical and mental health (Wang et al., 2020). By March 2020, soon after the arrival of the coronavirus in the United States infants and toddlers were taken out of daycares, and children and adolescents out of school; according to Education Week (May 2020), the pandemic led to a near total shutdown of schools, affecting those millions of U.S. public and private school students. Altogether, an estimated 1.5 billion children around the globe (87 percent of Earth's student population) were removed from childcare or school due to COVID-19 (UNESCO, 2020). All were therefore deprived of significant growth-promoting experiences which such situations offer from curricular education to extracurricular activities to peer relationships.

Interruptions of normal in-school instruction threaten to create educational deficits. In the era of COVID-19, learning experiences for many children transferred to digital platforms which can be less efficacious and advantageous to instruction than are in-person didactic experiences (Barr, 2019; Barr & Linebarger, 2017; Barr, McClure, & Palarkian, 2019; Snape & Viner, 2020). These privations by themselves promised to impede children's mental and socioemotional growth and development. (In a 1951 short story, *The Fun They Had,* Isaac Asimov tells a science-fiction tale set in the 2150s of the prevailing education program in which children learn individually, at home, from a robot teacher. Through the daydreams of 11-year-old Margie Jones about her grandfather's school experience, the story underscores the pleasures that children once enjoyed being in school together.) In addition, digital platforms are subject to known inequities and disparities (e.g., availability of computers, access to the Internet) by socioeconomic class, ethnic group, and nation state (Magnuson & Duncan, 2019; UNESCO, 2020). An on-the-spot survey completed online by more than 4,000 parents of children aged 4–15 in April to May 2020 in England found that half or more of parents found it quite or very hard to support their children's learning at home, that 64 percent of pupils in state schools from the richest households were being offered active help from schools, such as online teaching, compared with 47 percent from the poorest households, and that children from better-off families were spending 30 percent more time on home learning than those from poorer families (Andrew et al., 2020b). In the United States, according to Curriculum Associates 60 percent of low-income students are regularly logging into online instruction, even as 90 percent of high-income students do. In Mexico, only 60 percent of students have access to the Internet. Around the world, perhaps as many as 463 million schoolchildren lack Internet, television, or radio, leaving them with almost no access to education (UNICEF, 2020a).

In South Korea, Norway, and Turkey, K-12 students learn from national curricula; in the United States, each of thousands of school districts offers its own curriculum. In October 2020, Peru claimed the world's highest coronavirus mortality rate, and Peruvian children 14 and under are permitted out of their homes only one hour per day. The Peruvian government's distance learning program, "I Learn at Home," offers only a 30-minute state TV televised class for each grade per weekday. These inequities challenge distance learning gravely and foster the "K" distribution of opportunities and advancement that reify the "Matthew effect" whereby the "rich get richer and the poor poorer" (Matthew 25:29).

With respect to infants and toddlers in daycare, on average, childcare facility enrollment dropped 67 percent (Rampell, 2020) as about 60 percent of childcare programs in the United States alone temporarily closed (Bipartisan Policy Center, 2020). In consequence, the childcare industry in the United States (not in great shape pre-COVID) sustained large numbers of layoffs but continued to incur fixed costs (e.g., rent) even as COVID-19 introduced new expenses (e.g., for health guidelines and safety requirements and for smaller class sizes and so more staff per child, plus added costs for cleaning supplies, personal protective equipment, thermometers, disposable food implements, and extra sets of toys). An estimated 40 percent of the childcare facilities that existed pre-COVID-19 were expected to close permanently (NAEYC, 2020). In the face of this mounting crisis, parents of infants and toddlers who would normally turn to family, friends, and neighbors (so-called FFN) for childcare determined that option as unsafe, and so closed off yet another potential support and relief.

As underscored several times in this chapter, the course and future of the COVID-19 pandemic have been uncertain. Thus, with respect to children and adolescents in school, as the fall term approached in 2020, parents around the United States (where the epidemic was still rising) were gripped with indecision about whether children should return to school or should continue with forms of distance-learning. For teachers and school administrators at all levels, debates over "reopening" revolved around what measures must be in place to bring back students safely.

Should children return to school?

Pros	Cons
The Executive Branch of the U.S. Government and other organizations, such as the American Academy of Pediatrics (2020d), advocated for school openings and full in-person attendance.	The CDC and other organizations, such as the National Teachers Association, counseled against a "one size fits all" approach in deciding if and when schools should open. The American Federation of Teachers (AFT) recommended 100 percent virtual instruction and threatened strikes where schools and districts failed to adhere to CDC safety rules and regulations.
Children benefit most from in-person academic learning.	Children spread the coronavirus and so may infect one another, teachers, parents, and other family members living at home.
There are social and health benefits when children interact with their teachers and each other, and reciprocally social isolation is thought to lead to mental and physical harm.	The full health effects of COVID-19 on children are still unknown.
There are hardships to working families when children stay at home, as working parents need childcare to return to work.	Public health recommendations for making school spaces safe include physical distancing, good ventilation, mask wearing, frequent sanitizing, hand washing, etc. The logistics for implementing these measures with children and adolescents of different ages are daunting and financially prohibitive.
Families may be unskilled with requisite distance-learning technology and have sporadic or no access to internet connectivity.	To be safe from the coronavirus schools need more buses, computers, personal protective equipment, cleaning supplies, better ventilation, etc. The Council of Chief State School Officers estimated safely reopening schools could cost $158 billion to $245 billion; the AFT put the figure at $116.5 billion.
Schools offer free or reduced-cost meals for children from low household incomes.	
Children from low-income families and those with disabilities need the special services schools offer and face particular challenges learning from home.	

Pandemics and school attendance are incompatible in the absence of adequate testing, personal protective equipment, contact tracing, appropriate physical spacing, and proper ventilation. Given the realities of the COVID-19 pandemic, parents face no good options. Not surprisingly, national polling of different constituencies resulted in starkly different preference profiles for different reasons.

- In July 2020, some parents opined that schools should not open at all, others favored delaying the openings, and still others asserted that schools should only open with "major adjustments" (Miller & Benz, 2020). By August 2020, most U.S. American parents thought it would be unsafe to send their children back to school given the risks posed by the novel coronavirus, and more than 80 percent favored holding school at least partly online (Meckler & Guskin, 2020). Given three options, 44 percent of parents wanted their schools to offer a mix of online and in-person classes; 39 percent voted for all-virtual education; and 16 percent favored fully in-person school (1 percent had no opinion). Echoing other ethnic differences noted here, a national survey conducted in July found that twice as many European American parents (57 percent) thought in-person instruction was safe and so would send their children back to classrooms than African American and Latin American parents (21 and 27 percent, respectively; Ipsos & George Mason University Schar School of Policy and Government, 2020).
- Teachers evenly split between those who favored in-person instruction and those who wanted an all-virtual approach (Iannelli, 2020). Teachers' unions warned that adults in school buildings are at risk of infection. One poll found that 1 in 5 teachers was unlikely to return to reopened classrooms (Page, 2020).
- Students evenly split between those who favored in-person instruction and those who wanted an all-virtual approach (PFT, 2020).
- Only about 1 in 10 U.S. Americans at large thought daycare centers, preschools, or K-12 schools should open without restrictions (Miller & Benz, 2020), and Americans at large voiced concerns that reopening schools for in-person learning would lead to a coronavirus surge.

What is a parent to do? Some parents, in the face of needs to return to work and afford their child developmentally appropriate peer- and school-based experiences, opted to return their children to daycares and schools; others established "pandemic pods" which brought small numbers of infection-free children into privately financed bubbles with specially hired teachers; still others sacrificed their own employment to homeschool their children. Amidst this frantic decision making, a report appeared that confirmed high rates of coronavirus in children 1–17 years of age and warned, "Behavioral habits of young children and close quarters in school and day care settings raise concern for SARS-CoV-2 amplification in this population as public health restrictions are eased" (Heald-Sargent et al., 2020).

Generally speaking, experiences of others who have earlier confronted the same decision can be instructive. Believing it had beaten the virus, the Israeli government reopened its entire school system without restrictions on 17 May 2020. Soon after, at least 1,335 students and 691 staff members contracted the coronavirus (Schwartz & Lieber, 2020). This spike in infections among children then spread to the general population, according to epidemiological surveys by Israel's Health Ministry. By mid-July 2020, 125 schools and 258 kindergartens had been re-closed because of infections. Apparently, the disease spread quickly at a high school, affecting more than 260 people during a heat wave when mask rules were suspended and air conditioning was in constant use (Stein-Zamir et al., 2020). Summer camps for children are a long-standing tradition in the United States and gave rise to a similar lesson. In the wake of the long winter lockdown and in advance of the fall 2020 school year, many parents opted to send their children to summer camp. The outbreak at one Georgia overnight summer camp in late June 2020 (in the same state as the CDC) proved illustrative as 76 percent of campers and staff subsequently tested positive: Among those ages 6–10, 51 percent contracted the virus, among 11- to 17-year-olds 44 percent, and among 18- to 21-year-olds 33 percent. Although other precautions were taken, campers did a lot of singing, cheering, and shouting and did not wear face masks, and cabin windows were not opened for ventilation (Janes, 2020; Szablewski et al., 2020). Thus, despite efforts by camp officials to implement most recommended CDC strategies to prevent transmission, high COVID-19 attack rates appeared among persons in all age groups in this youth-centric overnight setting.

Infants and toddlers out of daycare, and children and adolescents out of school, directly anticipate economic consequences of the COVID-19 pandemic, as economists and business leaders alike have contended that returning children to daycares and schools is critical to reviving an economy. Many parents find it difficult to impossible to return to work if their children are not in childcare or classes. In essence, the argument goes, the childcare industry supports all others for without the childcare industry other industries are not able to return to where they need to be. In early 2020, 13 percent of U.S. parents had to quit a job or reduce their working hours due to a lack of childcare (Long, 2020), and parents lost an average of eight hours of work a week – the equivalent of a full day – because they had to address their children's needs. Some 17.5 million workers – 11 percent of the U.S. workforce – take care of young children on their own and were unlikely to return to work full time until daycares and schools fully reopened (Dingel, Patterson, & Vavra, 2020). Census data show that most employed mothers of young children are ages 30 to 49, prime working years (Christnacht & Sullivan, 2020), and any economy missing so many people in that age bracket from work will falter. Where there are insufficient daycare spots for children, there is a 12 percentage point drop in mothers' labor force participation (Schochet, 2020). One economist likened this situation to a "doughnut economy."

The U.S. 2020 Cares Act provided $3.5 billion in relief for childcare centers and $13.5 billion for K-12 schools (U.S. Department of the Treasury, 2020). That same bill authorized $25 billion for U.S. airlines, manifestly more generous assistance than awarded institutions that care for and educate U.S. children. Which is more critical to a country's economic infrastructure? As of fall 2020, ultimate relief for parents and employers still depended on the uncertain arrival of a vaccine (Johnson, 2020).

Even if children and adolescents show few or mild or brief symptoms, if any at all, they may still be infection vectors. A large study using contact tracing reported that adolescents in the 10- to 19-year-old range could spread the virus as efficiently as do adults; children younger than 10 were half as likely to transmit the virus, but still presented a risk (Park, Choe et al., 2020a). Indeed, children younger than 5, even with mild or moderate illness, were found to have higher levels of virus in the nose compared with older children and adults (Heald-Sargent et al., 2020). These developments gave pause to the impetus to open camps in the summer and daycares and schools in the fall of 2020, as it came to be commonly understood that infected youngsters may still spread the virus to teachers at school and to parents and grandparents at home. Confirming reports then began to abound: In June and July 2020, 12 children who acquired COVID-19 in Utah childcare facilities then transmitted the infection to at least 26 percent of non-facility contacts (Lopez et al., 2020); an asymptomatic child attending a family in-home daycare in New York led to four families becoming ill with infection, including six children at the daycare, one sibling, seven parents, and two grandmothers (Doran, 2020); and a 13-year-old girl at a three-week gathering of five households infected 12 family members from four states (Schwartz et al., 2020). By August 2020, the WHO (2020g) warned that young people were becoming primary spreaders of the virus in many countries. In the United States, approximately 3.3 million adults ages 65 and older live in a household with school-age children (Singh & Lee, 2020); put another way, about 20 percent of the U.S. population resides in homes with at least two adult generations or grandparents and grandchildren under 25 (Cohn & Passel, 2018). These statistics paint a worrisome picture of children's role in the pandemic for families and parent-child relationships (Yonker et al., 2020).

. . . for parent-child relationships

As parents and children were individually affected by the COVID-19 pandemic, parent-child relationships have not escaped their own idiosyncratic detrimental consequences. On a mundane level, parents and young children have needed to cope together constructively with imposed confinement, boredom, and frustration (Cluver et al., 2020). Of course, parents are children's primary socializers, and parent-child everyday interactions while under quarantine and stay-at-home conditions improved in salutary ways mentioned earlier but they also suffered in other ways. First, parents influence children by the models they present for coping during a crisis (White-Cummings, 2020). Parents demonstrate constructive or avoidant coping strategies and provide leadership to children about ways to manage novel or myriad disruptions to daily life or to withdraw. For example, parents must guide children in personal safety and disease-related infection management (Davis, 2020; Yoon, Newkirk, & Perry-Jenkins, 2015) such as adherence to prevention guidelines (e.g., hand washing, face covering, and physical distancing). Outcomes following a disaster (e.g., PTSD) are especially poor among children of highly distressed caregivers or caregivers who fail to cope adequately with their own negative mental health outcomes (Kerns et al., 2014; Kiliç, Kiliç, & Aydin, 2011). Second, parents critically buffer stress and negative mental health sequelae in their children: Parental emotional support mediates children's emotional symptoms following a disaster (Sprague et al., 2015), and parental confidence is protective against stress-related symptoms in children (Carpenter et al., 2017). As in excess of 50 million cases of coronavirus have been diagnosed and the world has fast exceeded 1.2 million deaths in the COVID-19 pandemic, parents everywhere must help their children cope with the illness or hospitalization or untimely demise of a family member. In these extraordinary times, saying goodbye to loved ones over cellphone screens, foregoing proper funerals, and dealing with hasty burials, with barely a chance to mourn have become tragically commonplace. Some children must cope with grief at the loss of one or both parents and, then, with how to make house payments, keep a car running, and meet terrifying hospital bills (Cox, 2020). Acknowledging the primacy of family relationships for nearly all youth, Hamilton et al. (2016, in this volume) commend the significance of youth relationships with adults who are not family members as sources of strength to help young people cope even in the face of stressful economic and social change.

Finally, as whole families and, in many circumstances around the globe, extended families are housebound together, an unintended, untoward, and unavoidable consequence of the pandemic is structural crowding. Crowding in the home has long been a concern to scholars interested in the health and adaptive functioning of families, parents, and children (Evans, 2006). Crowded conditions are systematically associated with respiratory illnesses, meningitis, and gastrointestinal problems in children (Baker, Taylor, & Henderson, 1998; Essen, Fogelman, & Head, 1978; Galpin, Whitaker, & Dubiel, 1992; Marsh, Gordon, Pantazis, & Heslop, 1999; Stanwell et al., 1994). Crowding encourages the spread of infection and increases the likelihood of injury and death as a consequence of lifestyle choices, like co-sleeping which has been identified as a factor in sudden infant death syndrome (Baker et al., 2000; Blair et al., 1999; Jaine, Baker, & Venugopal, 2011). Living in crowded quarters risks poor overall health among family members, partly as a consequence of having more direct exposure to viral and bacterial pathogens (Solari & Mare, 2012). Living in a confined space also increases stress and poor treatment in the household: For example, parents living in crowded conditions are less responsive to and involved with their children and engage in less effective monitoring and lower levels of individual supervision (Bradley & Caldwell, 1984; Evans, Maxwell, & Hart, 1999; Gove, Hughes, & Style, 1983; Wachs & Camli, 1991). Confinement and/or crowded conditions are also associated with increases in domestic violence and harsh and inconsistent discipline (see more on this topic later in this chapter). To compound this circumstance, on account of the pandemic-induced economic downturn young adults were more likely than other age groups to lose their jobs or take a pay cut; by July 2020, perhaps expectedly, a majority (52 percent) of 18- to 29-year-olds in the United States found themselves living with their parents, surpassing the previous peak reached during the Great Depression (Pew Research Center, 2020). Additional economic consequences of the COVID-19 pandemic are discussed next.

Economic consequences . . .

The COVID-19 pandemic also wreaked havoc with family micro- and world macroeconomies. As towns and cities, provinces and states, and regions and countries went into public-health mandated stay-at-home lockdowns, businesses shuttered. For example, people stopped dining out and shopping, so restaurants and malls closed; people ceased travelling, so hotels shut down and flying only "ghost planes" airlines operated at an average 10 percent passenger load capacities (Slotnick, 2020). These events had reverberating economic consequences for individuals and families and governments. As of mid-July 2020, 55 percent of pandemic-era closures on Yelp became permanent, and permanent business closures began to outnumber temporary ones as bankruptcies proliferated (Bhattaral, 2020; Yelp, 2020). In the United States alone, at least 4 million private-sector workers had their pay cut, and more than 6 million were forced into part-time positions during just the first months of the pandemic. In the United States, the COVID-19 pandemic produced the worst monthly unemployment figures since the Great Depression, and in the United Kingdom perhaps the steepest annual decline in output since 1706 (Bank of England, 2020; U.S. Department of Labor, 2020b). Altogether, nearly one-third of U.S. American workers took a direct hit from the coronavirus-related recession, in jobs lost, hours cut, or salaries slashed. By the end of July 2020, the U.S. Commerce Department announced, by advance estimate a second quarter change of −9.5 percent that would translate into a "real gross domestic product . . . decrease at an annual rate of 32.9 percent," potentially representing the loss of one-third of the U.S. economy (Mataloni, Wasshausen, Strassner, & Aversa, 2020).

Such labor market volatility resonates through families, parents, and children in multiple ways. Nearly one-third (31 percent) of households in the United States reported having expended most or all of their savings, and nearly one-half (46 percent) facing serious financial problems during the coronavirus outbreak (NPR et al., 2020). In September 2020, 36 percent of U.S. Americans who had lost a job or had a reduction in take-home pay due to COVID-19 reported that they could not last more than one month on savings (SimplyWise, 2020). Through August 2020, 46 percent reported that some adult household member lost a job or business, was furloughed, or had wages or hours cut. Of course unemployment erodes self-esteem and is known to manifest in personal depression as well as violence in the family (Han, Hetzner, & Brooks-Gunn, 2019, in this volume). Job loss undermines mental health (Benach et al., 2014): Individualized unemployment is followed by increases in psychological distress, depression, anxiety, alcohol consumption, illegal drug use, and even suicidal ideation (Catalano et al., 2011; Gassman-Pines, Ananat, & Gibson-Davis, 2014; Nagelhout et al., 2017) as well as interpersonally argumentative and violent behavior (Dooley & Catalano, 1988; Dooley, Catalano, & Wilson, 1994). Parent job loss and insecurity likewise threaten family safekeeping and harm child well-being and development; unemployment is even associated with increased rates of child mortality (Duncan et al., 2017; Li, Page, Martin, & Taylor, 2011). As Han et al. (2019) review, negative economic events that result in low or reduced wages and family financial hardships precipitate increased economic pressures on the family. Families that experience such economic pressures suffer material needs and food insecurity (by May 2020, an estimated 25 percent of U.S. Americans reported that they or a member of their household went without meals or relied on charities or government programs to obtain groceries; Hamel et al., 2020) as well as unpaid mortgage, rent, automobile, credit card, and utility bills (electric and gas debts alone were estimated to exceed $24.3 billion by the end of 2020; National Energy Assistance Directors' Association, 2020). These and other cutbacks subsequently lead to emotional distress, diminished supportive behaviors, and compromised quality and stability of family relationships. At a minimum, job losses or salary cuts translate into fewer resources to spend on children, but also amplify parenting stresses and compromise the quality of the family environment, as a study of 5,500 U.K. parents found (Andrew et al., 2020a). Financial privations in turn can undermine children's socioemotional competencies, cognitive development, and academic success, simultaneously risking depression and anxiety, and limiting access to potentially enriching and diverting extracurricular activities and opportunities that promote social, emotional, and mental well-being (Conger et al., 2010; Vandell, Simpkins, & Wegemer, 2019). As Ananat et al. (2017, p. 1128) concluded, "[M]acrolevel job losses are . . . community-level traumas that harm the mental health of both children and adults, and of both families who experience job loss and those who only witness it."

Of the nearly 1.1 million people who stopped working or looking for work in the United States in September 2020, almost 80 percent were women, a "clear sign" of the childcare burden that falls principally on working mothers (Van Dam & Long, 2020). Mothers (working or not) are much more likely than fathers to handle a majority of childcare and housework (Andrew et al., 2020c; Bornstein, 2015; McKinsey & Company, 2020). Even parents (especially mothers) who retained part- or full-time work during the COVID-19 pandemic still incurred costs of role strain from persistent attempts to balance work with their need to care for children (even with both work and children at home) and contend with disruptions to normal family life and routines. Especially heavy demands fell on dual-wage earner families, parents caring for children with healthcare or special needs, and single parents without a parenting partner, who sacrificed their own well-being to meet competing needs of their children (Martinez-Marcos & De la Cuesta-Benjumea, 2015; Weinraub & Kaufman, 2019). For women who are mothers without flexible or remote work plans, and who could not return to work on account of childcaring, future economic prospects loomed in even greater jeopardy (Modestino, 2020).

More devastating still, unemployment endangered access to a wide range of services and institutions vital to wholesome and well-functioning family life, such as childcare and early education facilities (many daycares closed, and those that did not serviced only a fraction of the number they enrolled before the pandemic and became unaffordable; Stein, 2020), family health care (job-based coverage accounts for 55 percent of U.S. Americans' health insurance, so job loss eliminates access to affordable and necessary health care; Goldstein, 2020), basic supplies and food security (in Washington, District of Columbia, the capital of the United States, the number of children without stable food options was expected to grow to 29 percent by the end of 2020; DC Food Policy Council, 2020), and in extreme cases housing (for some threatening eviction and homelessness). To gain a deeper understanding of the looming threat to families, parents, and children, it is worthwhile to explore just one of these factors in greater depth. In the United States, a federal eviction ban, included in the $2 trillion Cares Act legislation (U.S. Department of the Treasury, 2020) passed by Congress in March 2020, covered all tenants living in buildings with mortgages guaranteed by the U.S. Government. Cares Act legislation did not help the 19–23 million people – about one in five renters in the United States – the majority of whom reside in buildings with privately backed mortgages (McKay, Neumann, & Gilman, 2020). Renters in publicly financed rentals came under the risk of eviction at the end of August 2020. Once a family falls over the "eviction cliff," it is challenging to recover. Eviction is devastating with no good outcomes. If not precipitated by unemployment, eviction leads to unemployment as well as to family residential instability and homelessness and to children's academic decline. Eviction has well-studied negative health consequences for children and adults alike. It is an ACE, and so can result in chronic health problems for children that endure well into adulthood, including cardiac, pulmonary, and (ironically) respiratory disease. Once a person has a record of eviction, their credit scores plummet. This "scarlet E" is associated with increased depression and suicide. There are further knock-on consequences to evictions as when rent payments stop, so do mortgage disbursements, building maintenance, and employee salaries. On top of that, whenever the U.S. eviction moratorium ends renters will still owe millions of dollars in back rent, which they may be unable to pay, leaving renters under the continuing threat of eviction, landlords with mortgages still to pay, and building employees continuing without salaries.

In addition to individual and family hazards and their sequelae, the COVID-19 pandemic has precipitated local and far-reaching economic consequences for families, parents, and children on account of financial turmoil wrought to their communities. Towns, cities, and states have lost sales and income tax revenues creating steep fiscal challenges and the withdrawal or re-direction of critical resources away from personal and family supports (e.g., libraries, museums, parks, and transportation). As most U.S. localities and states are legally required to balance their budgets, local governments furloughed teachers, police, firefighters, and sanitation workers (Fishman, 2020). The loss of employment-related health insurance is estimated in turn to cost hospitals $13.9 billion to $41.8 billion (Goldstein, 2020).

On an international scale, tentacles of the COVID-19 pandemic are strangling populations now and threatening economies into the future. On account of the coronavirus pandemic, widespread starvation is forecasted, especially in at-risk nations (Chotiner, 2020); the 2020 Nobel Peace Prize (Nobel Peace Prize, 2020) was awarded to the World Food Program in recognition of its past and current "efforts to combat hunger" worldwide. Around the globe, certain businesses and entertainments – notably, hotels, airlines, restaurants, commercial offices, and the arts – have been ravaged. COVID-19 is challenging the UN Sustainable Development Goal of ending poverty by 2030 because global monetary poverty is increasing for the first time since 1990 through contractions in per capita household income or consumption (Reinhart & Reinhart, 2020; Sumner, Hoy, & Ortiz-Juarez, 2020). The World Bank (2020b) estimates a possible increase of 150 million people to the ranks of the world's poorest by the end of 2020. During the April-June 2020 lockdown, school children in England spent an average of 4.5 hours a day on home learning, including time spent on online classes, other school work, private tutoring, and other educational activities; however, that 4.5 hours represents a 25–30 percent reduction in pre-COVID-19 learning time (Andrew et al., 2020a). Such mutations in education even in a high-income country likely have substantial downstream economic implications. In a fall 2020 report, the Organization for Economic Cooperation and Development estimated that global economic output could conservatively decline by 1.5 percent over the rest of the 21st century because of disruptions to schooling caused by the pandemic (Schleicher, 2020). That might mean, for example in the United States, a total economic loss equivalent to $15.3 trillion. More dire still, the WHO, UNAIDS, and the Stop TB Partnership anticipate that the combined annual death toll from HIV, tuberculosis, and malaria could nearly double on account of chaos caused by COVID-19 (Global Fund, 2020).

Recommendations and supports for families, parents, and children during and after the SARS-CoV-2 pandemic

Families, parents, and children need supports during the SARS-CoV-2 pandemic just as they will need them after the pandemic subsides. The most effective supports will come by way of coordinated messages and interventions delivered at multiple levels. In accord with the prevailing contextual bioecological model in developmental science, such supports and interventions would take place at the parent and family level, at the community level, and at the level of nations. As families, parents, and children confront new uncertainties of the coronavirus epidemic, the risks to their wholesome functioning are many, and so supports from many quarters will be welcome. As examples, adolescents must be counseled to exercise greater vigilance in their risk behaviors, employers need to find creative ways to reopen their businesses safely, and governments ought to support families financially and institute moratoriums on evictions.

Consider in depth one domain of family functioning that is put at risk by the multiple adverse consequences of the COVID-19 pandemic and how that risk might be obviated or mitigated at different bioecological levels. One of the most important ways that parents meet their responsibilities and shape their children's behavior is through the use of proactive discipline to encourage desired behaviors in the future and reactive discipline to respond to misbehaviors after they occur with the overarching goal of teaching children moral behavior and socializing them. Parents hold a wide range of attitudes regarding the acceptability and advisability of different forms of discipline and deploy a wide range of actions to manage their children's behaviors. Many such parenting attitudes and actions are shaped by the situations in which parents find themselves. Thus, understandably, several of the preceding home life and economic consequences of the COVID-19 pandemic – stress, depression, deprivation of supports, unemployment – could accumulate and coordinate to exert adverse effects on parenting in the form of harsh and inconsistent discipline of children through physiological (HPA axis), emotional (negative affect, undermined regulation), and cognitive mechanisms (hostile attributions; Nemeroff, 2016). For example, a study in the United Kingdom reported a marked increase in the incidence of abusive head trauma to children in the period March–April 2020 compared with the same period in 2017–2019 (Sidpra, Abomelli, Hameed, Baker, & Mankad, 2020). In the United States a surge in physical intimate partner violence during the pandemic was documented radiologically in nearly double the number of victims sustaining injuries due to strangulation, stabbings, burns, or use of weapons such as knives, guns, and other objects in March–April 2020 compared with the same period during 2017–2019 (Gosangi et al., 2020). Before concluding this introduction, it may be illustrative to re-visit this issue and explore effective supports to address potential harsh treatment of children under the stressful conditions of the pandemic at the levels of parent, community, and nation.

Consequences of the SARS-COV-2 pandemic for parenting discipline and abuse

With respect to harsh discipline and violence against children, parents can be protectors or perpetrators. The consequences of both for children are far-reaching (United Nations Foundation, 2014). For example, less gray matter (structural elements of the brain that are important in processing emotions and decision making) in the prefrontal cortex has been measured in young adults who report that, as children, they experienced corporal punishment at least one time a month and corporal punishment with an object at least one time a year compared to young adults who were not chronically corporally punished when they were children (Tomoda et al., 2009). Meta-analyses and longitudinal work indicate that hostile/aggressive parent behavior is associated pan-culturally with deleterious effects on child mental health (Khaleque, 2017). Although the magnitude of these effects may differ (based on how normative corporal punishment is in a particular culture, for example), overall greater parent use of corporal punishment with children predicts greater child externalizing problems (including aggression) and internalizing problems (including anxiety) in many cultures (Lansford et al., 2014). Experiencing harsh and inconsistent discipline increases children's fearfulness, irritability, and negative emotionality (Lengua & Kovacs, 2005). Moreover, these factors instigate a "devil's cycle" as parents' uses of harsh verbal discipline and corporal punishment predict subsequent adolescent behavior problems, and adolescents with more behavior problems elicit harsher verbal discipline and corporal punishment from their parents (Lansford et al., 2011). In consequence of the pandemic, the numbers of children affected by harsh discipline and violence are thought to have increased (Fore et al., 2020; Noveck, 2020). However, actual levels of abuse during the pandemic may be hidden because many children are not seeing teachers or pediatricians, whom children could previously rely on to report abuse, and child protection agencies have curtailed caseworker home visits (Ingram, 2020).

Before COVID-19, an estimated 1 billion children between the ages of 2 and 17 experienced physical, sexual, or emotional abuse in a year (Hillis, Mercy, Amobi, & Kress, 2016; WHO, 2018a), costing perhaps 2–5 percent of global GDP (Pereznieto, Montes, Routier, & Langston, 2014). Monitoring violence against children, and understanding risk factors and consequences of such violence, are key parts of the action plan for the UN Sustainable Development Goals (SDGs). Specifically, SDG Target 16.2 is to end abuse, exploitation, trafficking, and all forms of violence against and torture of children, and Indicator 16.2.1 concerns the proportion of children aged 1–17 years who experience any physical punishment and/or psychological aggression by caregivers in the past month. From a human rights perspective, corporal punishment is not just an inadvisable disciplinary strategy because it is related to worse child outcomes, it is also unacceptable because using corporal punishment is disrespectful and a violation of the right to protection all people enjoy, regardless of age. Given the knowledge we possess about the likely corrosive effects on positive parenting provoked by the COVID-19 pandemic, it is imperative somehow to overcome the spread of this insidious social disease. Coordinated interventions at multiple levels will help to accomplish this goal.

Multilevel interventions: parents and families

Most government agencies and public service organizations whose responsibilities include the health and well-being of children have stepped up to provide support for parents and families in coping with the pandemic. Locally, parents want to do what they can to help their children cope with threatening circumstances created by the pandemic and take away from the experience positive life lessons. Supportive parenting and a quality parent–child relationship are vital to children's coping and positive development. In the aftermath of a cyclone in Australia, parents who rated their family as more functional, effective, and responsive had children with lower levels of internalizing behavior (McDermott & Cobham, 2012);

following the 2004 tsunami in southeast Asia, supportive parenting in terms of spending time with their children, being attuned to their behaviors, and even simple sharing of everyday events proved critical to resilience in Norwegian children (Hafstad et al., 2012); and following a major hurricane in Puerto Rico, adolescents with these experiences reported lower levels of internalizing symptoms (Felix et al., 2013). What can parents do to ensure that their children's memories of this time will be more genial than cheerless, to maximize children's thanks for their health and minimize indignation about limitations on their lives? Cognitive scientists contend that children's memories of the pandemic will be shaped by the positive (shared values) or negative (family contentiousness) experiences that repeat now.

Also in the short run, parents need to attend to their own needs. Mental health experts refer to a set of important skills as "psychological first aid" (Everly & Lating, 2017). The World Health Organization, War Trauma Foundation, and World Vision International (2011) recommend developing skills that help one be safe, connected to others, calm, and hopeful; gain access to social, physical, and emotional supports; and enable one able to help oneself and one's community.

Internationally UNICEF and the WHO, and in the United States the CDC, the American Academy of Pediatrics, and national PTA, as well as hundreds more (international, national, and local) organizations offer guidance and tips on all aspects of parenting during the pandemic https://tiltparenting.com/recommended-resources/. Resources include how to keep a child physically healthy, how to address children's fears and anxieties, how to ameliorate parents' own fears and anxieties, how to help children with distance learning, suggestions for academic and entertaining activities, self-care, and more. To access and vet all this information became a full-time job for parents.

In the longer run, there is a body of knowledge on parent interventions that work. The United Nations Foundation (2018) identified parenting as a key contributor to progress towards numerous SDGs, including Goals 1 (Ending Poverty in All Its Forms), 3 (Ensuring Healthy Lives and Promoting Well-Being for All at All Ages), and 11 (Create Safe, Secure, and Sustainable Cities and Communities). Given their worldwide missions, UNICEF and the WHO as global health organizations have increasingly emphasized parenting as a centerpiece for interventions aimed at fostering child physical well-being and mental health (Britto, Ponguta, Reyes, & Karnati, 2015; United Nations Foundation, 2017). Furthermore, in accord with specificity (as detailed earlier with respect to parents' responsibilities), different domains of parenting can be expected to respond to uniquely tailored parenting interventions: Parent warmth is promoted by parents providing positive attention and praising children (McMahon & Forehand, 2003); parent neglect/indifference and perceived rejection by children are diminished by prompting child-led parent–child play (McMahon & Forehand, 2003); and parent hostility/aggression is replaced by parents and children engaging in emotion regulation exercises (McMahon & Forehand, 2003; Rothenberg et al., 2020).

Parents can adopt two routes to foster more wholesome parent-child relationships and child developmental outcomes: They may emphasize the positive or they may de-emphasize the negative. Emphasizing and nurturing positive parent-child relationships, parent demonstrations of warmth provide children with positive attention for appropriate behavior (McMahon & Forehand, 2003). When children are not provided with such attention for appropriate behavior, they may seek attention by falling back on inappropriate behaviors such as arguing, yelling, or tantruming in bids for attention (i.e., externalizing behaviors) or withdrawing from interactions (internalizing behaviors; McMahon & Forehand, 2003). Triple P, the Positive Parenting Program, is a preventively oriented multilevel family intervention which aims to promote positive and caring relationships between parents and their children and help parents develop effective management strategies for dealing with a variety of childhood behavioral and emotional problems and common developmental issues (Sanders, Turner, & McWilliam, 2015, in this volume). Triple P draws on social learning theory, applied behavior analysis, research in developmental science and developmental psychopathology, social information processing models, and public health principles. Triple P teaches parents strategies to encourage their child's social and language skills, emotional self-regulation, independence, and problem-solving ability. Attainment of those skills promotes family harmony, reduces parent–child conflict and risk of child maltreatment, fosters flourishing peer relationships, and prepares children for successful experiences at school and later in life.

Such parent programs exist in many cultures around the world that effectively build parent positive attention and improve children's behavior (Gardner, Montgomery, & Knerr, 2016). For example, parent-child play for just 5 minutes a day is a proven strategy to address child abuse and neglect (McMahon & Forehand, 2003). These programs teach parents positive attention and appropriate discipline strategies using live coaching and have been demonstrated to be effective in numbers of cultures around the world with minimal adaptation. By contrast, a coercive process of interaction is instantiated in mutual hostility and aggression and is reinforced if it somehow leads to goal attainment. Coercive processes have been observed in many different cultures, and behavioral parent training interventions that target such coercive cycles of interaction have proven to be effective in many cultures as well (Gardner et al., 2016).

Thinking systematically about enduring family change, Fosco, Bumbarger, and Bamberger (2015, in this volume) examine delivery, support capacity, and infrastructure barriers which constrain the population-level impact of prevention programs. At the family level, they discuss the importance of testing guiding theories of prevention programs by assessing both processes and mechanisms that account for enduring changes in individual and family outcomes. Intervention studies support the effectiveness of targeting parents and families. In one study, families that were randomized to an intervention that improved positive parenting practices reduced young children's behavior problems, whereas children's behavior problems did not change in families randomized to a control group (Dishion et al., 2008). In another study, mothers who were randomized to an intervention, rather than control, group improved in their use of positive discipline strategies, which, in turn, attenuated children's externalizing behavior problems (Tein, Sandler, MacKinnon, & Wolchik, 2004). Evidence-based parenting programs provide effective strategies to improve relationships, reduce conflict, manage family finances, and relieve parenting stress (Ward et al., 2020). Randomized controlled trials have shown that families accessing such parenting programs benefit from diminished violence, mental health problems, alcohol use, and extreme poverty (Cluver et al., 2018; Puffer, Annan, Sim, Salhi, & Betancourt, 2017). There is also mounting evidence of the efficacy of such programs across high-, middle-, and low-income countries.

Which would be the better intervention target, parents' cognitions or parents' practices? Interventions aimed at reducing parents' use of punishment often include components focused first on changing parents' beliefs about the effectiveness and appropriateness of punishment as a prelude to teaching parents how to implement more child-friendly approaches to discipline. Data from the UNICEF Multiple Indicator Cluster Survey, a nationally representative survey delivered to more than 50 low- and middle-income countries, reveal that more children experience corporal punishment than have caregivers who believe using corporal punishment is necessary (Lansford & Deater-Deckard, 2012). Therefore, interventions that bypass attitudes and focus on changing parent behaviors directly may be advisable. Moreover, parents often resort to corporal punishment out of anger in the heat of the moment, rather than as part of any cognitively planned discipline strategy. This observation suggests that interventions aimed to train parents to stop, bring their emotions under control, and deploy alternate non-violent approaches to discipline could be effective. So, specific interventions that change actions (rather than trying to change attitudes) may be concrete and simpler for parents to comprehend and execute. Likewise, investments in parenting supports for emotion regulation and non-violent approaches to childrearing may prove rewarding.

Who is best positioned to implement such parent-focused interventions? In the immediacy of the moment, it is probably frontline providers of childcare – teachers, pediatricians, and social workers who often are consulted about how to manage children's behavior problems (Bornstein & Cote, 2004) – who can help parents best navigate these challenges. They may be regarded as trusted sources of information about discipline (Taylor, Moeller, Hamvas, & Rice, 2013). On this argument, providing information to these frontline workers in digestible form seems imperative.

Multilevel interventions: communities

Community policies can also be brought to bear to mitigate short- and long-term impacts of the COVID-19 pandemic on families, parents, and children. Community-level policies would include supports for caregivers' well-being, mental health, and capacity to provide nurturing care. Community frontline workers can be trained to address the mental health status of parents through, for example, Caring for the Caregiver initiatives (AHRQ, 2020). At the same level, effective mass media can be helpful: Triple P Online, the e-version of a parenting program for parents of children with elevated behavior problems, uses social media and games of parenting content to improve parents' behavior management skills

(Baker, Sanders, Turner, & Morawska, 2017). These community-based programs teach parents positive attention and appropriate discipline strategies using live coaching and have been demonstrated to work in numerous communities around the world with minimal adaptation (Gardner et al., 2016). It has been estimated that delivery costs of scaled up non-commercial parenting programs to a community level can be rendered ultimately affordable. New initiatives have proved capable of providing evidence-based parenting support through remote delivery, reaching tens of millions of families across 180 countries within the first 12 weeks of the COVID-19 pandemic (Cluver et al., 2020).

Accurate and timely information and confidence in government are also vital to parent and child coping and mental health during and after community-level emergencies. During the H1N1 (swine flu) epidemic in the United Kingdom, individuals who believed the information they were receiving about the outbreak were more likely to comply with suggestions to protect personal and public health (Rubin et al., 2009). High school students who reported feeling less safe and protected by the government eight months after the 9/11 terrorist attack in the United States were 4 times more likely to report PTSD symptoms compared to those who did not report a lack of trust in the government (Calderoni et al., 2006), and confidence in government responses was correlated with feelings of hope for the future immediately following those attacks as well as up to nine months later (Gross, Brewer, & Aday, 2009).

Multilevel interventions: nations

The cultural spillover theory of violence asserts that, in countries in which violence is more accepted, corporal punishment of children may be caregivers' default response (Baron & Straus, 1989). Anthropological studies demonstrate that corporal punishment of children is more frequent and sanctioned in societies that also endorse other forms of interpersonal violence (Lansford & Dodge, 2008). The *Global Status Report on Preventing Violence Against Children 2020* documented that just 25 percent of 155 participating governments reported that their support to parenting programs was adequate to reach all who needed them – in low- and middle-income countries the reach dropped to just 15 percent. Altogether, 139 countries do not yet have laws protecting children from corporal punishment in the home (Global Initiative to End All Corporal Punishment of Children, 2020). Significantly, in European countries where corporal punishment is legal, parents are 1.7 times more likely to report using corporal punishment.

Systematic investigation of a national corporal punishment ban was conducted in Sweden, the first country to outlaw corporal punishment (banning corporal punishment in 1979). The legal ban of corporal punishment was widely publicized (with, e.g., announcements on milk cartons). Swedish efforts proved successful in promoting knowledge of the law. More than 90 percent of the Swedish population was aware of the law one year after it passed (Ziegert, 1983). After the legal ban, endorsement and use of corporal punishment declined. Finland offers a second case study. Twenty-eight years after the 1983 legal ban in Finland (see Husa, 2011, for a review of legal reforms leading up to the ban), a representative sample of

4,609 15- to 80-year-olds reported whether they had been corporally punished. Finns who were born after the legal ban were significantly less likely to have been slapped and beaten as children than Finns who were born before the legal ban, with no significant decline in corporal punishment in the 39 years prior to the legal ban. These findings suggest that the law itself marked a turning point in the national use of corporal punishment by parents. Other countries might benefit from the Swedish and Finnish experiences.

Of course, changing a national law is not always sufficient to change individual behavior. A number of public awareness campaigns have been developed to promote awareness of laws involving child corporal punishment, to impart knowledge regarding the negative effects of corporal punishment, and to build capacity in using non-violent forms of discipline. Just as under the weight of a deadly pandemic, typical coping strategies and protective measures once utilized to manage adversity may not be as accessible as they were before the pandemic. Although there may be commonalities in the effects on children across geographies, public health strategies adopted by countries to reduce harsh treatment are likely to be moderated by local contextual factors such as cultural norms, laws, and human, technical, infrastructural, and financial resources (Bornstein, 2017).

With UNICEF and other partners, the WHO developed several evidence-based resources aimed at assisting countries to strengthen supports for positive parenting. These include:

- The *Nurturing Care Framework*, which highlights support for good health and adequate nutrition in the first three years of life, responsive caregiving, opportunities for early learning, and safety and security as key aspects of good parenting practices (WHO, 2018b).
- The *INSPIRE: Seven Strategies for Ending Violence Against Children* program, in which parent and caregiver supports aim at reducing risk factors for child maltreatment and other forms of violence against children aged 0–17 years by reducing harsh parenting practices and creating positive parent-child relationships (WHO, 2016).
- The *RESPECT Women* framework for preventing violence against women, in which child and adolescent abuse prevention through parent and caregiver support is a key pillar for reducing the likelihood of intimate partner violence (RESPECT women, 2019).

In 2016, a World Health Assembly resolution endorsed a WHO (2018a, p. 3) global plan of action on "strengthening the role of the health system within a national multisectoral response to address interpersonal violence, in particular against women and girls, and against children." A number of international parenting programs also specifically aim to help parents reduce resorting to corporal punishment and increase utilizing alternate forms of discipline (United Nations Foundation, 2014): Nurturing Care for Children, Parent Management Training, Positive Parenting and Sensitive Discipline, and the Positive Discipline in Everyday Parenting Program which has been adapted for use in 13 countries. A summary can be found at www.blueprintsprograms.com. International intervention efforts have turned to ways to promote parents' use of non-punitive forms of discipline and eliminate parents' reliance on corporal punishment (Britto et al., 2015). Vitally important to ensure the validity of all these international efforts is to follow canons for culturally adapting evidence-based family prevention and intervention programs as detailed in Kumpfer, Magalhães, Xie, and Kanse (2015, in this volume). UNICEF (2020b) has taken an omnibus approach to addressing family, parent, and child interests in the COVID-19 pandemic.

Looking to the future

According to the Editor of the *Lancet*, the British medical journal of record, even a vaccine will not eradicate the coronavirus. No vaccine is 100 percent effective, 100 percent safe, and available to 100 percent of people. Only non-pregnant adults have participated in early trials, not children, so a COVID-19 vaccine would not be recommended for children when it first becomes available (CDC, 2020i). The U.S. National Academies of Sciences, Engineering and Medicine (2020) reported that only 10–15 million doses of a vaccine would be available initially, which may cover only 3–5 percent of the U.S. population. Following its recommendations, children and young adults would receive the vaccine in a fourth tier of immunizations, before it is passed on to the remaining population. It would be God's work to get a vaccine to the 7+ billion people on the planet; the massive logistical challenges that confront manufacturing and distribution efforts are unimaginable (Zhang, 2020). Moreover, all 7+ billion people on the planet would not submit to vaccination anyway (Booth, 2020). A late September 2020 Gallup poll asked 2,730 adults, 18 years and older, "If a vaccine approved by the Food and Drug Administration were available right now at no cost, would you get vaccinated?" Only 50 percent said yes (Saad, 2020; see also Elbeshbishi & King, 2020). Indeed, epidemiological models suggest about 70 percent of the population would need to be vaccinated to inhibit spread of the coronavirus (Clemente-Suárez et al., 2020). According to the WHO (2020h), as of October 2020 fewer than 10 percent of people in most countries have contracted COVID-19.

Therefore, at the level of the individual, *behavior* is the first line of defense and resistance. Between the emergence and identification of an infectious disease like the novel coronavirus and the development and deployment of even a partially effective vaccine (the land speed record is the 1960s vaccine for mumps . . . four years, Eisele, 2020 . . . and that swift success relied heavily on extensive groundwork), what matters most to halt the spread of a person-to-person infection like the coronavirus is adherence to a remarkably short list of rather simple behaviors that relate back to the 3Vs:

- Covering mouth and nose.
- Washing hands.
- Avoiding poorly ventilated closed spaces.
- Keeping physically distant from others.

As has been well established for over a century since the 1918 influenza pandemic (Barry, 2005), these mitigation efforts are effective. Recall that the coronavirus originated in Wuhan, China, at the end of December 2019. The city of Wuhan, which instituted all these measures in force successfully stamped out the virus. After months without a confirmed case of domestic transmission, around 1.4 million children in the city returned to their classrooms at the start of September 2020 (Xinhua, 2020). In the first global projection of the COVID-19 pandemic by nation, the University of Washington Institute for Health Metrics and Evaluation (2020) predicted that nearly 770,000 lives worldwide could be saved between September 2020 and January 2021 through proven measures such as mask wearing and physical distancing. No one of these behaviors is at all difficult to execute, even if small children present a bit of a challenge (Davis, 2020). But, as 2020 unfolded what became remarkable was how peoples in different countries, and those within the same country, either adhered to these simple admonitions or neglected, avoided, flouted, or even belittled them at an extraordinary cost.

Conclusions

Parenthood ultimately means facilitating a child's happiness and optimism, self-confidence and purpose, capacity for intimacy and friendships, adaptive behaviors and achievement motivation, pleasure in play and work, and continuing academic success and educational fulfillment – all positive characteristics. Even before the COVID-19 pandemic, 43 percent of all children under 5 years of age in the world were estimated to be at risk of not achieving their developmental potential (Black et al., 2017). Today, the COVID-19 pandemic has profoundly altered trajectories of children's future development everywhere. A better understanding of disaster-specific stressors and their psychological sequelae is critical to redressing the many damaging impacts of the COVID-19 pandemic on families, parents, and children.

The CDC (2020e), WHO (2020i), and innumerable NGOs have launched interventions and offered specific resources that underscore the need to protect physical and mental health in families, parents, and children during the COVID-19 pandemic (e.g., guides for how to keep parent-child interactions positive). Clearly, supportive resources are required to protect families, parents, and children against the spreading coronavirus. Moreover, investigators in the medical, social, and behavioral sciences have responded to the COVID-19 pandemic by launching protocols and gathering data on all facets of family, parent, and child health and development. (A probe of Google Scholar using the search term "COVID 19" brought 56,500 results since 2019 in 0.09 seconds, and by the fall of 2020 the Wikimedia Foundation, 2020, reported that more than 82,000 editors had collaborated to create more than 5,000 Wikipedia articles about COVID-19 in 175 different languages that were viewed more than 500 million times.) In consequence, the contemporary literatures in multiple scientific fields are rapidly developing a broad body of empirical research that will document the course and consequences of COVID-19 around the world. Hopefully, many evidence-based findings will be brought to bear to support families, parents, and children during this unprecedented time.

Yet, at this writing in mid-October 2020 fundamental questions and deep uncertainties which have dominated the pandemic at all levels through the first ten months of 2020 persist. As the numbers of infections in the United States, Europe, Russia, and elsewhere rise, is the world experiencing an extended first or entering a second new wave of viral spread . . . and does a so-called second wave involve those not previously infected or those who were, recovered, and become reinfected? (Some public health authorities contend that it no longer makes sense to talk about "waves" of virus spread, but instead "spikes followed by plateaus.") Is the coronavirus mutating and how infectious are different sub-strains? (Decoding the coronavirus genome to identify sub-strains could specify infection origins, track transmission, and pinpoint contact tracing to control outbreaks.) What exactly is the fatality rate of COVID-19? (Case fatality rates are the percentage of deaths among confirmed cases; infection fatality rates are estimates of deaths as a proportion of all those believed to be infected. Epidemiologists also calculate fatality rates as deaths per 100,000 people in a population. Clearly, fatality rates also vary dramatically over time, age, region, country, and other factors.) Are lockdowns and shutdowns or their opposites in opening-up and achieving herd immunity the better future course of action to mitigate viral spread? (National and international public health officials today offer starkly contrasting opinions, as evidenced in the Great Barrington Declaration, 2020.) Can a person once infected and cleared of the virus be re-infected? (Albeit exceptional so far, multiple instances of people being infected for a second time after recovering from COVID-19 have been documented.) Should children return to school? (Parents still do not know whether it is best to maintain distance learning at home, sign up for a hybrid solution, or enroll their children back at in-person schooling.) When will a treatment finally arrive? (In September and October 2020 two main late-stage vaccine trials and one monoclonal antibody drug trial were paused.) Will vaccination require one, two, or even three doses, with what is the duration of protection, and at what cost? (There are currently more than 100 COVID-19 vaccine candidates under development, and all have different requirements.) When all is said and done, will the world just have to learn to live with the coronavirus? (After years of effort, there is still no vaccine for the rhinovirus common cold or the human immunodeficiency virus.) Etc.

A final note about scientific research in the era of SARS-CoV-2

This chapter draws heavily on published scientific research, but (as noted consistently) a hallmark of the COVID-19 pandemic has been uncertainty. Science itself is probabilistic. On top of that inherent degree of uncertainty, the COVID-19 pandemic so captured the attention of the world – scientists included – that the discipline as a whole began to fracture and in some cases (some would argue against better judgment) to abandon long-standing and hard-won canons of scientific research, vetting, and publication. So, the results from a drug trial with six rhesus monkeys on one day became international news the very next day (Kirkpatrick, 2020). No quantitative documentation. No written paper. No peer review. No archival publication.

Examples of this rush to publish are edifying and ring the cautionary note *caveat lector*.

- On 25 June 2020, the 67,000-member American Academy of Pediatrics (Camera, 2020) opined that children do not contract or spread the coronavirus the way adults do (in contrast, say, to how children spread influenza). That advice seemed sage until 16 July 2020, when reports for 59,073 contacts of 5,706 coronavirus disease index patients concluded that 10- to 19-year-old adolescents spread the virus as efficiently as do adults (Park, Choe et al., 2020a); children younger than 10 were half as likely to transmit the virus, but still posed a risk. By 30 July 2020, a Research Letter replicated that SARS-CoV-2 in children 5–17 years leads to similar levels of viral nucleic acid as adults, but detected up to 100-fold greater amount of the virus in the upper respiratory tracts of children younger than 5 years than in adults 18–65 years (Heald-Sargent et al., 2020). Still another study (Armann et al., 2020), only in preprint review by the *Lancet*, reported very low seropraevalence and transmission rates from adolescent students to their teachers, but the authors quickly cautioned that the study took place in Saxony, Germany, where the prevalence of coronavirus at the time was low and that their results therefore should not be used to guide clinical practice.
- Authors of a 14 July 2020 case report in *Nature Communications* "confirmed" by comprehensive virological and pathological investigations the transplacental transmission of SARS-CoV-2 in a neonate born to a mother infected in the last trimester of pregnancy and that the child presented with neurological compromise similar to that described in adult patients (Vivanti et al., 2020; see also Chen et al., 2020). Same day(!) 14 July expert reaction to the report was supportive but also divided and skeptical on methodological and statistical grounds (Chakkarapani et al., 2020). As of 25 September 2020, more than 20,000 pregnant women in the United States had tested positive for the coronavirus (CDC, 2020j). At this writing, it is unclear whether and how SARS-CoV-2 is transmitted from mother to fetus and what the long-term effects on child development may be.
- A non-peer-reviewed study posted to a preprint server on 11 July 2020 concluded that coronavirus-fighting antibodies drop off steeply two to three months after infection (Seow et al., 2020). A second study posted on 17 July 2020, also not peer-reviewed, concluded that coronavirus-fighting antibodies were stable and even increased in patients who started with lower levels right after their infections (Wajnberg et al., 2020).

The COVID-19 pandemic descended on the world as normally would be the case when untold numbers of academics and governmental and non-governmental scientists were in the middle of an equally untold number of research projects. Institutional closures and individuals sheltering in place brought to an abrupt halt much biomedical and social and behavioral science research. COVID-19 more than simply paused all this work; additionally, data from the time of the virus can be expected to be colored by extraordinary circumstances that thoroughgoingly changed almost all aspects of personal and societal behavior.

Finally, despite the surge of publications documented on Google Scholar, a study of 4,500 scientists in the United States and Europe reported an overall sharp decline in research productivity during the pandemic (Myers et al., 2020). It will come as no surprise to attentive readers of this chapter that the authors of this study attributed "the largest disruptions [of the scientific enterprise] . . . to a usually unobserved dimension: childcare."

References

Bolded references are reprinted in this volume

Abgrall, G., Akhounak, S., & Neff, E. (2020). Prise en charge medico-psychologique de nombreuses victimes lors de feux urbains. *Médecine de Catastrophe-Urgences Collectives, 4*(2), 145–147. Retrieved from https://www.sciencedirect.com/science/article/pii/ S1279847920300604?casa_token=CTZjKLKYd58AAAAA:NruXnXFRwJKtK2YbR9 orNQJUhK1dG1uhMgy3t23MTC3dbDDauioXW7JbjcUeCgU_b0s6G0C9x4s

Abgrall, G., Neff, E., Deloche-Gaudez, F., & Akhounak, S. (2020). *Le poste d'urgence médicopsychologique téléphonique: un nouvel outil dans la prise en charge du trauma par les CUMP*. Cachan: Lavoisier. Retrieved from http://cn2r.fr/wp-content/uploads/2020/03/ COVID_PEC_Psy_Final_notes3.pdf

Academy of Medical Sciences. (2020, April). *Survey results: Understanding people's concerns about the mental health impacts of the COVID-19 pandemic*. London: The Academy of Medical Sciences.

Achenbach, J., & Dupree, J. (2020). U.S. tops 60,000 daily coronavirus infections for first time since early August. *The Washington Post*. Retrieved from https://www.washington-post.com/health/2020/10/15/coronavirus-cases-surging/

Agency for Healthcare Research and Quality. (2016, reviewed 2017). *Care for the caregiver program implementation guide*. Rockville, MD: Agency for Healthcare Research and Quality. Retrieved from www.ahrq.gov/patient-safety/capacity/candor/modules/guide6.html

Almond, D. (2006). Is the 1918 influenza pandemic over? Long-term effects of in utero influenza exposure in the post-1940 US population. *Journal of Political Economy, 114*(4), 672–712. https://doi.org/10.1086/507154

American Academy of Pediatrics. (2020a). Children and COVID-19: State data report. American Academy of Pediatrics, Children's Hospital Association. Retrieved from https://services.aap.org/en/pages/2019-novel-coronavirus-covid-19-infections/ children-and-covid-19-state-level-data-report/

American Academy of Pediatrics. (2020b). Multisystem inflammatory syndrome in children (MIS-C) interim guidance. *Critical Updates on COVID-19*. Retrieved from https://services. aap.org/en/pages/2019-novel-coronavirus-covid-19-infections/clinical-guidance/ multisystem-inflammatory-syndrome-in-children-mis-c-interim-guidance/

American Academy of Pediatrics. (2020c). *Guidance on providing pediatric well-care during COVID-19*. Washington, DC: American Academy of Pediatrics. Retrieved from https://services.aap.org/en/pages/2019-novel-coronavirus-covid-19-infections/ clinical-guidance/guidance-on-providing-pediatric-well-care-during-covid-19/

American Academy of Pediatrics. (2020d). *COVID-19 planning considerations: Guidance for school re-entry*. Washington, DC: American Academy of Pediatrics. Retrieved from https://services.aap.org/en/pages/2019-novel-coronavirus-covid-19-infections/clinical-guidance/covid-19-planning-considerations-return-to-in-person-education-in-schools/

American College of Emergency Physicians. (2020). *ACEP COVID-19 field guide: Signs and symptoms.* Retrieved from www.acep.org/corona/covid-19-field-guide/patient-presentation/signs-and-symptoms/

American Psychological Association (APA). (2020). Stress in the time of COVID-19. *Stress in America, 2,* 1–2. Retrieved from https://www.apa.org/news/press/releases/stress/2020/stress-in-america-covid-june.pdf

Ananat, E. O., Gassman-Pines, A., Francis, D. V., & Gibson-Davis, C. M. (2017). Linking job loss, inequality, mental health, and education. *Science, 356*(6343), 1127–1128. Retrieved from https://science.sciencemag.org/content/356/6343/1127.summary?casa_token=HqhkFYqnH7YAAAAA:MZvycQczD7pM4yt0EQ8xp3jMFwqYnxver6C_sQQaZyH_Tb7OnKPauwZwQVH0KAsk3gkCqZW6cLf7J5g

Anand, S., Montez-Rath, M., Han, J., Bozeman, J., Kerschmann, R., Beyer, P., . . . & Chertow, G. M. (2020). Prevalence of SARS-CoV-2 antibodies in a large nationwide sample of patients on dialysis in the USA: A cross-sectional study. *The Lancet.* Retrieved from https://www.thelancet.com/action/showPdf?pii=S0140-6736%2820%2932009-2

Anda, R. F., Felitti, V. J., Bremner, J. D., Walker, J. D., Whitfield, C. H., Perry, B. D., . . . & Giles, W. H. (2006). The enduring effects of abuse and related adverse experiences in childhood. *European Archives of Psychiatry and Clinical Neuroscience, 256*(3), 174–186. https://doi.org/10.1007/s00406-005-0624-4

Andrew, A., Cattan, S., Costa-Dias, M., Farquharson, C., Kraftman, L., Krutikova, S., . . . & Sevilla, A. (2020a). *Family time use and home learning during the COVID-19 lockdown.* London: Institute for Fiscal Studies. Retrieved from https://www.ifs.org.uk/publications/15038

Andrew, A., Cattan, S., Costa-Dias, M., Farquharson, C., Kraftman, L., Krutikova, S., . . . & Sevilla, A. (2020b). *Learning during the lockdown: real-time data on children's experiences during home learning.* London: Institute for Fiscal Studies. Retrieved from https://www.ifs.org.uk/uploads/Edited_Final-BN288%20Learning%20during%20the%20lockdown.pdf

Andrew, A., Cattan, S., Costa-Dias, M., Farquharson, C., Kraftman, L., Krutikova, S., . . . & Sevilla, A. (2020c). *The gendered division of paid and domestic work under lockdown.* London: Institute for Fiscal Studies. Retrieved from https://www.ifs.org.uk/publications/14943

Armann, J. P., Unrath, M., Kirsten, C., Lueck, C., Dalpke, A., & Berner, R. (2020). Anti-SARS-CoV-2 IgG antibodies in adolescent students and their teachers in Saxony, Germany (SchoolCoviDD19): Very low seropraevalence and transmission rates. *medRxiv.* https://doi.org/10.1101/2020.07.16.20155143v3

Armstrong, R. A., Kane, A. D., & Cook, T. M. (2020). Outcomes from intensive care in patients with COVID-19: A systematic review and meta-analysis of observational studies. *Anaesthesia, 75*(10), 1340–1349. Retrieved from https://associationofanaesthetists-publications.onlinelibrary.wiley.com/doi/full/10.1111/anae.15201

Asimov, I. (1951). The fun they had. https://archive.org/stream/Fantasy_Science_Fiction_v006n02_1954-02/Fantasy__Science_Fiction_v006n02_1954-02" \l "page/n125/mode/2up

Baker, D., Taylor, H., & Henderson, J. (1998). Inequality in infant morbidity: Causes and consequences in England in the 1990s. ALSPAC Study Team. Avon Longitudinal Study of Pregnancy and Childhood. *Journal of Epidemiology & Community Health, 52*(7), 451–458. http://doi.org/10.1136/jech.52.7.451

46 *Marc H. Bornstein*

Baker, M., McNicholas, A., Garrett, N., Jones, N., Stewart, J., Koberstein, V., & Lennon, D. (2000). Household crowding a major risk factor for epidemic meningococcal disease in Auckland children. *The Pediatric Infectious Disease Journal, 19*(10), 983–990. Retrieved from https://journals.lww.com/pidj/Abstract/2000/10000/Household_crowding_a_major_risk_factor_for.9.aspx

Baker, S., Sanders, M. R., Turner, K. M., & Morawska, A. (2017). A randomized controlled trial evaluating a low-intensity interactive online parenting intervention, Triple P. Online Brief, with parents of children with early onset conduct problems. *Behaviour Research and Therapy, 91*, 78–90. https://doi.org/10.1016/j.brat.2017.01.016

Bank of England. (2020). *Monetary policy report: May 2020.* Bank of England Monetary Policy Committee. Retrieved from https://www.bankofengland.co.uk/-/media/boe/files/monetary-policy-report/2020/may/monetary-policy-report-may-2020

Baron, L., & Straus, M. A. (1989). *Four theories of rape in American society: A state-level analysis.* New Haven, CT: Yale University Press.

Barr, R. (2019). Growing up in the digital age: Early learning and family media ecology. *Current Directions in Psychological Science, 28*(4), 341–346.

Barr, R., & Linebarger, D. N. (Eds.). (2017). *Media exposure during infancy and early childhood: The effect of content and context on learning and development.* New York: Springer.

Barr, R., McClure, E., & Palarkian, R. (2019). Maximizing the potential for learning from screen experiences in early childhood: What the research says. *Zero to Three, 40*(2), 29–36.

Barry, J. M. (2005). *The great influenza: The story of the deadliest pandemic in history.* New York: Penguin Books.

Beigel, J. H., Tomashek, K. M., Dodd, L. E., Mehta, A. K., Zingman, B. S., Kalil, A. C., . . . the ACTT-1 Study Group Members. (2020). Remdesivir for the treatment of Covid-19: Preliminary report. *The New England Journal of Medicine.* https://doi.org/10.1056/NEJMoa2007764

Benach, J., Vives, A., Amable, M., Vanroelen, C., Tarafa, G., & Muntaner, C. (2014). Precarious employment: Understanding an emerging social determinant of health. *Annual Review of Public Health, 35*, 229–253. https://doi.org/10.1146/annurev-publhealth-032013-182500

Bernstein, L. (2020). 'Nobody has very clear answers for them': Doctors search for treatments for covid-19 long-haulers. The *Washington Post.* Retrieved from https://www.washingtonpost.com/health/covid-long-haulers-treatment/2020/10/15/207b4af8-098f-11eb-9be6-cf25fb429f1a_story.html

Bhattaral, A. (2020). Pandemic bankruptcies: A running list of retailers that have filed for Chapter 11. *The Washington Post.* Retrieved from www.washingtonpost.com/business/2020/05/27/retail-bankrupcy-chapter11/

Bipartisan Policy Center. (2020). *Nationwide survey: Child care in the time of coronavirus.* Washington, DC: Bipartisan Policy Center. Retrieved from https://bipartisanpolicy.org/blog/nationwide-survey-child-care-in-the-time-of-coronavirus/

Birnir, B. (2020). Ventilation and the SARS-CoV-2 Coronavirus analysis of outbreaks in a restaurant and on a bus in China, and at a Call Center in South Korea. *medRxiv.* Retrieved from https://www.medrxiv.org/content/10.1101/2020.09.11.20192997v1

Bixler, D., Miller, A. D., Mattison, C. P., Taylor, B., Komatsu, K., . . . & Pediatric Mortality Investigation Team. (2020). SARS-CoV-2–associated deaths among persons aged 21 years: United States, February 12–July 31, 2020. *Centers for Disease Control and Prevention: Morbidity and Mortality Weekly Report, 69*(37), 1324–1329. Retrieved from https://www.cdc.gov/mmwr/volumes/69/wr/mm6937e4.htm?s_cid=mm6937e4_w

Black, M. M., Walker, S. P., Fernald, L. C., Andersen, C. T., DiGirolamo, A. M., Lu, C., . . . & Devercelli, A. E. (2017). Early childhood development coming of age: Science through the life course. *The Lancet, 389*(10064), 77–90. https://doi.org/10.1016/S0140-6736(16)31389-7

Blair, P. S., Mitchell, E., Fleming, P. J., Smith, I. J., Platt, M. W., Young, J., . . . & Golding, J. (1999). Babies sleeping with parents: Case-control study of factors influencing the risk of the sudden infant death syndrome. Commentary: Cot death – The story so far. *British Medical Journal, 319*(7223), 1457–1462. https://doi.org/10.1136/bmj.319.7223.1457

Bolt, M. A., Helming, L. M., & Tintle, N. L. (2018). The associations between self-reported exposure to the Chernobyl nuclear disaster zone and mental health disorders in Ukraine. *Frontiers in Psychiatry, 9*, 32. https://doi.org/10.3389/fpsyt.2018.00032

Booth, W. (2020). Lancet editor Richard Horton has harsh words for Trump, hope for science. *The Washington Post*. Retrieved from www.washingtonpost.com/world/europe/lancet-richard-horton-trump-vaccines/2020/07/29/1209b610-d048-11ea-826b-cc394d824e35_story.html

Bornstein, M. H. (2015). Children's parents. In M. H. Bornstein & T. Leventhal (Eds.), *Ecological settings and processes in developmental systems*. Volume 4 of the *Handbook of child psychology and developmental science* (7th ed., pp. 55–132). Editor-in-Chief: R. M. Lerner. Hoboken, NJ: Wiley. https://doi.org/10.1002/9781118963418.childpsy403

Bornstein, M. H. (2017). The specificity principle in acculturation science. *Perspectives on Psychological Science, 12*(1), 3–45. https://doi.org/10.1177/1745691616655997

Bornstein, M. H. (Ed.). (2019). *Handbook of parenting* (3rd ed.). New York: Routledge.

Bornstein, M. H., & Cote. L. (2004). Who is sitting across from me? Immigrant mothers' knowledge about children's development. *Pediatrics, 114*, 557–564. https://doi.org/10.1542/peds.2004-0713

Bornstein, M. H., Cote, L. R., Haynes, O. M., Hahn, C.-S., & Park, Y. (2010). Parenting knowledge: Experiential and sociodemographic factors in European American mothers of young children. *Developmental Psychology, 46*, 1677–1693. Retrieved from https://psycnet.apa.org/buy/2010-18950-001

Bradley, R. H., & Caldwell, B. M. (1984). The relation of infants' home environments to achievement test performance in first grade: A follow-up study. *Child Development, 55*(3), 803–809. https://doi.org/10.2307/1130131

Britto, P. R., Ponguta, L. A., Reyes, C., & Karnati, R. (2015). *A systematic review of parenting programs for young children*. New York: UNICEF.

Bronfenbrenner, U., & Morris, P. A. (2006). The bioecological model of human development. In R. M. Lerner & W. Damon (Eds.), *Handbook of child psychology: Theoretical models of human development* (Vol. 1, pp. 793–828). Hoboken, NJ: Wiley.

Brooks, S. K., Webster, R. K., Smith, L. E., Woodland, L., Wessely, S., Greenberg, N., & Rubin, G. J. (2020). The psychological impact of quarantine and how to reduce it: Rapid review of the evidence. *Lancet, 395*, 912–920. https://doi.org/10.1016/S0140-6736(20)30460-8

Burki, T. (2020). England and Wales see 20,000 excess deaths in care homes. *The Lancet, 395*(10237), P1602. Retrieved from https://www.thelancet.com/journals/lancet/article/PIIS0140-6736(20)31199-5/fulltext

Calderoni, M. E., Alderman, E. M., Silver, E. J., & Bauman, L. J. (2006). The mental health impact of 9/11 on inner-city high school students 20 miles north of Ground Zero. *Journal of Adolescent Health, 39*(1), 57–65. https://doi.org/10.1016/j.jadohealth.2005.08.012

Camera, L. (2020). Pediatric group calls for children to return to schools despite coronavirus. *US News*. Retrieved from https://www.usnews.com/news/education-news/articles/2020-06-29/pediatric-group-calls-for-children-to-return-to-schools-despite-coronavirus

Cárdenas Castro, M., Arnoso Martínez, M., & Faúndez Abarca, X. (2019). Deliberate rumination and positive reappraisal as serial mediators between life impact and posttraumatic growth in victims of state terrorism in Chile (1973–1990). *Journal of Interpersonal Violence, 34*(3), 545–561. https://doi.org/10.1177/0886260516642294

Carleton, R. N. (2016). Into the unknown: A review and synthesis of contemporary models involving uncertainty. *Journal of Anxiety Disorders, 39*, 30–43. https://doi.org/10.1016/j.janxdis.2016.02.007

Carpenter, A. L., Elkins, R. M., Kerns, C., Chou, T., Greif Green, J., & Comer, J. S. (2017). Event-related household discussions following the Boston Marathon bombing and associated posttraumatic stress among area youth. *Journal of Clinical Child & Adolescent Psychology, 46*(3), 331–342. https://doi.org/10.1080/15374416.2015.1063432

Catalano, R., Goldman-Mellor, S., Saxton, K., Margerison-Zilko, C., Subbaraman, M., LeWinn, K., & Anderson, E. (2011). The health effects of economic decline. *Annual Review of Public Health, 32*, 431–450. https://doi.org/10.1146/annurev-publhealth-031210-101146

Centers for Disease Control and Prevention (CDC). (2020a). *Using antibody tests for COVID-19*. Atlanta, GA: Centers for Disease Control and Prevention. Retrieved from https://www.cdc.gov/coronavirus/2019-ncov/lab/resources/antibody-tests.html#:~:text=These%20tests%20look%20for%20the,off%20a%20specific%20infection

Centers for Disease Control and Prevention (CDC). (2020b). *CDC updates COVID-19 transmission webpage to clarify information about types of spread*. Atlanta, GA: Centers for Disease Control and Prevention. Retrieved from https://www.cdc.gov/media/releases/2020/s0522-cdc-updates-covid-transmission.html

Centers for Disease Control and Prevention (CDC). (2020c). *How COVID-19 spreads*. Atlanta, GA: Centers for Disease Control and Prevention. Retrieved from https://www.cdc.gov/coronavirus/2019-ncov/prevent-getting-sick/how-covid-spreads.html

Centers for Disease Control and Prevention (CDC). (2020d). *Social distancing: Keep a safe distance to slow the spread*. Atlanta, GA: Centers for Disease Control and Prevention. Retrieved from https://www.cdc.gov/coronavirus/2019-ncov/prevent-getting-sick/social-distancing.html

Centers for Disease Control and Prevention (CDC). (2020e). *People with certain medical conditions*. Atlanta, GA: Centers for Disease Control and Prevention. Retrieved from https://www.cdc.gov/coronavirus/2019-ncov/need-extra-precautions/people-with-medical-conditions.html?CDC_AA_refVal=https%3A%2F%2Fwww.cdc.gov%2Fcoronavirus%2F2019-ncov%2Fneed-extra-precautions%2Fgroups-at-higher-risk.html#obesity

Centers for Disease Control and Prevention (CDC). (2020f). *CDC updates, expands list of people at risk of severe COVID-19 illness*. Atlanta, GA: Centers for Disease Control and Prevention. Retrieved from https://www.cdc.gov/media/releases/2020/p0625-update-expands-covid-19.html

Centers for Disease Control and Prevention (CDC). (2020g). *Older adults*. Atlanta, GA: Centers for Disease Control and Prevention. Retrieved from https://www.cdc.gov/coronavirus/2019-ncov/need-extra-precautions/older-adults.html

Centers for Disease Control and Prevention (CDC). (2020h). *Health department: Reported cases of multisystem inflammatory syndrome in children (MIS-C) in the United States*. Atlanta, GA: Centers for Disease Control and Prevention. Retrieved from https://www.cdc.gov/mis-c/cases/index.html

Centers for Disease Control and Prevention (CDC). (2020i). *8 things to know about vaccine planning*. Atlanta, GA: Centers for Disease Control and Prevention. Retrieved from https://www.cdc.gov/coronavirus/2019-ncov/vaccines/8-things.html

Centers for Disease Control and Prevention (CDC). (2020j). *Data on COVID-19 during pregnancy*. Atlanta, GA: Centers for Disease Control and Prevention. Retrieved from https://www.cdc.gov/coronavirus/2019-ncov/cases-updates/special-populations/pregnancy-data-on-covid-19.html

Cha, A. E. (2020). Forty percent of people with coronavirus infections have no symptoms. Might they be the key to ending the pandemic? *The Washington Post*. Retrieved from www.washingtonpost.com/health/2020/08/08/asymptomatic-coronavirus-covid/

Chakkarapani, E., Heazell, A., Lewis, R., Khan, R., Lees, C., Shennan, A., & Knight, M. (2020). Expert reaction to a case study which finds evidence for the potential transmission of SARS-CoV-2 via the placenta from a mother to her baby. *Science Media Centre.* Retrieved from https://www.sciencemediacentre.org/expert-reaction-to-a-case-study-which-finds-evidence-for-the-potential-transmission-of-sars-cov-2-via-the-placenta-from-a-mother-to-her-baby/

Chen, H., Guo, J., Wang, C., Luo, F., Yu, X., Zhang, W., . . . & Liao, J. (2020). Clinical characteristics and intrauterine vertical transmission potential of COVID-19 infection in nine pregnant women: A retrospective review of medical records. *The Lancet, 395*(10226), 809–815. https://doi.org/10.1016/S0140-6736(20)30360-3

Chidambaram, P. (2020). *Rising cases in long-term care facilities are cause for concern*. Kaiser Family Foundation. Retrieved from https://www.kff.org/coronavirus-covid-19/issue-brief/rising-cases-in-long-term-care-facilities-are-cause-for-concern/

Chotiner, I. (2020). COVID-19 will lead to "catastrophic" hunger. *The New Yorker*. Retrieved from www.newyorker.com/news/q-and-a/the-coronavirus-crisis-will-lead-to-catastrophic-hunger

Christnacht, C., & Sullivan, B. (2020). *About two-thirds of the 23.5 million working women with children Under 18 worked full-time in 2018*. United States Census Bureau: The choices working mothers make. Retrieved from www.census.gov/library/stories/2020/05/the-choices-working-mothers-make.html

Clemente-Suárez, V. J., Hormeño-Holgado, A., Jiménez, M., Benitez-Agudelo, J. C., Navarro-Jiménez, E., Perez-Palencia, N., . . . & Tornero-Aguilera, J. F. (2020). Dynamics of population immunity due to the Herd effect in the COVID-19 pandemic. *Vaccines, 8*(2), 236. https://doi.org/10.3390/vaccines8020236

Cleveland Clinic. (2020). What it means to be a coronavirus "long-hauler": A Q&A about lingering symptoms of COVID-19. *Cleveland Clinic: Health Essentials.* Retrieved from https://health.clevelandclinic.org/what-it-means-to-be-a-coronavirus-long-hauler/

Cluver, L. D., Lachman, J. M., Sherr, L., Wessels, I., Krug, E., Rakotomalala, S., . . . & McDonald, K. (2020). Parenting in a time of COVID-19. *The Lancet, 395*(10231), E64. https://doi.org/10.1016/S0140-6736(20)30736-4

Cluver, L. D., Meinck, F., Steinert, J. I., Shenderovich, Y., Doubt, J., Romero, R. H., . . . & Nzima, D. (2018). Parenting for lifelong health: A pragmatic cluster randomised controlled trial of a non-commercialised parenting programme for adolescents and their families in South Africa. *British Medical Journal Global Health, 3*(1). Retrieved from https://gh.bmj.com/content/3/1/e000539.abstract

Cohn, D., & Passel, J. S. (2018). *A record 64 million Americans live in multigenerational households*. Washington, DC: Pew Research Center. Retrieved from www.pewresearch.org/fact-tank/2018/04/05/a-record-64-million-americans-live-in-multigenerational-households/

Conger, R. D., Conger, K. J., & Martin, M. J. (2010). Socioeconomic status, family processes, and individual development. *Journal of Marriage and Family, 72*(3), 685–704. https://doi.org/10.1111/j.1741-3737.2010.00725.x

Conrad, A., Paschall, K. W., & Johnson, V. (2019). Persistent economic insecurity and harsh parenting: A latent transition analysis. *Children and Youth Services Review, 101,* 12–22. https://doi.org/10.1016/j.childyouth.2019.03.036

Coronavirus Anxiety Project. (2020). Retrieved from https://sites.google.com/cnu.edu/coronavirusanxietyproject/home

COVID Alliance. (2020). 2020 Sturgis motorcycle rally analysis: Mobility-based risk, geographic impacts, and quarantine compliance. *COVID Alliance.* Retrieved from https://www.washingtonpost.com/context/sturgis-motorcycle-rally-analysis/3cbcecc2-a142-473d-b626-0c20089710c0/?itid=lk_inline_manual_24

Cox, J. W. (2020). They depended on their parents for everything: Then the virus took both. *The Washington Post.* Retrieved from www.washingtonpost.com/graphics/2020/local/coronavirus-orphans-kids-lose-parents/

Crnic, K. A., & Coburn, S. S. (2019). Stress and parenting. In M. H. Bornstein (Ed.), *Handbook of parenting. Volume 4: Social conditions and applied parenting* (3rd ed., pp. 421–448). New York: Routledge. https://doi.org/10.4324/9780429398995-14

Czeisler, M. É., Lane, R. I., Petrosky, E., Wiley, J. F., Christensen, A., Njai, R., . . . & Howard, M.E. (2020). Mental health, substance use, and suicidal ideation during the COVID-19 pandemic: United States, June 24–30, 2020. *Morbidity and Mortality Weekly Report, 69*(32), 1049–1057. Retrieved from https://www.cdc.gov/mmwr/volumes/69/wr/mm6932a1.htm

Czeisler, M. É., Marynak, K., Clarke, K. E., Salah, Z., Shakya, I., Thierry, J. M., . . . & Howard, M. E. (2020). Delay or avoidance of medical care because of COVID-19–related concerns: United States, June 2020. *Centers for Disease Control and Prevention: Morbidity and Mortality Weekly Report, 69*(36), 1250–1257. Retrieved from https://www.cdc.gov/mmwr/volumes/69/wr/mm6936a4.htm?s_cid=mm6936a4_w

Dalton, L., Rapa, E., & Stein, A. (2020). Protecting the psychological health of children through effective communication about COVID-19. *The Lancet Child & Adolescent Health, 4*(5), 346–347. Retrieved from www.thelancet.com/journals/lanchi/article/PIIS2352-4642(20)30097-3/fulltext

Davis, J. (2020). How to help children adjust to masks, according to experts and parents. *The Washington Post.* Retrieved from www.washingtonpost.com/lifestyle/on-parenting/how-to-help-children-adjust-to-masks-according-to-experts-and-parents/2020/08/05/c431c45c-cb7c-11ea-bc6a-6841b28d9093_story.html

DC Food Policy Council. (2020). Food security report. *DC Food Policy Council.* Retrieved from https://dcfoodpolicy.org/foodsecurity2020/

de Best, R. (2020). Coronavirus (COVID-19) deaths worldwide per one million population as of October 12, 2020, by country. *Statista.* Retrieved from https://www.statista.com/statistics/1104709/coronavirus-deaths-worldwide-per-million-inhabitants/

DeFilippis, E., Impink, S. M., Singell, M., Polzer, J. T., & Sadun, R. (2020). *Collaborating during coronavirus: The impact of COVID-19 on the nature of work.* Working Paper 27612. Cambridge, MA: National Bureau of Economic Research. Retrieved from www.nber.org/papers/w27612.pdf

Dingel, J. I., Patterson, C., & Vavra, J. (2020). *Childcare obligations will constrain many workers when reopening the US economy.* Chicago, IL: University of Chicago, Becker Friedman Institute for Economics Working Paper, (2020–46). Retrieved from https://bfi.uchicago.edu/wp-content/uploads/BFI_WP_202046.pdf

Dishion, T. J., Shaw, D., Connell, A., Gardner, F., Weaver, C., & Wilson, M. (2008). The family check-up with high-risk indigent families: Preventing problem behavior by increasing parents' positive behavior support in early childhood. *Child Development, 79*(5), 1395–1414. https://doi.org/10.1111/j.1467-8624.2008.01195.x

Dong, Y., Mo, X., Hu, Y., Qi, X., Jiang, F., Jiang, Z., & Tong, S. (2020). Epidemiology of COVID-19 among children in China. *Pediatrics, 145*, e20200702. Retrieved from https://pediatrics.aappublications.org/content/145/6/e20200702

Dooley, D., & Catalano, R. (1988). Recent research on the psychological effects of unemployment. *Journal of Social Issues, 44*(4), 1–12. https://doi.org/10.1111/j.1540-4560.1988.tb02088.x

Dooley, D., Catalano, R., & Wilson, G. (1994). Depression and unemployment: Panel findings from the Epidemiologic Catchment Area study. *American Journal of Community Psychology, 22*(6), 745–765. https://doi.org/10.1007%2FBF02521557

Doran, E. (2020). At least 16 sick after coronavirus exposure at DeWitt in-home day care: "Take this seriously . . . stay home if sick at all". *Syracuse.* Retrieved from www.syracuse.com/coronavirus/2020/07/at-least-16-sick-after-coronavirus-exposure-at-dewitt-in-home-day-care-take-this-seriously-stay-home-if-sick-at-all.html?utm_source=twitter&utm_campaign=syracuse_sf&utm_medium=social

Duffin, E. (2020). How often do you attend church or synagogue – At least once a week, almost every week, about once a month, seldom, or never? *Statista.* Retrieved from www.statista.com/statistics/245491/church-attendance-of-americans/#:~:text=According%20to%20a%202019%20survey,Americans%20who%20attend%20every%20week.&text=Despite%20only%20about%20a%20fifth,themselves%20to%20be%20very%20religious

Duncan, G. J., Magnuson, K., & Votruba-Drzal, E. (2017). Moving beyond correlations in assessing the consequences of poverty. *Annual Review of Psychology, 68*, 413–434. https://doi.org/10.1146/annurev-psych-010416-044224

Education Week. (2020). Retrieved from www.edweek.org/ew/index.html?cmp=cpc-googew-branding&ccid=branding&ccag=branding&cckw=edweek&cccv=branding+ad&s_kwcid=AL!6416!3!101329662899!b!!g!!edweek&gclid=EAIaIQobChMIuvOOucjy6gIVywiICR3kwgrKEAAYASAAEgLyLfD_BwE

Eisele, J. (2020). How a new vaccine was developed in record time in the 1960s. *History.* Retrieved from www.history.com/news/mumps-vaccine-world-war-ii

Elbeshbishi, S., & King, L. (2020). Exclusive: Two-thirds of Americans say they won't get COVID-19 vaccine when it's first available, USA Today/Suffolk poll shows. *USA Today.* Retrieved from https://www.usatoday.com/story/news/politics/2020/09/04/covid-19-two-thirds-us-wont-take-vaccine-right-away-poll-shows/5696982002/

Essen, J., Fogelman, K., & Head, J. (1978). Childhood housing experiences and school attainment. *Child: Care, Health and Development, 4*(1), 41–58. https://doi.org/10.1111/j.1365-2214.1978.tb00070.x

Evans, G. W. (2006). Child development and the physical environment. *Annual Review of Psychology, 57*, 423–451. Retrieved from www.annualreviews.org/doi/abs/10.1146/annurev.psych.57.102904.190057?casa_token=pouXGwG0-jIAAAAA:dp3TgKnkHq8idddxCi2CuvGHcVD3sQ0k8iqkxM2zWVKFWuix3nFyXluss5LagMoxdRX0TjgBE1OoWA

Evans, G. W., Maxwell, L. E., & Hart, B. (1999). Parental language and verbal responsiveness to children in crowded homes. *Developmental Psychology, 35*(4), 1020–1023. https://doi.org/10.1037/0012-1649.35.4.1020

Evans, S. (2020). Analysis: Coronavirus set to cause largest ever fall in annual CO2 emissions. *CarbonBrief.* Retrieved from https://www.carbonbrief.org/analysis-coronavirus-set-to-cause-largest-ever-annual-fall-in-co2-emissions

Everly, G. S. J., & Lating, J. M. (2017). *The Johns Hopkins guide to psychological first aid.* Johns Hopkins University Press.

Express Scripts. (2020). America's state of mind report. *Express Scripts.* Retrieved from https://www.express-scripts.com/corporate/americas-state-of-mind-report

52   *Marc H. Bornstein*

Federal Reserve Bank of New York. (2020). *Quarterly report on household debt and credit.* New York: Federal Reserve Bank of New York. Retrieved from www.newyorkfed.org/ medialibrary/interactives/householdcredit/data/pdf/HHDC_2020Q2.pdf

Felix, E., You, S., Vernberg, E., & Canino, G. (2013). Family influences on the long term post-disaster recovery of Puerto Rican youth. *Journal of Abnormal Child Psychology, 41,* 111–124. https://doi.org/10.1007/s10802-012-9654-3

Ferguson, N., Laydon, D., Nedjati-Gilani, G., Imai, N., Ainslie, K., Baguelin, M., . . . & Ghani, A. C. (2020). Report 9: Impact of non-pharmaceutical interventions (NPIs) to reduce COVID19 mortality and healthcare demand. *Imperial College London, 10,* 77482. Retrieved from https://www.imperial.ac.uk/mrc-global-infectious-disease-analysis/ covid-19/report-9-impact-of-npis-on-covid-19/

Fifield, K. (2020). Your lungs, heart, brain, and more: How coronavirus attacks the body. *Health: Conditions and Treatments.* Retrieved from www.aarp.org/health/conditions-treatments/info-2020/covid-19-and-your-body.html

Fisher, K. A., Tenforde, M. W., Feldstein, L. R., Lindsell, C. J., Shapiro, N. I., Files, D. C., . . . & Self, W.H. (2020). Community and close contact exposures associated with COVID-19 among symptomatic adults ≥18 years in 11 outpatient health care facilities: United States, July 2020. *Centers for Disease Control and Prevention: Morbidity and Mortality Weekly Report, 69*(36), 1258–1264. Retrieved from https://www.cdc.gov/ mmwr/volumes/69/wr/mm6936a5.htm

Fisher, P., Lombardi, J., & Kendall-Taylor, N. (2020). Why households with young children warrant our attention and support during (and after) the COVID-19 pandemic. *Rapid-EC Project.* Retrieved from https://medium.com/rapid-ec-project/why-house holds-with-young-children-warrant-our-attention-and-support-during-and-after-the-b7cee9b76184

Fishman, T. C. (2020). America's next crisis is already here: State and local governments are being hit hard by the pandemic, and the consequences could be dangerous for democracy. *The Atlantic.* Retrieved from www.theatlantic.com/ideas/archive/2020/05/ state-and-local-governments-are-plunging-crisis/611932/

Food and Drug Administration (FDA). (2020). Fact sheet for healthcare providers: New York SARS-CoV-2 real-time RT-PCR diagnostic panel. *FDA: Coronavirus Disease 2019 (COVID-19).* Retrieved from https://www.fda.gov/media/135662/download

Fore, H. et al. (2020). *Joint leaders' statement – Violence against children: A hidden crisis of the COVID-19 pandemic.* Geneva, Switzerland: World Health Organization.

Fosco, G. M., Bumbarger, B., & Bamberger, K. T. (2015). Thinking systematically for enduring family change. In M. J. Van Ryzin, K. L. Kumpfer, G. M. Fosco, & M. T. Greenberg (Eds.), *Family-based prevention programs for children and adolescents: Theory, research, and large-scale dissemination* (pp. 308–328). New York: Psychology Press.

Fussell, E., & Lowe, S. R. (2014). The impact of housing displacement on the mental health of low-income parents after Hurricane Katrina. *Social Science & Medicine, 113,* 137–144. https://doi.org/10.1016/j.socscimed.2014.05.025

Galea, S., Merchant, R. M., & Lurie, N. (2020). The mental health consequences of COVID-19 and physical distancing: The need for prevention and early intervention. *JAMA Internal Medicine, 180*(6), 817–818. https://doi.org/10.1001/jamainternmed.2020.1562

Galpin, O. P., Whitaker, C. J., & Dubiel, A. J. (1992). Helicobacter pylori infection and overcrowding in childhood. *Lancet, 339*(8793), 619. Retrieved from http://pascal-francis.inist.fr/vibad/index.php?action=getRecordDetail&idt=5219770

Gardner, F., Montgomery, P., & Knerr, W. (2016). Transporting evidence-based parenting programs for child problem behavior (age 3–10) between countries: Systematic review and meta-analysis. *Journal of Clinical Child & Adolescent Psychology*, *45*(6), 749–762. https://doi.org/10.1080/15374416.2015.1015134

Gassman-Pines, A., Ananat, E. O., & Gibson-Davis, C. M. (2014). Effects of state-wide job losses on adolescent suicide-related behaviors. *American Journal of Public Health*, *104*(10), 1964–1970. Retrieved from https://ajph.aphapublications.org/doi/abs/10.2105/AJPH.2014.302081

Gelkopf, M., Berger, R., Bleich, A., & Silver, R. C. (2012). Protective factors and predictors of vulnerability to chronic stress: A comparative study of 4 communities after 7 years of continuous rocket fire. *Social Science & Medicine*, *74*(5), 757–766. https://doi.org/10.1016/j.socscimed.2011.10.022

#GivingTuesday. (2020). *#GivingTuesdayNow creates global wave of generosity in response to COVID-19 crisis*. Retrieved from www.givingtuesday.org/blog/2020/05/givingtuesdaynow-creates-global-wave-generosity-response-covid-19-crisis

Gjelten, T. (2020). Several churches announce they won't reopen this year. *NPR: Religion*. Retrieved from www.npr.org/2020/07/17/892195734/several-churches-announce-they-wont-reopen-this-year

Global Fund. (2020). *Mitigating the impact of COVID-19 on countries affected by HIV, tuberculosis and malaria*. Geneva, Switzerland: The Global Fund to Fight AIDS, Tuberculosis and Malaria. Retrieved from www.theglobalfund.org/media/9819/covid19_mitigatingimpact_report_en.pdf

Global Initiative to End All Corporal Punishment of Children. (2020). Retrieved from https://endcorporalpunishment.org/

Godfred-Cato, S., Bryant, B., Leung, J., et al. (2020, March–July). COVID-19 – Associated multisystem inflammatory syndrome in children – United States. *MMWR and Morbidity and Mortality Weekly Report*, ePub: 7 August 2020. http://doi.org/10.15585/mmwr.mm6932e2external icon

Goldstein, A. (2020). First, the coronavirus pandemic took their jobs: Then, it wiped out their health insurance. *Washington Post*. Retrieved from https://www.washingtonpost.com/health/first-the-coronavirus-pandemic-took-their-jobs-then-it-wiped-out-their-health-insurance/2020/04/18/1c2cb5bc-7d7c-11ea-8013-1b6da0e4a2b7_story.html

Gorbalenya, A. E., Baker, S. C., Baric, R. S., Baker, S. C., Baric, R. S., de Groot, R. J., . . . & Ziebuhr, J. (2020). Severe acute respiratory syndrome-related coronavirus: The species and its viruses – A statement of the Coronavirus Study Group. *Nature Microbiology*, *5*, 536–544. https://doi.org/10.1038/s41564-020-0695-z

Gosangi, B., Park, H., Thomas, R., Gujrathi, R., Bay, C. P., Raja, A. S., . . . & Khurana, B. (2020). Exacerbation of physical intimate partner violence during COVID-19 lockdown. *Radiology*, 202866. Retrieved from https://pubs.rsna.org/doi/10.1148/radiol.2020202866

Government. (2020). Coronavirus (COVID-19). *Governo Italiano: Presidenza del Consiglio dei Ministri*. Retrieved from http://www.governo.it/it/coronavirus

Götzinger, F., Santiago-García, B., Noguera-Julián, A., Lanaspa, M., Lancella, L., Calò Carducci, I., . . . ptbnet COVID-19 Study Group. (2020). COVID-19 in children and adolescents in Europe: A multinational, multicentre cohort study. *Lancet Child and Adolescent Health*, *S2352–4642*(20), 30177. Retrieved from www.thelancet.com/journals/lanchi/article/PIIS2352-4642(20)30177-2/fulltext

Gould, S. J. (1977). *Ontogeny and phylogeny*. Cambridge, MA: Harvard University Press.

Gove, W. R., Hughes, M., & Style, C. B. (1983). Does marriage have positive effects on the psychological well-being of the individual? *Journal of Health and Social Behavior*, *24*(2), 122–131. https://doi.org/10.2307/2136639

Great Barrington Declaration. (2020). https://gbdeclaration.org/

Greenhalgh, T., Knight, M., A'Court, C., Buxton, M., & Husain, L. (2020). Management of post-acute covid-19 in primary care. *BMJ, 370*, m3026. https://doi.org/10.1136/bmj.m3026

Griffith, D. M., Sharma, G., Holliday, C. S., Enyia, O. K., Valliere, M., Semlow, A. R., . . . & Blumenthal, R. S. (2020). Men and covid-19: A biopsychosocial approach to understanding sex differences in mortality and recommendations for practice and policy interventions. *Centers for Disease Control and Prevention: Preventing Chronic Disease, 17*, E63. Retrieved from https://www.cdc.gov/pcd/issues/2020/20_0247.htm

Gross, K., Brewer, P. R., & Aday, S. (2009). Confidence in government and emotional responses to terrorism after September 11, 2001. *American Politics Research, 37*(1), 107–128. https://doi.org/10.1177/1532673X08319954

Guarino, B., Janes, C., & Cha, A. E. (2020). Spate of new research supports wearing masks to control coronavirus spread. *The Washington Post*. Retrieved from www.washingtonpost.com/health/2020/06/13/spate-new-research-supports-wearing-masks-control-coronavirus-spread/

Hafstad, G. S., Haavind, H., & Jensen, T. K. (2012). Parenting after a natural disaster: A qualitative study of Norwegian families surviving the 2004 tsunami in Southeast Asia. *Journal of Child and Family Studies, 21*(2), 293–302. https://doi.org/10.1007/s10826-011-9474-z

Hallsten, L. (2005). 'Burnout' and 'wornout': Concepts and data from a national survey. In A. S. G. Antoniou & C. L. Cooper (Eds.), *Research companion to organizational health psychology* (pp. 516–537). Cheltenham, England: Edward Elgar.

Hamel, L., Kearney, A., Kirzinger, A., Lopes, L., Muñana, C., & Brodie, M. (2020). *Impact of coronavirus on personal health, economic and food security, and Medicaid*. Kaiser Family Foundation. Retrieved from https://www.kff.org/report-section/kff-health-tracking-poll-may-2020-health-and-economic-impacts/

Hamilton, S. F., Hamilton, M. A., DuBois, D. L., Martínez, M. L., Cumsille, P., Brady, B . . . & Sellers, D. E. (2016). Youth-adult relationships as assets for youth: Promoting positive development in stressful times. In A. C. Peterson, S. H. Koller, F. Motti-Stefanidi, & S. Verma (Eds.), *Positive youth development in global contexts of social and economic change* (pp. 157–182). New York: Routledge.

Hamner, L., Dubbel, P., Capron, I., Ross, A., Jordan, A., . . . & Leibrand, H. (2020). High SARS-CoV-2 attack rate following exposure at a choir practice: Skagit County, Washington, March 2020. *Centers for Disease Control and Prevention: Morbidity and Mortality Weekly Report, 69*(19), 606–610. Retrieved from https://www.cdc.gov/mmwr/volumes/69/wr/mm6919e6.htm

Han, W. J., Hetzner, N. P., & Brooks-Gunn, J. (2019). Employment and parenting. In M. H. Bornstein (Ed.), *Handbook of parenting. Volume 4: Social conditions and applied parenting* (3rd ed., pp. 274–300). New York: Routledge. https://doi.org/10.4324/9780429398995-8

Harlan, C., & Pitrelli, S. (2020). Italy's Bergamo is calling back coronavirus survivors: About half say they haven't fully recovered. *Washington Post*. Retrieved from https://www.washingtonpost.com/world/2020/09/08/bergamo-italy-covid-longterm/?arc404=true

Harris, R. (2020). Advances in ICU care are saving more patients who have COVID-19. *Shots: Health News from NPR*. Retrieved from https://www.npr.org/sections/health-shots/2020/09/20/914374901/advances-in-icu-care-are-saving-more-patients-who-have-covid-19

Harris, R. (2020). Coronavirus update: Convalescent plasma treatment and risks of reinfection. *NPR: Health*. Retrieved from https://www.npr.org/2020/08/24/905536105/coronavirus-update-convalescent-plasma-treatment-and-risks-of-reinfection

Harvard Medical School. (2020). *If you've been exposed to the coronavirus.* Harvard Health Publishing. Retrieved from https://www.health.harvard.edu/diseases-and-conditions/if-youve-been-exposed-to-the-coronavirus#:~:text=We%20know%20that%20 a%20person,start%20to%20experience%20symptoms

Haseltine, W. A. (2020). *A family guide to Covid* (2nd ed). ACCESS Health International. Retrievd from https://read.amazon.com/kp/embed?asin=B08C95DPQM&preview= newtab&linkCode=kpe&ref_=cm_sw_r_kb_dp_B3CeFbHACGDS7&tag=thewaspos 09-20&reshareId=6TZCD96HM3HP0AKXKY3M&reshareChannel=system

Havers, F. P., Reed, C., Lim, T., Montgomery, J. M., Klena, J. D., Hall, A. J., . . . & Thornburg, N. J. (2020). Seroprevalence of antibodies to SARS-CoV-2 in 10 sites in the United States. *JAMA Internal Medicine.* https://doi.org/10.1001/ jamainternmed.2020.4130

Hawryluck, L., Gold, W. L., Robinson, S., Pogorski, S., Galea, S., & Styra, R. (2004). SARS control and psychological effects of quarantine, Toronto, Canada. *Emerging Infectious Diseases, 10*(7), 1206–1212. https://doi.org/10.3201/eid1007.030703

Heald-Sargent, T., Muller, W. J., Zheng, X., Rippe, J., Patel, A. B., & Kociolek, L. K. (2020). Age-related differences in nasopharyngeal severe acute respiratory syndrome coronavirus 2 (SARS-CoV-2) levels in patients with mild to moderate coronavirus disease 2019 (COVID-19). *JAMA Pediatrics, 174*(9), 902–903. Retrieved from https:// jamanetwork.com/journals/jamapediatrics/fullarticle/2768952

Hendricks, C., & Bornstein, M. H. (2007). Ecological analysis of early adolescents' stress responses to 9/11 in the Washington, DC, area. *Applied Development Science, 11*(2), 71–88. https://doi.org/10.1080/10888690701384905

Hillis, S., Mercy, J., Amobi, A., & Kress, H. (2016). Global prevalence of past-year violence against children: A systematic review and minimum estimates. *Pediatrics, 137*(3), e20154079. https://doi.org/10.1542/peds.2015-4079

Holman, E. A., Thompson, R. R., Garfin, D. R., & Silver, R. C. (2020). The unfolding COVID-19 pandemic: A probability-based, nationally representative study of mental health in the US. *Science Advances*, eabd5390. Retrieved from https://advances.sciencemag.org/content/early/2020/09/23/sciadv.abd5390.1

Honig, A. S. (2019). Choosing childcare for young children. In M. H. Bornstein (Ed.), *Handbook of parenting. Volume 5. The practice of parenting* (3rd ed., pp. 319–346). New York: Routledge. https://doi.org/10.4324/9780429401695-11

Horesh, D., & Brown, A. D. (2020). Traumatic stress in the age of COVID-19: A call to close critical gaps and adapt to new realities. *Psychological Trauma: Theory, Research, Practice, and Policy, 12*(4), 331–335. http://doi.org/10.1037/tra0000592

Hoynes, H., Schanzenbach, D. W., & Almond, D. (2016). Long-run impacts of childhood access to the safety net. *American Economic Review, 106*(4), 903–934. https://doi. org/10.1257/aer.20130375

Huang, L., Zhang, X., Zhang, X., Wei, Z., Zhang, L., Xu, J., . . . & Xu, A. (2020). Rapid asymptomatic transmission of COVID-19 during the incubation period demonstrating strong infectivity in a cluster of youngsters aged 16–23 years outside Wuhan and characteristics of young patients with COVID-19: A prospective contact-tracing study. *Journal of Infection, 80*, e1–13. Retrieved from www.journalofinfection.com/article/ S0163-4453(20)30117-1/fulltext

Hubler, S., Fuller, T., Singhvi, A., & Love, J. (2020). Many Latinos couldn't stay home. Now virus cases are soaring in their communities. *The New York Times.*

Huckins, J. F., DaSilva, A. W., Wang, W., Hedlund, E., Rogers, C., Nepal, S. K., . . . & Wagner, D. D. (2020). Mental health and behavior of college students during the early phases of the COVID-19 pandemic: Longitudinal smartphone and ecological momentary assessment study. *Journal of Medical Internet Research, 22*(6), e20185. Retrieved from www.jmir.org/2020/6/e20185/

Husa, S. (2011). Finland: Children's right to protection. In J. E. Durant & A. B. Smith (Eds.), *Global pathways to abolishing physical punishment* (pp. 122–133). New York, NY: Routledge.

Iannelli, N. (2020). Fairfax Co. teachers split 50–50 on returning to school buildings. WTOP News. Retrieved from https://wtop.com/fairfax-county/2020/07/fairfax-co-teachers-split-50-50-on-returning-to-school-buildings/

Igielnik, R. (2020). *Most Americans say they regularly wore a mask in stores in the past month; fewer see others doing it.* Pew Research Center. Retrieved from https://www. pewresearch.org/fact-tank/2020/06/23/most-americans-say-they-regularly-wore-a-mask-in-stores-in-the-past-month-fewer-see-others-doing-it/

Ingram, J. (2020). Has child abuse surged under COVID-19? Despite alarming stories from ERs, there's no answer. *NBC News*. Retrieved from https://www.nbcnews.com/health/kids-health/has-child-abuse-surged-under-covid-19-despite-alarming-stories-n1234713

Institute for Health Metrics and Evaluation. (2020). First COVID-19 global forecast: IHME projects three-quarters of a million lives could be saved by January 1. HealthData. Retrieved from http://www.healthdata.org/news-release/first-covid-19-global-forecast-ihme-projects-three-quarters-million-lives-could-be

Ipsos & George Mason University Schar School of Policy and Government. (2020). Poll. *The Washington Post*. Retrieved from https://context-cdn.washingtonpost. com/notes/prod/default/documents/83793df5-694a-46f3-b9b0-6eb3934fef90/note/2e3fcf2d-d320-4847-b4f2-44da53baf170.#page=1

Jaine, R., Baker, M., & Venugopal, K. (2011). Acute rheumatic fever associated with household crowding in a developed country. *The Pediatric Infectious Disease Journal, 30*(4), 315–319. Retrieved from https://journals.lww.com/pidj/Abstract/2011/04000/Acute_Rheumatic_Fever_Associated_With_Household.9.aspx

Janes, C. (2020). Report: Coronavirus infected scores of children and staff at Georgia sleep-away camp. *The Washington Post*. Retrieved from www.washingtonpost.com/health/2020/07/31/georgia-children-covid-outbreak/

Jiao, W. Y., Wang, L. N., Liu, J., Fang, S. F., Jiao, F. Y., Pettoello-Mantovani, M., & Somekh, E. (2020). Behavioral and emotional disorders in children during the COVID-19 epidemic. *The Journal of Pediatrics, 221*, 264–266. Retrieved from https://www.ncbi. nlm.nih.gov/pmc/articles/PMC7127630/

Johns Hopkins University of Medicine. (2020). *Mortality analyses*. Coronavirus Resource Center. Retrieved from https://coronavirus.jhu.edu/data/mortality

Johnson, C. Y. (2020). A coronavirus vaccine won't change the world right away. *The Washington Post*. Retrieved from www.washingtonpost.com/health/2020/08/02/covid-vaccine/

Jose, R., Holman, E. A., & Silver, R. C. (2019). Community organizations and mental health after the 2013 Boston Marathon bombings. *Social Science & Medicine, 222*, 367–376. https://doi.org/10.1016/j.socscimed.2018.08.019

Juth, V., Silver, R. C., Seyle, D. C., Widyatmoko, C. S., & Tan, E. T. (2015). Post-disaster mental health among parent – Child dyads after a major earthquake in Indonesia. *Journal of Abnormal Child Psychology, 43*(7), 1309–1318. https://doi.org/10.1007/s10802-015-0009-8

Kerns, C. E., Elkins, R. M., Carpenter, A. L., Chou, T., Green, J. G., & Comer, J. S. (2014). Caregiver distress, shared traumatic exposure, and child adjustment among area youth following the 2013 Boston Marathon bombing. *Journal of Affective Disorders, 167*, 50–55. https://doi.org/10.1016/j.jad.2014.05.040

Khaleque, A. (2017). Perceived parental hostility and aggression, and children's psychological maladjustment, and negative personality dispositions: A meta-analysis. *Journal of Child and Family Studies, 26*(4), 977–988. Retrieved from https://link.springer.com/content/pdf/10.1007/s10826-016-0637-9.pdf

Kiliç, C., Kiliç, E. Z., & Aydin, I. O. (2011). Effect of relocation and parental psychopathology on earthquake survivor-children's mental health. *The Journal of Nervous and Mental Disease, 199*(5), 335–341. https://doi.org/10.1097/NMD.0b013e3182174ffa

Kim, L., Whitaker, M., O'Halloran, A., et al. (2020). Hospitalization rates and characteristics of children aged <18 years hospitalized with laboratory-confirmed COVID-19 – COVID-NET, 14 States, March 1 – July 25, 2020. *MMWR and Morbidity and Mortality Weekly Report*. http://doi.org/10.15585/mmwr.mm6932e3

King, S., & Laplante, D. P. (2015). Using natural disasters to study prenatal maternal stress in humans. In M. C. Antonelli (Ed.), *Perinatal programming of neurodevelopment* (pp. 285–313). New York, NY: Springer. https://doi.org/10.1007/978-1-4939-1372-5_14

Kirkpatrick, D. D. (2020). In race for a coronavirus vaccine, an Oxford group leaps ahead. *New York Times*. Retrieved from www.nytimes.com/2020/04/27/world/europe/coronavirus-vaccine-update-oxford.html

Kitchener, C. (2020). "The mom shame is so real": There's no way to win in this pandemic. *The Lily: Work*. Retrieved from www.thelily.com/the-mom-shame-is-so-real-theres-no-way-to-win-in-the-pandemic/

Koralnik, I. J., & Tyler, K. L. (2020). COVID-19: A global threat to the nervous system. *Annals of Neurology, 88*(1), 1–11. https://doi.org/10.1002/ana.25807

Kumpfer, K. L., Magalhães, C., Xie, J., & Kanse, S. (2015). Cultural and gender adaptations of evidence-based family interventions. In M. J. Van Ryzin, K. L. Kumpfer, G. M. Fosco, & M. T. Greenberg (Eds.), *Family-based prevention programs for children and adolescents* (pp. 256–281). New York: Psychology Press.

Labarda, C. E., Jopson, Q. D. Q., Hui, V. K., & Chan, C. S. (2020). Long-term displacement associated with health and stress among survivors of Typhoon Haiyan. *Psychological Trauma: Theory, Research, Practice and Policy*. https://doi.org/10.1037/tra0000573

Lansford, J. E., Criss, M. M., Laird, R. D., Shaw, D. S., Pettit, G. S., Bates, J. E., & Dodge, K. A. (2011). Reciprocal relations between parents' physical discipline and children's externalizing behavior during middle childhood and adolescence. *Development and Psychopathology, 23*(1), 225–238. https://doi.org/10.1017/S0954579410000751

Lansford, J. E., & Deater-Deckard, K. (2012). Childrearing discipline and violence in developing countries. *Child Development, 83*(1), 62–75. https://doi.org/10.1111/j.1467-8624.2011.01676.x

Lansford, J. E., & Dodge, K. A. (2008). Cultural norms for adult corporal punishment of children and societal rates of endorsement and use of violence. *Parenting: Science and Practice, 8*(3), 257–270. https://doi.org/10.1080/15295190802204843

Lansford, J. E., Sharma, C., Malone, P. S., Woodlief, D., Dodge, K. A., Oburu, P., . . . & Tirado, L. M. U. (2014). Corporal punishment, maternal warmth, and child adjustment: A longitudinal study in eight countries. *Journal of Clinical Child & Adolescent Psychology, 43*(4), 670–685. https://doi.org/10.1080/15374416.2014.893518

Layne, S. P., Hyman, J. M., Morens, D. M., & Taubenberger, J. K. (2020). New coronavirus outbreak: Framing questions for pandemic prevention. *Science: Translational Medicine, 12*(534). https://doi.org/10.1126/scitranslmed.abb1469

Leeb, R. T., Price, S., Sliwa, S., Kimball, A., Szucs, L., Caruso, E., . . . & Lozier, M. (2020). COVID-19 trends among school-aged children: United States, March 1–September 19, 2020. *Centers for Disease Control and Prevention: Morbidity and Mortality Weekly*

Report, 69(39), 1410–1415. Retrieved from https://www.cdc.gov/mmwr/volumes/69/wr/mm6939e2.htm?s_cid=mm6939e2_w

Lengua, L. J., & Kovacs, E. A. (2005). Bidirectional associations between temperament and parenting and the prediction of adjustment problems in middle childhood. *Journal of Applied Developmental Psychology, 26*(1), 21–38. https://doi.org/10.1016/j.appdev.2004.10.001

Lerner, R. M. (2018). *Concepts and theories of human development* (4th ed.). New York: Routledge.

Li, Z., Page, A., Martin, G., & Taylor, R. (2011). Attributable risk of psychiatric and socioeconomic factors for suicide from individual-level, population-based studies: A systematic review. *Social Science & Medicine, 72*(4), 608–616. https://doi.org/10.1016/j.socscimed.2010.11.008

Liang, L., Ren, H., Cao, R., Hu, Y., Qin, Z., Li, C., & Mei, S. (2020). The effect of COVID-19 on youth mental health. *Psychiatric Quarterly, 91*, 841–852. Retrieved from https://link.springer.com/article/10.1007%2Fs11126-020-09744-3

Liu, J. J., Bao, Y., Huang, X., Shi, J., & Lu, L. (2020). Mental health considerations for children quarantined because of COVID-19. *The Lancet Child & Adolescent Health, 4*(5), 347–349. Retrieved from https://www.thelancet.com/journals/lanchi/article/PIIS2352-4642(20)30096-1/fulltext?luicode=10000011&lfid=10760366554755 36&u=https%3A%2F%2Fwww.thelancet.com%2Fjournals%2Flanchi%2Farticle%2FP IIS2352-4642%2820%2930096-1%2Ffulltext

Long, H. (2020). The big factor holding back the US economic recovery: Child care. *The Washington Post.* Retrieved from www.washingtonpost.com/business/2020/07/03/big-factor-holding-back-us-economic-recovery-child-care/

Long, S. W., Olsen, R. J., Christensen, P. A., Bernard, D. W., Davis, J. J., Shukla, M., . . . & Musser, J. (2020). Molecular architecture of early dissemination and massive second wave of the SARS-CoV-2 Virus in a major metropolitan area. *medRxiv.* Retrieved from https://www.medrxiv.org/content/10.1101/2020.09.22.20199125v3

Lopez, A. S., Hill, M., Antezano, J., Vilven, D., Rutner, T., Bogdanow, L., . . . & Tran, C.H. (2020). Transmission dynamics of COVID-19 outbreaks associated with child care facilities: Salt Lake City, Utah, April–July 2020. *Centers for Disease Control and Prevention: Morbidity and Mortality Weekly Report, 69*(37), 1319–1323. Retrieved from https://www.cdc.gov/mmwr/volumes/69/wr/mm6937e3.htm?s_cid=mm6937e3_w

Lu, X., Zhang, L., Du, H., Zhang, J., Li, Y. Y., Qu, J., . . . & Wu, C. (2020). SARS-CoV-2 infection in children. *New England Journal of Medicine, 382*(17), 1663–1665. https://doi.org/10.1056/NEJMc2005073

Ludvigsson, J. F. (2020). Systematic review of COVID-19 in children shows milder cases and a better prognosis than adults. *Acta Paediatrica, 109*(6), 1088–1095. https://doi.org/10.1111/apa.15270

Lumey, L. H., Stein, A. D., Kahn, H. S., Van der Pal-de Bruin, K. M., Blauw, G. J., Zybert, P. A., & Susser, E. S. (2007). Cohort profile: The Dutch Hunger Winter families study. *International Journal of Epidemiology, 36*(6), 1196–1204. https://doi.org/10.1093/ije/dym126

Lynch, D. J. (2020). In a bleak economy, these companies are flourishing. *The Washington Post.* Retrieved from www.washingtonpost.com/business/2020/08/10/recession-coronavirus-pandemic-winners/

Maeda, M., & Oe, M. (2017). Mental health consequences and social issues after the Fukushima disaster. *Asia Pacific Journal of Public Health, 29*(2_suppl), 36S–46S. https://doi.org/10.1177/1010539516689695

Magnuson, K. A., & Duncan, G. J. (2019). Parents in poverty. In M. H. Bornstein (Ed.), *Handbook of parenting. Volume 4: Social conditions and applied parenting* (3rd ed., pp. 301–328). New York: Routledge. https://doi.org/10.4324/9780429398995-9

Mahoney, A., & Boyatzis, C. J. (2019). Parenting, religion, and spirituality. In M. H. Bornstein (Ed.), *Handbook of Parenting. Volume 5: The practice of parenting* (3rd ed., pp. 515–552). New York: Routledge. https://doi.org/10.4324/9780429401695-18

Mäkelä, M. J., Puhakka, T., Ruuskanen, O., Leinonen, M., Saikku, P., Kimpimäki, M., . . . & Arstila, P. (1998). Viruses and bacteria in the etiology of the common cold. *Journal of Clinical Microbiology*, *36*, 539–542.

Mallapaty, S. (2020). The coronavirus is most deadly if you are older and male: New data reveal the risks. *Nature*, *585*(7823), 16–17. Retrieved from https://www.nature.com/articles/d41586-020-02483-2

Mandavilli, A., & Tully, T. (2020). White House is not tracing contacts for "super-spreader" Rose Garden event. *New York Times*. Retrieved from https://www.nytimes.com/2020/10/05/health/contact-tracing-white-house.html

Marsh, A., Gordon, D., Pantazis, C., & Heslop, P. (1999). *Home sweet home? The impact of poor housing on health*. Bristol: The Policy Press.

Martinez-Marcos, M., & De la Cuesta-Benjumea, C. (2015). Women's self-management of chronic illnesses in the context of caregiving: A grounded theory study. *Journal of Clinical Nursing*, *24*(11–12), 1557–1566. https://doi.org/10.1111/jocn.12746

Masarik, A. S., & Conger, R. D. (2017). Stress and child development: A review of the Family Stress Model. *Current Opinion in Psychology*, *13*, 85–90. https://doi.org/10.1016/j.copsyc.2016.05.008

Masten, A. S., Narayan, A. J., Silverman, W. K., & Osofsky, J. D. (2015). Children in war and disaster. In M. H. Bornstein & T. Leventhal (Eds.), *Ecological settings and processes. Volume 4: Handbook of child psychology and developmental science* (7th ed., pp. 704–745). Editor-in-chief: R. M. Lerner. Hoboken, NJ: Wiley.

Masten, A. S., & Palmer, A. R. (2019). Parenting to promote resilience in children. In M. H. Bornstein (Ed.), *Handbook of parenting. Volume 5: The practice of parenting* (3rd ed., pp. 156–188). New York: Routledge. https://doi.org/10.4324/9780429401695-6

Mataloni, L., Wasshausen, D., Strassner, E., & Aversa, J. (2020). Gross domestic product, second quarter 2020: (Advance estimate) and annual update. *Bureau of Economic Analysis*, *20*(37). Retrieved from www.bea.gov/sites/default/files/2020-07/gdp2q20_adv.pdf

McDermott, B. M., & Cobham, V. E. (2012). Family functioning in the aftermath of a natural disaster. *BMC Psychiatry*, *12*(1), 1–7. https://doi.org/10.1186/1471-244X-12-55

McKay, K. L., Neumann, Z., & Gilman, S. (2020). *20 Million renters are at risk of eviction; policymakers must act now to mitigate widespread hardship*. Washington, DC: The Aspen Institute. Retrieved from www.aspeninstitute.org/blog-posts/20-million-renters-are-at-risk-of-eviction/

McKinsey & Company. (2020). *Women in the workplace 2020: Corporal American is at a critical crossroads*. Retrieved from https://wiw-report.s3.amazonaws.com/Women_in_the_Workplace_2020.pdf

McMahon, R. J., & Forehand, R. (2003). *Helping the noncompliant child: A clinician's guide to effective parent training*. New York: Guilford.

Meckler, L., & Guskin, E. (2020). Fearing coronavirus and missed classes, many parents prefer mixing online and in-person school, poll finds. *The Washington Post*. Retrieved from www.washingtonpost.com/education/post-poll-schools-parents-covid-trump/2020/08/05/f04ae490-d722-11ea-9c3b-dfc394c03988_story.html

Mervosh, S., Lu, D., & Swales, V. (2020). See which states and cities have told residents to stay at home. *New York Times*. Retrieved from www.nytimes.com/interactive/2020/us/coronavirus-stay-at-home-order.html

Michaud, J., & Kates, J. (2020). *What do we know about children and coronavirus transmission*? Retrieved from www.kff.org/coronavirus-covid-19/issue-brief/what-do-we-know-about-children-and-coronavirus-transmission/

Mikolajczak, M., Brianda, M. E., Avalosse, H., & Roskam, I. (2018). Consequences of parental burnout: Its specific effect on child neglect and violence. *Child Abuse & Neglect, 80*, 134–145. https://doi.org/10.1016/j.chiabu.2018.03.025

Mikolajczak, M., Gross, J. J., & Roskam, I. (2019). Parental burnout: What is it, and why does it matter? *Clinical Psychological Science, 7*(6), 1319–1329. https://doi.org/10.1177/2167702619858430

Miller, S., & Benz, J. (2020). *Concerns about reopening schools loom large*. University of Chicago: AP NORC. Retrieved from https://apnorc.org/projects/concerns-about-school-re-openings-loom-large/

Modestino, A. S. (2020). Coronavirus child-care crisis will set women back a generation. *The Washington Post*. Retrieved from www.washingtonpost.com/us-policy/2020/07/29/childcare-remote-learning-women-employment/

Morawska, L., & Milton, D. K. (2020). It is time to address airborne transmission of coronavirus disease 2019 (COVID-19). *Clinical Infectious Diseases*, ciaa939. https://doi.org/10.1093/cid/ciaa939

Moriarty, L. F., Plucinski, M. M., Marston, B. J., Kurbatova, E. V., Knust, B., Murray, E. L., . . . & Solano County COVID-19 Team. (2020). Public health responses to COVID-19 outbreaks on cruise ships: Worldwide, February–March 2020. *Centers for Disease Control and Prevention: Morbidity and Mortality Weekly Report, 69*(12), 347–352. Retrieved from https://www.cdc.gov/mmwr/volumes/69/wr/mm6912e3.htm

Morin, C. M., & Carrier, J. (2020). The acute effects of the COVID-19 pandemic on insomnia and psychological symptoms. *Sleep Medicine*, S1389-9457(20)30261-6. https://doi.org/10.1016/j.sleep.2020.06.005

Myers, K., Tham, W. Y., Yin, Y., Cohodes, N., Thursby, J. G., Thursby, M., . . . & Wang, D. (2020). *Quantifying the immediate effects of the COVID-19 pandemic on scientists*. Retrieved from SSRN 3608302. https://arxiv.org/pdf/2005.11358.pdf

Nagelhout, G. E., Hummel, K., de Goeij, M. C., de Vries, H., Kaner, E., & Lemmens, P. (2017). How economic recessions and unemployment affect illegal drug use: A systematic realist literature review. *International Journal of Drug Policy, 44*, 69–83. https://doi.org/10.1016/j.drugpo.2017.03.013

National Academies of Sciences, Engineering, and Medicine. (2020). *Framework for equitable allocation of COVID-19 vaccine*. Washington, DC: The National Academies Press.

National Association for the Education of Young Children (NAEYC). (2020). *Holding on until help comes: A survey reveals child care's fight to survive*. Washington, DC: National Association for the Education of Young Children. Retrieved from www.naeyc.org/sites/default/files/globally-shared/downloads/PDFs/our-work/public-policy-advocacy/holding_on_until_help_comes.survey_analysis_july_2020.pdf

National Center for Education Statistics. (2020). *Back to school statistics*. Washington, DC: National Center for Education Statistics. Retrieved from https://nces.ed.gov/fastfacts/display.asp?id=372

National Energy Assistance Directors' Association. (2020). *Electric and gas residential arrearages are growing rapidly projected to grow from $9.8 billion as of July 31 to*

$24.3 billion by year end. Retrieved from https://neada.org/wp-content/uploads/2020/10/covidarrearagespr.pdf

National Institutes of Health. (2020). *Study suggests new coronavirus may remain on surfaces for days*. Bethesda, MD: National Institutes of Health. Retrieved from www.nih.gov/news-events/nih-research-matters/study-suggests-new-coronavirus-may-remain-surfaces-days

Navajo Nation Department of Health. (2020). Positive cases of COVID-19. *Dikos Nstaaígíí COVID-19*. Retrieved from www.ndoh.navajo-nsn.gov/COVID-19

Nelson-Coffey, S. K., & Stewart, D. (2019). Well-being in parenting. In M. H. Bornstein (Ed.), *Handbook of parenting. Volume 3: Being and becoming a parent* (3rd ed., pp. 596–619). New York: Routledge. https://doi.org/10.4324/9780429433214-17

Nemeroff, C. B. (2016). Paradise lost: The neurobiological and clinical consequences of child abuse and neglect. *Neuron, 89*(5), 892–909. https://doi.org/10.1016/j.neuron.2016.01.019

Nobel Peace Prize. (2020). *All Nobel Peace Prizes*. Retrieved from https://www.nobelprize.org/prizes/peace/2020/wfp/facts

NORC at the University of Chicago. (2020). Historic shift in Americans' happiness amidst pandemic. *COVID Response Tracking Study Report*. Retrieved from https://www.norc.org/PDFs/COVID%20Response%20Tracking%20Study/Historic%20Shift%20in%20Americans%20Happiness%20Amid%20Pandemic.pdf

North, C. S. (2016). Disaster mental health epidemiology: Methodological review and interpretation of research findings. *Psychiatry, 79*(2), 130–146. https://doi.org/10.1080/00332747.2016.1155926

Noveck, J. (2020, March 24). With isolation, abuse activists fear an "explosive cocktail". *AP News*. Retrieved from https://apnews.com/7b9b15a1215611f69f02f4388100266d

NPR, Robert Johnson Wood Foundation, & Harvard T. H. Chan School of Public Health. (2020). The Impact of coronavirus on households across America. *Harvard National Report*. Retrieved from https://cdn1.sph.harvard.edu/wp-content/uploads/sites/94/2020/09/NPR-RWJF-Harvard-National-Report_092220_Final-1.pdf

Oshitani, H., & the Expert Members of the National COVID-19 Cluster Taskforce at Ministry of Health, Labour, and Welfare, Japan. (2020). Cluster-based approach to coronavirus disease 2019 (COVID-19) in Japan: February–April 2020. *Japanese Journal of Infectious Diseases*. https://doi.org/10.7883/yoken.JJID.2020.363

Ossola, A. (2020). What everyone should know about ventilation and preventing Covid-19. *Quartz*. Retrieved from https://qz.com/1907977/how-to-check-air-ventilation-to-prevent-covid-19-spread/

Page, S. (2020). Back to school? 1 in 5 teachers are unlikely to return to reopened classrooms this fall, poll says. *USA Today: Education*. Retrieved from www.usatoday.com/story/news/education/2020/05/26/coronavirus-schools-teachers-poll-ipsos-parents-fall-online/5254729002/

Palca, J. (2020). Five coronavirus treatments in development. *Shots: Health News from NPR*. Retrieved from https://www.npr.org/sections/health-shots/2020/06/11/873399184/five-coronavirus-treatments-in-development

Panchal, N., Kamal, R., Orgera, K., Cox, C., Garfield, R., Hamel, L. . . . & Chidambaram, P. (2020). The implications of COVID-19 for mental health and substance use. Kaiser Family Foundation. Retrieved from https://www.kff.org/report-section/the-implications-of-covid-19-for-mental-health-and-substance-use-issue-brief/

Park, C. L., Russell, B. S., Fendrich, M., Finkelstein-Fox, L., Hutchison, M., & Becker, J. (2020b). Americans' COVID-19 stress, coping, and adherence to CDC guidelines. *Journal of General Internal Medicine*, 1–8. https://doi.org/10.1007/s11606-020-05898-9

Park, Y. J., Choe, Y. J., Park, O., Park, S. Y., Kim, Y. M., Kim, J., . . . & Lee, J. (2020a). Early Release-Contact tracing during Coronavirus disease outbreak, South Korea, 2020. *Emerging Infectious Diseases*, *26*(10). Retrieved from https://wwwnc.cdc.gov/eid/article/26/10/20-1315_article

Pereznieto, P., Montes, A., Routier, S., & Langston, L. (2014). *The costs and economic impact of violence against children*. Richmond, VA: ChildFund. Retrieved from www.childfund.org/uploadedFiles/public_site/media/Articles/current/2014/ODI%20Report%20%20The%20cost%20and%20economic%20impact%20of%20violence%20against%20children.pdf

Pew Research Center. (2020). *COVID-19 disruptions associated with a large increase in the share of young adults living with parent(s)*. Pew Research Center. Retrieved from https://www.pewresearch.org/fact-tank/2020/09/04/a-majority-of-young-adults-in-the-u-s-live-with-their-parents-for-the-first-time-since-the-great-depression/ft_2020-09-04_livingwithparents_01a/

Philadelphia Federation of Teachers. (2020). *Second survey regarding reopening schools: June 29, 2020*. Philadelphia, PA: Philadelphia Federation of Teachers. Retrieved from https://pft.org/wp-content/uploads/2020/06/PFTReopening2_June292020.pdf

PR Newswire. (2020). Regeneron's REGN-COV2 antibody cocktail reduced viral levels and improved symptoms in non-hospitalized COVID-19 patients. *Regeneron: Investors and Media*. Retrieved from https://investor.regeneron.com/news-releases/news-release-details/regenerons-regn-cov2-antibody-cocktail-reduced-viral-levels-and

Puffer, E. S., Annan, J., Sim, A. L., Salhi, C., & Betancourt, T. S. (2017). The impact of a family skills training intervention among Burmese migrant families in Thailand: A randomized controlled trial. *PloS One*, *12*(3), e0172611. https://doi.org/10.1371/journal.pone.0172611

Puntmann, V. O., Carerj, M. L., Wieters, I., Fahim, M., Arendt, C., Hoffamnn, J., . . . & Nagel, E. (2020). Outcomes of cardiovascular magnetic resonance imaging in patients recently recovered from coronavirus disease 2019 (COVID-19). *JAMA Cardiology*. Retrieved from https://jamanetwork.com/journals/jamacardiology/fullarticle/2768916

Ragab, D., Salah Eldin, H., Taeimah, M., Khattab, R., & Salem, R. (2020). The COVID-19 cytokine storm; what we know so far. *Frontiers in Immunology*, *11*, 1446. https://doi.org/10.3389/fimmu.2020.01446

Rampell, C. (2020). Child-care centers have already been reopening. The results are troubling. *The Washington Post*. Retrieved from www.washingtonpost.com/opinions/child-care-centers-have-already-been-reopening-the-results-are-troubling/2020/07/13/3ce91a00-c53b-11ea-b037-f9711f89ee46_story.html

RECOVERY Collaborative Group. (2020). Dexamethasone in hospitalized patients with Covid-19 – Preliminary report. *New England Journal of Medicine*. Retrieved from https://www.nejm.org/doi/10.1056/NEJMoa2021436

Reinhart, C., & Reinhart, V. (2020). The pandemic depression: The global economy will never be the same. *Foreign Affairs*, September/October. Retrieved from https://www.foreignaffairs.com/articles/united-states/2020-08-06/coronavirus-depression-global-economy

RESPECT women. (2019). *Preventing violence against women*. Geneva: World Health Organization. (WHO/RHR/18.19). Licence: CC BY-MC-SA 3.0 IGO. Retrieved from https://www.unwomen.org/-/media/headquarters/attachments/sections/library/publications/2019/respect-women-preventing-violence-against-women-en.pdf?la=en&vs=5901

Revival Outside the Walls. (2020). Almost two-thirds of Americans (62%) believe the coronavirus is a message from God to humanity to change the way they live. *This Week's Shocking Stat*. Retrieved from www.rotw.com/this-weeks-shocking-stat?mwm_id=314

025773220&gclid=EAIaIQobChMI4OqVrYv46gIVhCmzAB3pTAaREAAYASAAEgL
QGvD_BwE

Rodriguez-Diaz, C. E., Guilamo-Ramos, V., Mena, L., Hall, E., Honermann, B., Crowley, J. S., . . . & Sullivan, P. S. (2020). Risk for COVID-19 infection and death among
Latinos in the United States: Examining heterogeneity in transmission dynamics. *Annals of Epidemiology*. Retrieved from www.sciencedirect.com/science/article/
pii/S1047279720302672

Roose, K. (2020). The week in tech: How to stop coronavirus "doomsurfing." *New York
Times*. Retrieved from https://www.nytimes.com/2020/03/20/technology/coronavirus-
doomsurfing.html

Rothenberg, W. A., Lansford, J. E., Bornstein, M. H., Chang, L., Deater-Deckard, K., Di
Giunta, L., . . . & Skinner, A. T. (2020). Effects of parental warmth and behavioral con-
trol on adolescent externalizing and internalizing trajectories across cultures. *Journal of
Research on Adolescence*. https://doi.org/10.1111/jora.12566

Roubinov, D., Bush, N. R., & Boyce, W. T. (2020). How a pandemic could advance the science
of early adversity. *JAMA Pediatrics*. https://doi.org/10.1001/jamapediatrics.2020.2354

Rubin, G. J., Amlôt, R., Page, L., & Wessely, S. (2009). Public perceptions, anxiety, and
behaviour change in relation to the swine flu outbreak: Cross sectional telephone survey. *British Medical Journal, 339*, b2651. https://doi.org/10.1136/bmj.b2651

Saad, L. (2020). Americans' readiness to get COVID-19 vaccine falls to 50%. *Gallup*.
Retrieved from https://news.gallup.com/poll/321839/readiness-covid-vaccine-falls-past-
month.aspx

**Sanders, M. R., Turner, K. M. T., & McWilliam, J. (2015). The Triple P – Positive
parenting program: A community-wide approach to parenting and family support.
In M. J. Van Ryzin, K. L. Kumpfer, G. M. Fosco, & M. T. Greenberg, (Eds.), *Family
based prevention programs for children and adolescents* (pp. 134–159). New York:
Psychology Press.**

Santoli, J. M., Lindley, M. C., DeSilva, M. B., Kharbanda, E. O., Daley, M. F., Galloway,
L., . . . & Weintraub, E. (2020). Effects of the COVID-19 pandemic on routine pediatric
vaccine ordering and administration: United States, 2020. *Centers for Disease Control
and Prevention: Morbidity and Mortality Weekly Report, 69*(19), 591–593. Retrieved
from https://www.cdc.gov/mmwr/volumes/69/wr/mm6919e2.htm

Schleicher, A. (2020). The impact of COVID-19 on education: Insights from *Education at a
Glance 2020. OECD*, 3–30. Retrieved from https://www.oecd.org/education/the-impact-
of-covid-19-on-education-insights-education-at-a-glance-2020.pdf

Schochet, L. (2020). The child care crisis is keeping women out of the workforce.
Center for America Progress: Early Childhood. Retrieved from www.american
progress.org/issues/early-childhood/reports/2019/03/28/467488/child-care-crisis-
keeping-women-workforce/

Schofield, T. J., Conger, R. D., Gonzales, J. E., & Merrick, M. T. (2016). Harsh parenting,
physical health, and the protective role of positive parent-adolescent relationships. *Social
Science & Medicine, 157*, 18–26. https://doi.org/10.1016/j.socscimed.2016.03.027

Schuchat, A. (2020). Public Health response to the initiation and spread of pandemic
COVID-19 in the United States, February 24 – April 21, 2020. *MMWR and Morbidity
Mortality Weekly Report, 69*, 551–556. http://doi.org/10.15585/mmwr.mm6918e2external
icon

Schwartz, F., & Lieber, D. (2020). Israelis fear schools reopened too soon as Covid-
19 cases climb. *The Wall Street Journal*. Retrieved from www.wsj.com/articles/
israelis-fear-schools-reopened-too-soon-as-covid-19-cases-climb-11594760001

Schwartz, N. G., Moorman A. C., Makaretz, A., Chang, K. T., Chu, V. T., Szablewski, C. M., . . . Stewart, R. J. (2020). Adolescent with COVID-19 as the source of an outbreak at a 3-week family gathering – four states, June–July 2020. *MMWR Morbidity and Mortality Weekly Report, 69*, 1457–1459. http://dx.doi.org/10.15585/mmwr.mm6940e2 external icon

Schwedel, H. (2020). An interview with the scientist and mom who had a little secret during her CNN appearance. *Slate*. Retrieved from https://slate.com/human-interest/2020/09/cnn-mom-pants-interview.html

Seow, J., Graham, C., Merrick, B., Acors, S., Steel, K. J., Hemmings, O., . . . & Betancor, G. (2020). Longitudinal evaluation and decline of antibody responses in SARS-CoV-2 infection. *medRxiv*. Retrieved from www.medrxiv.org/content/10.1101/2020.07.09.20148429v1

Seto, S., Imamura, F., & Suppasri, A. (2019). Challenge to build the science of human survival from disaster starting from analysis for the 2011 Tohoku tsunami. *Journal of Disaster Research, 14*(9), 1323–1328. Retrieved from www.jstage.jst.go.jp/article/jdr/14/9/14_1323/_article/-char/ja/

Sidpra, J., Abomeli, D., Hameed, B., Baker, J., & Mankad, K. (2020). Rise in the incidence of abusive head trauma during the COVID-19 pandemic. *Archives of Disease in Childhood*. Retrieved from https://adc.bmj.com/content/early/2020/06/30/archdischild-2020-319872

SimplyWise. (2020). *Retirement confidence index*. SimplyWise. Retrieved from https://www.simplywise.com/blog/retirement-confidence-index/-savingsimpact

Singh, R., & Lee, C. (2020). More than 3 million people age 65 or older live with school-age children, and could be at heightened risk of COVID-19 infection if children bring the virus home from school. KFF: Newsroom. Retrieved from www.kff.org/coronavirus-covid-19/press-release/more-than-3-million-people-age-65-or-older-live-with-school-age-children-and-could-be-at-heightened-risk-of-covid-19-infection-if-children-bring-the-virus-home-from-school/

Sisk, B., Cull, W., Harris, J. M., Rothenburger, A., & Olson, L. (2020). National trends of cases of COVID-19 in children based on US State Health Department Data. *Pediatrics*. Retrieved from https://pediatrics.aappublications.org/content/pediatrics/early/2020/09/23/peds.2020-027425.full.pdf

Skinner, A. T., Goodwin, J., Alampay, L. P., Lansford, J. E., Bacchini, D., Bornstein, M. H. . . . & Yotanyamaneewong, S. (2020). *Parenting during adolescence as a moderator of links between COVID-19 disruption and reported changes in parents' and young adults' adjustment in five countries*. Unpublished manuscript, Duke University.

Slef, K. (2020). Coronavirus surprise: Remittances to Mexico rise during pandemic. *The Washington Post*. Retrieved from www.washingtonpost.com/world/the_americas/coronavirus-remittance-mexico-guatemala-salvador-honduras/2020/08/05/5a1bcdbe-d5be-11ea-930e-d88518c57dcc_story.html

Slotnick, D. (2020). Why airlines are required to keep flying "ghost planes" under the terms of the coronavirus bailout package. *Business Insider*. Retrieved from www.businessinsider.com/coronavirus-airlines-bailout-empty-flights-requirement-2020-4

Smeltz, D., Daalder, I. H., Friedhoff, K., Kafura, C., & Helm, B. (2020). Divided we stand: Democrats and Republicans diverge on US foreign policy. The Chicago Council on Global Affairs. Retrieved from https://www.thechicagocouncil.org/publication/lcc/divided-we-stand

Smith, A. (2020). What are the early symptoms of coronavirus (COVID-19)? *Medical News Today*. Retrieved from www.medicalnewstoday.com/articles/coronavirus-early-symptoms

Snape, M. D., & Viner, R. M. (2020). COVID-19 in children and young people. *Science*, eabd6165. https://doi.org/10.1126/science.abd6165

Solari, C. D., & Mare, R. D. (2012). Housing crowding effects on children's wellbeing. *Social Science Research, 41*(2), 464–476. https://doi.org/10.1016/j.ssresearch.2011.09.012

Spinelli, M., Lionetti, F., Pastore, M., & Fasolo, M. (2020). Parents and children facing the COVID-19 outbreak in Italy. *Frontiers in Psychology, 11*, 1713. https://doi.org/10.3389/fpsyg.2020.01713

Sprague, C. M., Kia-Keating, M., Felix, E., Afifi, T., Reyes, G., & Afifi, W. (2015). Youth psychosocial adjustment following wildfire: The role of family resilience, emotional support, and concrete support. *Child & Youth Care Forum, 44*(3), 433–450. https://doi.org/10.1007/s10566-014-9285-7

Sprang, G., & Silman, M. (2013). Posttraumatic stress disorder in parents and youth after health-related disasters. *Disaster Medicine and Public Health Preparedness, 7*, 105–110. https://doi.org/10.1017/dmp.2013.22

Stanwell, R. E., Stuart, J. M., Hughes, A. O., Robinson, P., Griffin, M. B., & Cartwright, K. (1994). Smoking, the environment and meningococcal disease: A case control study. *Epidemiology & Infection, 112*(2), 315–328. https://doi.org/10.1017/S0950268800057733

Stein, A., Dalton, L., Rapa, E., Bluebond-Langner, M., Hanington, L., Stein, K. F., . . . & Bland, R. (2019). Communication with children and adolescents about the diagnosis of their own life-threatening condition. *The Lancet, 393*(10176), 1150–1163. https://doi.org/10.1016/S0140-6736(18)33201-X

Stein, P. (2020). Day cares are reopening: But they can only serve small groups and fear for their survival. *Washington Post.* Retrieved from https://www.washingtonpost.com/local/education/day-cares-are-reopening-but-they-can-only-serve-small-groups-and-fear-for-their-survival/2020/09/28/cf7d321c-fd93-11ea-b555-4d71a9254f4b_story.html

Stein-Zamir, C., Abramson, N., Shoob, H., Libal, E., Bitan, M., Cardash, T., . . . & Miskin, I. (2020). A large COVID-19 outbreak in a high school 10 days after schools' reopening, Israel, May 2020. *Eurosurveillance, 25*(29), 2001352. Retrieved from www.eurosurveillance.org/content/10.2807/1560-7917.ES.2020.25.29.2001352#html_fulltext

Sumner, A., Hoy, C., & Ortiz-Juarez, E. (2020). Estimates of the impact of COVID-19 on global poverty. *UNU-WIDER*, April, 800–809. Retrieved from https://www.wider.unu.edu/sites/default/files/Publications/Working-paper/PDF/wp2020-43.pdf

Swallow, K. M., Zacks, J. M., & Abrams, R. A. (2009). Event boundaries in perception affect memory encoding and updating. *Journal of Experimental Psychology: General, 138*(2), 236–257. https://doi.org/10.1037/a0015631

Sweeny, K. (2018). On the experience of awaiting uncertain news. *Current Directions in Psychological Science, 27*, 281–285.

Szablewski, C. M., Chang, K. T., Brown, M. M., Chu, V. T., Yousaf, A. R., Anyale-chi, N., . . . & Stewart, R. J. (2020). SARS-CoV-2 transmission and infection among attendees of an overnight camp: Georgia, June 2020. *Morbidity and Mortality Weekly Report, 69*(31), 1023. Retrieved from https://context-cdn.washingtonpost.com/notes/prod/default/documents/497af396-19d9-4e92-9757-2f9c396279d1/note/c46d9483-5107-4cfc-8adc-17f27e02414d.#page=1

Szczerbińska, K. (2020). Could we have done better with COVID-19 in nursing homes? *European Geriatric Medicine, 11*, 639–643. Retrieved from https://link.springer.com/article/10.1007/s41999-020-00362-7

Taylor, C. A., Moeller, W., Hamvas, L., & Rice, J. C. (2013). Parents' professional sources of advice regarding child discipline and their use of corporal punishment. *Clinical Pediatrics, 52*(2), 147–155. https://doi.org/10.1177/0009922812465944

Tein, J.-Y., Sandler, I. N., MacKinnon, D. P., & Wolchik, S. A. (2004). How did it work? Who did it work for? Mediation in the context of a moderated prevention effect for children of divorce. *Journal of Consulting and Clinical Psychology, 72*(4), 617–624. https://doi.org/10.1037/0022-006X.72.4.617

Thebault, R., Ba Tran, A., & Williams, V. (2020). The coronavirus is infecting and killing black Americans at an alarmingly high rate. *The Washington Post.* Retrieved from www.washingtonpost.com/nation/2020/04/07/coronavirus-is-infecting-killing-black-americans-an-alarmingly-high-rate-post-analysis-shows/?arc404=true&tid=a_inl_manual

Thebault, R., & Fowers, A. (2020). Pandemic's weight falls on Hispanics and Native Americans, as death toll passes 150,000. *The Washington Post.* Retrieved from www.washingtonpost.com/health/2020/07/31/covid-us-death-toll-150k/?arc404=true

Thompson, D. (2020, July 27). Hygiene theatre is a huge waste of time. *The Atlantic.* Retrieved from www.theatlantic.com/ideas/archive/2020/07/scourge-hygiene-theater/614599/

Tomoda, A., Suzuki, H., Rabi, K., Sheu, Y. S., Polcari, A., & Teicher, M. H. (2009). Reduced prefrontal cortical gray matter volume in young adults exposed to harsh corporal punishment. *Neuroimage, 47,* T66–T71. https://doi.org/10.1016/j.neuroimage.2009.03.005

UNESCO. (2020). *1.37 billion students now home as COVID-19 school closures expand, ministers scale up multimedia approaches to ensure learning continuity.* Retrieved from https://en.unesco.org/news/137-billion-students-now-home-covid-19-school-closures-expand-ministers-scale-multimedia

UNICEF. (2020a). *COVID-19: Are children able to continue learning during school closures?* New York: United Nations. Retrieved from https://data.unicef.org/resources/remote-learning-reachability-factsheet/

UNICEF. (2020b). *Accelerated solutions to COVID-19: Societal impacts and responses for children, adolescents, families, and communities.* New York: United Nations.

United Nations Foundation. (2014). *Hidden in plain sight: A statistical analysis of violence against children.* New York: United Nations Foundation.

United Nations Foundation. (2017). *Standards for ECD parenting programmes in low and middle income countries.* New York, NY: United Nations Foundation. Retrieved from the UNICEF website: www.unicef.org/earlychildhood/files/UNICEF-Standards_for_Parenting_Programs_6-8-17_pg.pdf

United Nations Foundation. (2018). *Sustainable development goals.* New York: United Nations Foundation. Retrieved from https://unfoundation.org/what-we-do/issues/sustainable-development-goals/?gclid=EAIaIQobChMI9a7nnNzy6gIVEpSzCh1WoAw-EAAYASAAEgKwhfD_BwE

United Nations Foundation. (2020). *Policy brief: The impact of COVID-19 on children.* New York: United Nations Foundation. Retrieved from https://unsdg.un.org/resources/policy-brief-impact-covid-19-children

U.S. Department of Labor. (2020a). *General facts on women and job-based health.* Washington, DC: U.S. Department of Labor. Retrieved from https://www.dol.gov/sites/dolgov/files/EBSA/about-ebsa/our-activities/resource-center/fact-sheets/women-and-job-based-health.pdf

U.S. Department of Labor. (2020b). *Unemployment insurance weekly claims.* Retrieved from www.dol.gov/ui/data.pdf

U.S. Department of the Treasury. (2020). *The CARES Act works for all Americans.* Retrieved from https://home.treasury.gov/policy-issues/cares

Van Damn, A., & Long, H. (2020). Moms, black Americans, and educators are in trouble as economy recovery slows. *Washington Post.* Retrieved from https://www.washingtonpost.com/business/2020/10/02/september-jobs-inequality/

Vandell, D. L., Simpkins, S. D., & Wegemer, C. M. (2019). Parenting and children's organized activities. In M. H. Bornstein (Ed.), *Handbook of parenting. Volume 5: The practice of parenting* (3rd ed., pp. 347–379). New York: Routledge.

Vivanti, A., Vauloup-Fellous, C., Prevot, S., Zupan, V., Suffee, C., Do Cao, J., . . . & De Luca, D. (2020). Transplacental transmission of SARS-CoV-2 infection. *Nature, 11*, 3572. Retrieved from https://www.nature.com/articles/s41467-020-17436-6

Volz, E. M., Hill, V., McCrone, J. T., Price, A., Jorgensen, D., O'Toole, A., . . . & Connor, T. R. (2020). Evaluating the effects of SARS-CoV-2 Spike mutation D614G on transmissibility and pathogenicity. *medRxiv*. Retrieved from https://www.medrxiv.org/content/10.1101/2020.07.31.20166082v2

Wachs, T. D., & Camli, O. (1991). Do ecological or individual characteristics mediate the influence of the physical environment upon maternal behavior. *Journal of Environmental Psychology, 11*(3), 249–264. https://doi.org/10.1016/S0272-4944(05)80186-0

Wajnberg, A., Amanat, F., Firpo, A., Altman, D., Bailey, M., Mansour, M., . . . & Stadlbauer, D. (2020). SARS-CoV-2 infection induces robust, neutralizing antibody responses that are stable for at least three months. *medRxiv*. Retrieved from www.medrxiv.org/content/10.1101/2020.07.14.20151126v1.full.pdf

Wang, G., Zhang, Y., Zhao, J., Zhang, J., & Jiang, F. (2020). Mitigate the effects of home confinement on children during the COVID-19 outbreak. *The Lancet, 395*(10228), 945–947. Retrieved from www.thelancet.com/journals/lancet/article/PIIS0140-6736(20)30547-X/fulltext?fbclid=IwAR393QgIUwsA8tLHX9xlJlwNzVqXbHtR1fBsTCMZ_pxBwVytKON2GzMv3KI

Ward, C. L., Wessels, I. M., Lachman, J. M., Hutchings, J., Cluver, L. D., Kassanjee, R., . . . & Gardner, F. (2020). Parenting for lifelong health for young children: A randomized controlled trial of a parenting program in South Africa to prevent harsh parenting and child conduct problems. *Journal of Child Psychology and Psychiatry, 61*(4), 503–512. https://doi.org/10.1111/jcpp.13129

Weaver, C. (2020). Why am I having weird dreams lately? *New York Times*. Retrieved from https://www.nytimes.com/2020/04/13/style/why-weird-dreams-coronavirus.html

Weiner, R., Alcantara, C., & Ba Tran, A. (2020). More cities and states are opening bars and restaurants despite mounting evidence of potential danger. *Washington Post*. Retrieved from https://www.washingtonpost.com/health/2020/09/14/covid-spread-restaurants-bars/

Weinraub, M., & Kaufman, R. (2019). Single parenthood. In M. H. Bornstein (Ed.), *Handbook of parenting. Volume 3: Being and becoming a parent* (3rd ed., pp. 271–310). New York: Routledge. https://doi.org/10.4324/9780429433214-8

White-Cummings, C. (2020). How parents can mentally prepare themselves for a school year like no other. *The Washington Post*. Retrieved from www.washingtonpost.com/lifestyle/on-parenting/how-parents-can-mentally-prepare-themselves-for-a-school-year-like-no-other/2020/08/06/1a6a023a-cb7d-11ea-bc6a-6841b28d9093_story.htmlWikimedia Foundation. (2020). *Wikipedia and COVID-19: Explore the data*. Retrieved from https://wikimediafoundation.org/covid19/data/

Williams, A., & Sedgwick, J. (2020). US has 4% of the world's population, but more than 25% of global coronavirus cases. *Fox5*. Retrieved from https://www.fox5ny.com/news/us-has-4-of-the-worlds-population-but-more-than-25-of-global-coronavirus-cases

Wilson, C. (2021). *Understanding children's worry: Clinical, developmental and cognitive psychological perspectives* (1st ed.). New York: Routledge.

Winnicott, D. W. (1965). *The maturational processes and the facilitating environment: Studies in the theory of emotional development*. New York: Routledge.

Wisner, B., Paton, D., Alisic, E., Eastwood, O., Shreve, C., & Fordham, M. (2018). Communication with children and families about disaster: Reviewing multi-disciplinary literature 2015–2017. *Current Psychiatry Reports, 20*(9), 73. https://doi.org/10.1007/s11920-018-0942-7

Witte, K., & Allen, M. (2000). A meta-analysis of fear appeals: Implications for effective public health campaigns. *Health Education & Behavior, 27*(5), 591–615. https://doi.org/10.1177/109019810002700506

Woodward, B. (2020). *Rage*. New York: Simon & Schuster.

World Bank. (2020a). *World Bank predicts sharpest decline of remittances in recent history*. Washington, DC: World Bank. Retrieved from www.worldbank.org/en/news/press-release/2020/04/22/world-bank-predicts-sharpest-decline-of-remittances-in-recent-history

World Bank. (2020b). *COVID-19 to add as many as 150 million extreme poor by 2021*. Washington, DC: World Bank. Retrieved from https://www.worldbank.org/en/news/press-release/2020/10/07/covid-19-to-add-as-many-as-150-million-extreme-poor-by-2021

World Health Organization (WHO). (2016). *INSPIRE: seven strategies for ending violence against children*. Geneva, Switzerland: World Health Organization.

World Health Organization (WHO). (2018a). *Violence against children*. Geneva, Switzerland: World Health Organization. https://www.who.int/health-topics/violence-against-children - tab=tab_1

World Health Organization (WHO). (2018b). *Nurturing care for early childhood development: A framework for helping children survive and thrive to transform health and human potential*. Geneva, Switzerland: World Health Organization. Retrieved from https://apps.who.int/iris/bitstream/handle/10665/272603/9789241514064-eng.pdf

World Health Organization (WHO). (2020a). *Novel Coronavirus (2019-nCoV)*. Situation Report – 22. Geneva, Switzerland: World Health Organization. Retrieved from https://www.who.int/docs/default-source/coronaviruse/situation-reports/20200211-sitrep-22-ncov.pdf?sfvrsn=fb6d49b1_2

World Health Organization (WHO). (2020b). *WHO Director-General's opening remarks at the media briefing on COVID-19 – 11 March 2020*. Geneva, Switzerland: World Health Organization. Retrieved from https://www.who.int/dg/speeches/detail/who-director-general-s-opening-remarks-at-the-media-briefing-on-covid-19---11-march-2020

World Health Organization (WHO). (2020c). *Modes of transmission of virus causing COVID-19: Implications for IPC precaution recommendations*. Geneva, Switzerland: World Health Organization. Retrieved from https://www.who.int/news-room/commentaries/detail/modes-of-transmission-of-virus-causing-covid-19-implications-for-ipc-precaution-recommendations

World Health Organization (WHO). (2020d). *Coronavirus disease (COVID-19) advice for the public: When and how to use masks*. Geneva, Switzerland: World Health Organization. Retrieved from https://www.who.int/emergencies/diseases/novel-coronavirus-2019/advice-for-public/when-and-how-to-use-masks

World Health Organization (WHO). (2020e). *Substantial investment needed to avert mental health crisis*. Geneva, Switzerland: World Health Organization. Retrieved from https://www.who.int/news/item/14-05-2020-substantial-investment-needed-to-avert-mental-health-crisis

World Health Organization (WHO). (2020f). *At least 80 million children under one at risk of diseases such as diphtheria, measles and polio as COVID-19 disrupts routine vaccination efforts, warn Gavi, WHO and UNICEF*. Geneva, Switzerland: World Health Organization. Retrieved from https://www.who.int/news/item/22-05-2020-at-least-80-million-children-under-one-at-risk-of-diseases-such-as-diphtheria-measles-and-polio-as-covid-19-disrupts-routine-vaccination-efforts-warn-gavi-who-and-unicef

World Health Organization (WHO). (2020g). *Virtual press conference on COVID-19 in the Western Pacific: Remarks by Dr. Takeshi Kasai.* Geneva, Switzerland: World Health Organization. Retrieved from https://www.who.int/westernpacific/news/speeches/detail/virtual-press-conference-on-covid-19-in-the-western-pacific

World Health Organization (WHO). (2020h). WHO Director-General's opening remarks at the media briefing on COVID-19 – 12 October 2020. Geneva, Switzerland: World Health Organization. Retrieved from https://www.who.int/dg/speeches/detail/who-director-general-s-opening-remarks-at-the-media-briefing-on-covid-19---12-october-2020

World Health Organization (WHO). (2020i). *Coronavirus disease (COVID-19) pandemic.* Geneva, Switzerland: World Health Organization. Retrieved from https://www.who.int/emergencies/diseases/novel-coronavirus-2019?gclid=Cj0KCQjwoJX8BRCZARIsAEWBFMLCsderEVPgzI9dl_oivQ21rplDs-izGV1F9tD5p0oKbYL0UtuakN8aAihuEALw_wcB

World Health Organization, War Trauma Foundation, & World Vision International. (2011). *Psychological first aid: Guide for field workers.* Geneva, Switzerland: WHO.

Xinhua. (2020). Schools in China's Wuhan start new semester. *Xinhuanet.* Retrieved from http://www.xinhuanet.com/english/2020-09/01/c_139334337.htm

Yelp. (2020). Yelp: Local economic impact report. *Yelp: Economic Average.* Retrieved from www.yelpeconomicaverage.com/yelp-coronavirus-economic-impact-report.html

Yonker, L. M., Neilan, A. M., Bartsch, Y., Patel, A. B., Regan, J., Arya, P., . . . & Fasano, A. (2020). Pediatric SARS-CoV-2: clinical presentation, infectivity, and immune responses. *The Journal of Pediatrics,* in press. Retrieved from https://www.jpeds.com/article/S0022-3476(20)31023-4/fulltext

Yoon, Y., Newkirk, K., & Perry-Jenkins, M. (2015). Parenting stress, dinnertime rituals, and child well-being in working-class families. *Family Relations, 64*(1), 93–107. https://doi.org/10.1111/fare.12107

Zdanowicz, C., Jackson, A., & Orjoux, A. (2020). Coronavirus cases tied to a Maine wedding reception hit 147, with 3 deaths. *CNN.* Retrieved from https://www.cnn.com/2020/09/05/us/maine-wedding-outbreak-covid-cases-trnd/index.html

Zhang, S. (2020). Vaccine chaos is looming. *The Atlantic.* Retrieved from https://www.theatlantic.com/health/archive/2020/09/covid-19-most-complicated-vaccine-campaign-ever/616521/

Zhou, S. J., Zhang, L. G., Wang, L. L., Guo, Z. C., Wang, J. Q., Chen, J. C., . . . & Chen, J. X. (2020). Prevalence and socio-demographic correlates of psychological health problems in Chinese adolescents during the outbreak of COVID-19. *European Child & Adolescent Psychiatry, 29,* 749–758. https://doi.org/10.1007/s00787-020-01541-4

Ziegert, K. A. (1983). The Swedish prohibition of corporal punishment: A preliminary report. *Journal of Marriage and the Family, 45*(4), 917–926. Retrieved from www.jstor.org/stable/351805

CHAPTER ONE

Children's worry and development

Charlotte Wilson

WORRY IN A DEVELOPMENTAL CONTEXT

The previous chapter explored the concept of worry and the definitions that have been used for adults and children. One of the criticisms that has been raised about our current understanding of children's worry is that it adapted from our understanding of adult worry. As Vasey and Daleiden noted back in 1994:

> While caution is necessary when applying adult-based models to children, their careful use can provide an important heuristic for initial research efforts. As research progresses, we expected that a more developmentally appropriate model of worry in children will emerge.
>
> Vasey and Daleiden (1994, p. 186)

Unfortunately, this model has not emerged. Applying adult models to children risks missing some of the key differences that may be present due to development. If we explore the different facets of worry we find that a number of these change across childhood and are predicated on cognitive, language, social, and emotional development. This chapter reviews these different facets of worry and details the literature to date that helps us understand the early development of worry.

DEVELOPMENT OF WORRY ACROSS CHILDHOOD

Throughout childhood there are changes and transitions that mark children's lives. These range from physical transitions such as growth spurts and puberty, to social transitions such as starting school, starting secondary school, dating, and making and breaking friendships. In addition to predictable transitions are those that are common across childhood that are more individual and unpredictable such as moving house or moving school, childhood illnesses, and the arrival of siblings. All these events can prompt children's worries, but other aspects of children's development also appear to impact what children worry about.

The interest in how worry changes across childhood dates back to the earliest studies of worry in children. Writing in 1953 Angelino and Shedd report:

> Very broadly and only with reservation can we state that at age 10, 11, and 12 we find a preponderance of fears connected with animals. At 13 we find a shift to school-connected content. At age 15 this content appears to give way to economic and political interest which increases through age 18.

Angelino and Shedd (1953)

Over 60 years later their findings are still relevant and represent a good description of what changes in children's worry over time. A number of studies have explored changes in children's worry, and these have used a wide variety of methodologies to determine such changes (see Chapter 1 for a review of these). Some studies have used lists of worries generated from pilot work and asked children to rate them on frequency and intensity (e.g. Brown et al., 2006). Others have used semi-structured interviews which combine open-ended questions with structured prompting about specific worries (e.g. Henker, Whalen, & O'Neil, 1995; Laing et al., 2009; Muris et al., 2000; Silverman, Greca, & Wasserstein, 1995). Only a small number of studies have used formal questionnaires of worry or worry processes to look at developmental changes (e.g. Barahmand, 2008; Chorpita et al., 1997; Pasarelu et al., 2017). From these studies it appears that there is some evidence that worry frequency increases to age ten (Caes et al., 2016; Muris, Merckelbach et al., 2000; Muris, Merckelbach, Meesters, et al., 2002) and then declines after that (Caes et al., 2016; Laing et al., 2009), but that the intensity of worries declines more in mid-childhood and increases after that (Caes et al., 2016; Silverman, Greca, & Wasserstein, 1995). However, the evidence isn't strong and with such varied methodologies, respondents, and age ranges it is hard to strongly support the idea of developmental changes in the frequency and intensity of worries (Cartwright-Hatton, 2006).

What is much clearer is that, as suggested by Angelino and Shedd, the content of children's worries changes over time. In young children the predominant worries, just like predominant fears, are physical and immediate. These include worries about animals, separation from parents, and bullying (Laing et al., 2009; Muris, Merckelbach, et al., 2000; Stevenson-Hinde & Shouldice, 1995). At older ages children become more worried about school, health, physical appearance, and personal harm (Brown et al., 2006; Caes et al., 2016; Henker, Whalen, & O'Neil, 1995; Muris, Merckelbach, et al., 2000), with only the oldest children worrying about social ills (Angelino & Shedd, 1953; Henker, Whalen, & O'Neil, 1995).

Alongside this development in the content of worry is development in children's ability to describe their worries with greater elaboration (Henker, Whalen, & O'Neil, 1995). Indeed, given the development of language and introspective capacity across childhood it is difficult to determine whether it is the experience of worry that changes or the ability to talk about it. Furthermore, given that worry is defined as primarily verbal it is difficult to determine whether it is increased language and cognitive ability that opens up the ability to think and therefore worry about different topics or whether the developmental shifts in the content of worry reflect children's widening experience of the world (Muris, Merckelbach, Meesters, et al., 2002). Given that many of our interventions for anxious and worried children are predominantly verbal exploring the inter-relationships between language development and worry development may be important. Examining whether there are developmental shifts in the components of worry and processes involved in worry may also help us understand whether the adult models of worry do really help us understand worry in children.

Another aspect of children's experience that is likely to impact the content of their worries is their cultural context. Several studies have concluded that anxiety symptoms in children do differ across different cultures (Essau et al., 2004; Silverman, Greca, & Wasserstein, 1995; Varela et al., 2008), with differences found in which anxiety disorders are most prevalent, which fear is most commonly reported, and which wider anxiety symptoms are reported. These of course represent different aspects of the experience of anxiety; the reporting, and even experiencing, of different symptoms is likely to be influenced by the social desirability of such symptoms in your society, with somatic symptoms being more socially accepted than emotional symptoms in some families and in some societies (e.g. Varela & Hensley-Maloney, 2009). The prevalence of individual worries also likely represents individual children's experiences. If you live in poverty with uncertain access to food and shelter, then your worries are more likely to be about hunger and safety. Whereas if you are wealthy and not living in precarious circumstances, your worries are more likely to be about friendships, school, and achievement. What appears to be the case, however, is that there are more differences between individuals in different cultures than there are between cultures. Furthermore, the content of worry does not appear to determine strongly whether it is becomes a problem. Chapter 4 will further review cross-cultural differences in the mechanisms involved in problematic worry.

COMPONENTS OF WORRY

As we saw in the previous chapter there are a number of different psychological processes involved in worry. Worry anticipates the future. This needs a child to be able to anticipate and think about the future and to think about hypothetical situations. Worry is iterative. This needs a child to be able to think repeatedly about one situation. This might involve sustained attention and might involve thinking about complex ideas where iteration of thought is possible. Worry involves or feels like problem solving and more often than not this will be social problem solving. This ability to solve social problems emerges throughout childhood and involves social and emotional skills, as well as cognitive and language skills. Problematic worry involves catastrophisation. This requires complex cognitive and language skills.

When worry is broken down into the different components, it is clear that all aspects of development are implicated, from cognitive and language development to emotional and social development. This chapter focuses on these four components, exploring what we know about how they develop across childhood and adolescence and then linking this to our understanding of the development of worry.

FUTURE THINKING

Future thinking has been described as one of the most important processes within human cognition, with some researchers suggesting that it distinguishes us from other species (Atance & O'Neill, 2005b). It is future thinking that allows us to prepare for and plan our own futures, whether explicitly or implicitly. Therefore, worry may be seen as future thinking that aims to prepare for and plan for the negative or catastrophic possible futures. Future thinking is a fundamental part of worry. Although you can worry about things past, it is usually the impact they may have on the future that is concerning. The focus on the future in worry may be one of the factors that distinguishes worry from rumination (Segerstrom et al., 2000), and therefore this future focus in worry needs consideration of the complex cognitive processes involved in putting ourselves into possible futures.

Much work has been done on children's ability to think about the future or mentally time travel. For example, Suddendorf (2010) asked three- and four-year-old children to say something that they would be doing tomorrow. Their parents were asked to rate whether these events were likely, and it was found that at four years of age, children almost always proposed realistic events, but younger than this, the ability was more unreliable. Across this age range (three to four years) a significant minority of children could not talk about something they would be doing tomorrow. In a slightly different paradigm, Atance and O'Neill

(2005a) gave children a number options of what to take with them on a future trip. They chose from a pool of desirable and helpful options and then justified their choices. The determination of whether the child was thinking about the future or not was on the basis of how they justified their choice. They found that at age three, about 40–50% children were justifying their choices using future focused language. Extending this Atance and Meltzoff (2005) asked three, four, and five year olds about a possible future event, but this time the event called for a specific item; for example, one prompt involved a snowy scene, and the options children could choose were a winter coat, arm bands (water wings), or a towel. All children chose the correct item at a level better than chance, but this approached a ceiling level with the four and five year olds (91% and 97% correct, respectively). Differences between the different ages were even more marked for using future language in justifying the choices, with 35%, 62%, and 71% of three, four, and five year olds using future state language in their justification. We replicated these findings using a different scene involving a tropical greenhouse full of insects (Barrett & Wilson, 2019). Once again we found that children chose appropriate items more often than they used future uncertain terms to justify them. This ability to justify choices using these future uncertain terms was related to age but not to verbal ability (Figure 2.1).

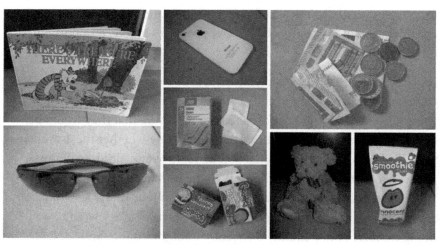

Figure 2.1 *Items used in the future thinking task.*

The reliance on language for determining future thinking has some limitations, especially as these future thinking skills are developing at the same time that language is at a basic level but is quickly advancing. Therefore other experimental paradigms haven't relied on language. For example, Suddendorf, Nielsen, and von Gehlen (2011) showed children a puzzle that they couldn't complete because they didn't have all the parts. They then showed the children into a different room for a different task. However, in this second room was the part that the child needed to complete the puzzle in the first room, along with other desirable objects. As they left this second room children were asked to choose an object that they would like to take back into the first room. The reasoning was that children who were thinking about the future would choose the object that was needed to complete the puzzle, but those who weren't would just choose a more desirable object. At three years of age children chose the correct object at a chance level, but by four years of age children more often chose an object that could help them solve the problem.

A different but related body of research focused on children's thinking about the future is counterfactual thinking. Worries can typically be viewed as hypothetical thinking about the future, whereas counterfactual thinking is when future possibilities are in contradiction to what is currently happening or known. So, if worry is asking 'what if?' counterfactual thinking is asking 'what if that hadn't happened?'.

> Alice got her exam results and was disappointed. She was worried about whether it might impact on her future choices and her future career. Very soon she was thinking to herself, 'if only I had studied harder', 'if only the right question had come up on that test paper' 'if only I had eaten a proper breakfast the morning of the exam'.

There is debate about what age children start being able to think counterfactually (Beck et al., 2014) that mirrors the debate about hypothetical future thinking. There is some evidence that a certain kind of counterfactual thinking is present from about three years of age (Harris, German, & Mills, 1996; Robinson & Beck, 2000), whereas other researchers suggest that it starts a little later, from four years old (Riggs et al., 1998). It does appear, like hypothetical future thinking, to develop through childhood into adolescence, with greater complexity and capacity for abstraction (Beck et al., 2014; Rafetseder & Perner, 2012).

Therefore it suggests that the ability to think into the future does start early, from age four to five or so but that the nature of the task might significantly impact this. Therefore another interesting question is not when children develop this ability to mentally time travel but in what circumstances. Atance and Meltzoff (2006) found that children's current state significantly impacted on their ability to predict their future desires. They randomised 48 three-, four-, and five-year-old children into four groups: two groups got lots of salty pretzels during their task, and the other two didn't. The children were then asked to nominate what they would like, pretzels or water, with one group in each condition asked what they wanted right now, and the other asked what they would like to accompany a different task tomorrow. The children who had eaten the pretzels reported that they would want water, whether or not they were choosing for right now or to have tomorrow. This has been replicated in different age groups (Mahy et al., 2014) and we find that even adults find it hard to overcome their current emotion when thinking about the future (Kramer et al., 2017; Wilson & Gilbert, 2005). Furthermore, emotion valence appears to influence the presence of spontaneous counterfactual thinking in both adults (Roese & Olson, 1997) and children (Guajardo, McNally, & Wright, 2016).

This has significant implications both for worry and more generally for self-report of anxiety. Many clinicians have had the experience of children in the clinic room denying any difficulties with their anxiety and reporting very convincingly that they will be able to stroke the dog/go to school/go to bed in their own bed. Furthermore, several trials have found significant changes when parent or clinician report are used, but much smaller, and often non-significant, changes when self-report is used. Instead of concluding that children are not very good respondents, maybe we need to consider that young children are much more influenced by their current feeling and mental state than older children and adults and that their reports that things are fine and will be fine indicate this limitation of ability.

> Philippa, aged 13 was just starting therapy. She had not been into school for about 7 months. She had experienced significant bullying and had not been able to return after a summer break. Every morning her mother and father tried to encourage her to return to school and every morning she cried, shouted, and sometimes vomited. Her parents were on the point of giving up and school wanted to know when she was going to be back. Following an assessment it was considered that Philippa might benefit from cognitive behaviour therapy and so the therapist and Philippa sat down to plan some goals for the therapy. Philippa categorically stated she wanted to get back to school. She wanted to do well and get a good job and she missed her friends. The therapist set up a hierarchy of activities where getting back to school was at the top, and thinking about entering the school doors was at the bottom. In therapy Philippa was able to tolerate the anxiety of thinking about entering the school and found that the anxiety went down to low levels whilst thinking about this. This gave her great confidence and she told the therapist that she was ready to go back to school. She said she wanted to skip to the top of the hierarchy and go back into school on Monday. The therapist talked with her about the fact she hadn't been in since before summer. Philippa dismissed this and said she was ready and she felt strong enough to do it. She told her parents this was what was going to happen despite the therapist's suggestion that it seemed unlikely. Philippa didn't manage to get into school on the Monday and was upset and disappointed when she came back to therapy.

In a series of studies we have extended these findings to explore some additional issues in future thinking (Wilson, Curtin, O'Brien, Skelton, & Easton, in prep.). For these studies, we recruited 65 children of 5–6 year olds, 55 children of 7–9 year olds, and 60 children of 14–15 year olds. These children were given Atance and Meltzoff's trip task (Atance &

Meltzoff, 2005) along with measures of verbal ability and anxiety and worry. Half of the children in each age group were randomised into a negative mood induction condition, where they were played slow sad music, the lights were lowered, and the researcher spoke in a low quiet voice. It was predicted that children might choose more comforting options for the trip and that sad mood might make the children's justifications more present-focused. Results were complicated by the fact that the mood manipulation worked differently in each age group. In the youngest age group the mood manipulation did not work at all. The researcher reported that children did remain quiet during the sad music, but as soon as the researcher spoke to them afterwards, their mood lifted immediately. For the seven- to nine-year-old age group the mood induction was successful, but it was short lived, whereas for the older age group, the mood induction was successful and lasted throughout the experimental procedure. However, the mood induction did not impact on the choices made or the justifications given for choices in any age group. On further examination, however, some subtle differences emerged. In the two youngest groups there was an impact of verbal ability (as measured by the BPVS; Dunn & Dunn, 2009) on justifications, with uncertainty terms and references to the future being related to higher vocabulary. To explore the role of mood further we explored time taken to make choices (14–16 year olds), with the hypothesis that rumination or worry about choices may lead to longer choice times and also the number of words used to justify the answer (seven to nine year olds), with the hypothesis that perseveration might lead to an increase in words used. We could not find evidence that negative mood led to increased time taken to choose the objects to take on the trip; however, we did find evidence in the seven to nine year olds that children in a low mood condition used more words to justify their answers, perhaps suggesting some level of perseveration. Furthermore, when split by group, the association between vocabulary skills and future/uncertainty terms used in the justification could only be found in the neutral mood group, suggesting that other factors, not just verbal ability, were impacting on the responses when the children were experiencing low mood.

Echoing this finding, Mahy et al. (2014) make the important distinction between 'hot' and 'cold' reasoning processes, suggesting that thinking about the future when it requires inhibition of a current mood or physiological state may require more 'hot' processing, whereas thinking about the future more generally does not. They found that in the 'cold' processing condition, seven year olds out-performed three year olds, but this was not the case in the 'hot' processing condition. In order to fully determine whether the ability to think into the future is impacted by mood, we must design a condition in which the future event is in conflict with the current mood, perhaps anticipating a positive event or outcome.

When thinking about the future, we may also need to consider children's organisation of memory more generally. Vasey (1993) argued that young children do not have the organisational structures that are required to propagate worry, and therefore context dependency may be crucial to understanding distress and worry in younger children.

> Kae was 3 when she went on holiday. She was used to travelling, having moved countries on her 1st birthday, and was usually a happy traveller. But this time she wasn't happy in the airport. Her parents checked in the larger luggage and the airport staff asked them whether they had followed the guidelines with regards our hand luggage. They replied that they had. They reminded Kae that she would have to put her beloved Lucie-Bear through the scanner and she looked very concerned. Her mother asked her what was wrong. Kae couldn't tell her. Her mother asked whether it was putting Lucie-Bear through the scanner. She said it was. Her mother asked her what she thought might happen. She shook her head to tell her mother she didn't know. When they approached the security check Kae reluctantly handed over Lucie-Bear to be put in a tray to be scanned. She was very upset and concerned. Her mother asked again what she thought might happen and she again shook her head. Her mother asked whether she thought Lucie-Bear might get lost and her eyes widened, filled with tears and she nodded. A combination of reassurance and the few minutes it took to get Lucie-Bear back was enough to put things right.

Lagatutta has carried out a series of studies on young children exploring their tendency to use past information when thinking about the future or 'life history theory of mind' (Lagattuta, Tashjian, & Kramer, 2018). All the studies suggest that no matter how you measure children's use of the past to think about the future, some children as young as four years old use this life history information, with greater numbers of children using this information as age increases. This includes using past information to predict future emotions (Lagattuta, Wellman, & Flavell, 1997; Lagattuta & Wellman, 2001), to predict future worries and behaviours (Lagattuta, 2007; Lagattuta & Sayfan, 2011, 2013b), and in their use of uncertainty ratings and language when thinking about the future (Lagattuta & Sayfan, 2011). The studies suggest that both general age-related development and executive functioning (EF) impact on children's ability to use past information to predict the future (Lagattuta, Tashjian, & Kramer, 2018), with children's verbal ability impacting on their use of language to talk about the future (Lagattuta, 2007; Lagattuta, Wellman, & Flavell, 1997). These studies also throw some light on the subtleties of future thinking. As well as differences across the age range, there were also some subtle gender differences, with female participants using uncertain ratings and using uncertainty in their language more than male participants (Lagattuta & Sayfan, 2011). There was some evidence that younger children required the past and the future to share exact details in order to be able to predict the future based on the past; however, older children managed to use this past information to predict the future even when it was only similar, rather than exactly the same (Lagattuta, 2007). Across the age range understanding the future emotion or behaviour of someone was easier when there was a contrast between the current emotion and the predicted emotion, for example, the predicted emotion being negative and the current emotion being positive, and in general negative emotions were easier to predict (Lagattuta & Wellman, 2001). Finally, there was a recency effect, with most recent past behaviours impacting more than behaviours previous to this (Lagattuta, Tashjian, & Kramer, 2018; Lagattuta & Sayfan, 2013a).

This studies suggest that using past events to think about the future may be possible for even very young children, but that certain individual and environmental factors may impact on whether this occurs spontaneously. Children with greater verbal and cognitive ability, perhaps specifically with greater EF capacity, may be more likely to use past information to think into the future. Furthermore, if there is a mismatch between current emotion and predictions about the future, these may prompt future thinking more than if the current mood matches the predicted future mood. Given the impact of worry on EF, we may also predict that when children are worried their capacity to think accurately into the future may be impaired and they may rush to more certain judgements about what might happen.

Despite the importance of future thinking in understanding worry, we are only just beginning to determine the parameters that might impact on this relationship and to understand how individual differences might impact on the ability to worry and how worry might impact on the ability to think into the future. What is clear however is that children as young as four do have rudimentary capacities to think about the future and to talk about possible future events, although this may not occur spontaneously, and it may be limited in some ways. If this is the case, then children should have the ability to worry about future possible outcomes from at least four years of age, if not earlier.

PROBLEM SOLVING

Another literature that might be relevant to think about here is the research on problem solving. Chapter 1 reviewed the research on the relationship between worry and problem solving, but can the developmental psychology literature help us understand the development of worry by understanding the development of problem solving?

Developmentally, it appears that children start problem solving very early in life (Keen, 2011). From infancy babies appear to be exploring their environment in order to solve the problems it poses. From age six months babies appear to use simple problem solving such as putting an object in the other hand to free up the hand that is needed. From age nine months they use objects for things they are not designed for, but that achieve a different end (Lockman, 2000), for example, using a toy to push something along or hit something, or later, when infants are able to walk, using a toy kitchen as a set of ladders to reach high shelves. We also have evidence that children use social problem solving very early in life. It could be argued that social referencing, whereby an infant uses the affective response of a parent or caregiver to determine information about the safety of the situation (Emde, 1992), is one of the earliest forms of social problem solving. In situations of uncertainty the ability to use non-verbal information from a trusted caregiver may be crucial to the determination of the situation as safe. As children get older, they may look to others to learn about the environment. In her classic studies, Smetana describes how children develop their social order in relation to other children through play in nursery and pre-school settings (Smetana, 1985, 1993). Similarly, Dunn systematically observed and described the verbal interactions between pre-schoolers that provided good evidence that even young children show social problem solving (Dunn, 1988).

Both problem solving in general and social problem solving more specifically continue to develop across childhood (Figure 2.2). As children understand the intentions of others better, develop a larger range of strategies to solve inter-personal problems, and develop skills in carrying these out, their ability in successful problem solving

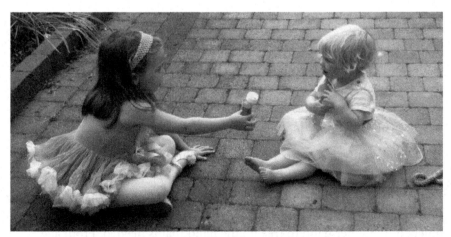

Figure 2.2 *Learning from each other: social problem solving in action.*

increases (Rubin & Rose-Krasnor, 1992). By adolescence, most young people are successfully negotiating complex social relationships, the emergence of romantic/intimate relationships, and developing into their adult identities (Blakemore, 2018). Indeed it has been suggested that in adolescence there is a rise in the importance of social relationships that can be seen in brain structures and function (Blakemore, 2008; Nelson et al., 2005; Steinberg, 2005).

A number of different processes are working concurrently to ensure the smooth development of these social problem-solving abilities. Some researchers (e.g. Leslie, 1994) have emphasised simple maturational processes whereby the development that occurs in brain structure and functioning allows for more complex information processing and behaviour to develop. These can also be framed within an evolutionary perspective (Belsky, Steinberg, & Draper, 1991), which highlights the key goals of the human organism at different life stages. Early life stages may be seen as aiming to understand when and how your needs are going to be met, with an early focus on survival, developing into a more generalised understanding of the availability and predictability of resources. These broad brush goals determine a variety of complex behaviours and it may be that a fine grained understanding of the mechanisms of social problem solving may need reference to behavioural or social learning models (Bandura, 1969, 2001). These learning models propose that we may learn much of our behaviour not only by differential reinforcement of our own behaviour – for example, being invited to play by being friendly, or being rejected by being loud and boisterous – but also that we learn by observing others. As Bandura notes 'learning would be exceedingly laborious, not to mention hazardous, if people had to rely solely on the effects of their own actions to inform them what to do'.

This developmental progression in the ability to socially problem solve is likely to be related to developments in metacognitive ability (Weil et al., 2013), which, in turn, is related to developments in executive functions (Roebers, 2017). It appears that all these functions predominantly involve the pre-frontal cortex (Dumontheil, 2014; Qiu et al., 2018). This is one of the later brain areas to develop, with significant changes occurring both in childhood and across adolescence (Dumontheil, 2014; Tsujimoto, 2008). It is also an area implicated in generalised anxiety disorder (GAD; Goossen, van der Starre, & van der Heiden, 2019), suggesting a link between problematic worry and deficits in social problem solving.

Finally, it is important to understand the impact of individual differences on these processes. For example, in her studies of pre-schoolers' social interactions, Hughes found strong associations between the ability to socially problem solve and other cognitive abilities, such as EF and theory of mind development (Astington & Hughes, 2013; Hughes & Leekam, 2004). Even if we are learning our social behaviour through our own experiences and by observing others, this is impacted by the cognitive capacity we have individually to do this.

> David was born with a significant learning disability and at eight years of age he had no spoken language. However, he used lots of different ways to communicate. In his family of origin there were many children and a lot of rough and tumble play which sometimes tipped over into aggression. On a school trip with a teacher David was keen to get the teacher's attention and started by pinching her arm. As he was safe, and he was not causing her pain she ignored this behaviour. He then tried to push her arm and started hitting her. Again, she ignored this behaviour. There was a short pause, and then David tried gently tickling her and making gentle vocalisations. David had observed how other children got attention, so started with the one that worked at home, moving through strategies he had seen other children try.

Much of the literature on social problem solving focuses on when it goes wrong. There are robust associations between problem-solving deficits and negative outcomes such as peer relationship difficulties (Warden & MacKinnon, 2003), aggression (Keltikangas-Jarvinen, 2002; Takahashi, Koseki, & Shimada, 2009), poor mental health such as anxiety and depression (Wright et al., 2010), and self-harm and suicide (Speckens & Hawton, 2011). These different outcomes interact with each other, with aggressive children having poor peer relationships and poor mental health (Werner & Crick, 2004), and young people who self-harm also showing poor peer relationships (Stallard et al., 2013). What these studies do not show is the direction of effect. Several studies indicate that poor problem solving leads to poor outcomes (e.g. Hawton et al., 1999; Spears et al., 2014), but few explore problem solving as an outcome. Given the cognitive capacity needed for successful problem solving, it might be expected that any psychological difficulty that takes up cognitive capacity, such as worry or rumination, might impact on problem solving. Indeed Guerreiro et al. (2013) call for more well-designed longitudinal studies to allow us to further explore the interactions between these mechanisms.

Therefore the developmental psychology literature on problem solving suggests that it does start very young, and interactive processes including simple maturation, social learning, and reciprocal reinforcement may play a role in its development. Furthermore, individual differences will impact on the child's ability to problem solve across a wide range of situations. Problem-solving deficits may well lead to a variety of poor outcomes for children and may interact with other processes, such as the development of peer relationships to mediate or moderate these outcomes.
However, poor problem solving is associated with difficulties with peer relationships, behaviour, and mental health, and therefore if worry is a poor way of problem solving, the reliance on worry to solve problems is likely to cause children further difficulties. Chapter 1 suggested that worried children may indeed not have problem-solving deficits, but rather may have poor confidence in their own ability to problem solve. Exploring the problem-solving theories may well help us explain how this poor confidence develops and how worry might impact on poor long-term outcomes for young people.

EXECUTIVE FUNCTIONS

By examining future thinking and problem solving it becomes clear that children's cognitive ability is important in our wider understanding of the development of worry. The aspect of cognitive ability that might be particularly important for understanding worry is those aspects of worry that allow us to sustain our attention, reflect on our own experiences, and our ability to iterate our thinking by following logical thought processes. Many of these cognitive abilities come under the umbrella of executive functions.

Like many cognitive abilities executive functions appear to develop throughout childhood. EF has been split into different components by different researchers, but it is widely accepted that inhibition, working memory, and cognitive flexibility are key components (Diamond, 2013). We know that these all develop across childhood, with a basic working memory ability being the first to mature, and certain aspects of inhibition being latest to mature. There is a significant literature on the relationships between anxiety and EF, testing, and developing Eysenck's attentional control theory (Eysenck et al., 2007). In this theory, and much of the empirical work supporting it, anxiety is seen to impair EF. This occurs across both adult and child populations (Kertz et al., 2016; Ursache & Raver, 2014; Visu-Petra, Miclea, & Visu-Petra, 2013), and in populations that do not have typical neurodevelopment (Hollocks et al., 2014; Ng-Cordell et al., 2018).

However, there is much less research that links these components to worry. In order to explore these links it might be relevant to draw on an adult model of worry. One of the key models that considers executive functions in worry has been developed and tested by Colette Hirsch and colleagues. Hirsch and Mathews (Hirsch & Mathews, 2012) detail a cognitive model of worry in adults. It draws strongly on cognitive psychology as well as being driven by a wealth of clinical experience. Hirsch and Mathews propose that it is both controlled or voluntary attentional processes and uncontrollable or involuntary attentional processes that contribute to the representation of the threat. These attentional processes can be considered part of the wider construct of executive functions. In the model if someone is unable to ignore or over-ride a negative representation of a threat then the top-down controlled attentional processes are allocated to dealing with the threat and this inevitably leads to prolonged worry. The model is built on evidence about cognitive biases in worriers. These biases include attention towards threat, with worriers more likely to attend to threat in their environment, and also more likely to have difficulties disengaging from thinking about threat. Research with both anxious adults and children suggest that anxiety is consistently associated with biased attention to threat (Bar-Haim et al., 2007; Dudeney, Sharpe, & Hunt, 2015). Furthermore, these biased attentional processes are specifically associated with worry and GAD in adults (Goodwin, Yiend, & Hirsch, 2017), with less evidence that they are specifically associated with worry and GAD in children; Waters, Bradley, and Mogg (2014) find evidence for increased attention towards threat in young people with GAD. Hirsch and Mathews also propose interpretation biases in GAD, with worriers more likely to interpret a situation as threatening. These interpretation biases are seen both in adults (Feng et al., 2019) and young people (Stuijfzand et al., 2018) with GAD and high levels of worry (for a review of the Hirsch and Mathews model in young people see Songco, Hudson, and Fox (2020)).

It appears then that cognitive biases are associated with anxiety and worry in children, but how do these relate more broadly to executive functions? One of the paradoxes of worry described by Hirsch and Mathews is that worry itself reduces our capacity for controlling our attention. Attention towards threat and negative threat interpretations' impact deplete our attentional processes (Hirsch, Hayes, & Mathews, 2009), but this process may be highly relevant to children. In young children attentional control is only just developing, and therefore there may be bi-directional relationships between attentional control and worry. Children who are just developing attentional control or have naturally poor attentional control may therefore struggle to inhibit worry, and in addition worry-prone children may have impaired attentional control due to their worry. Attentional control abilities do appear to be highly associated with worry in children (Gramszlo et al., 2018; Gramszlo & Woodruff-Borden, 2015) and may interact with meta-cognitions in predicting higher levels of worry (Reinholdt-Dunne et al., 2019), but there is less evidence about which directions of effect may be present.

Geronimi and colleagues (2016) explored the links between worry and EF in 7–12 year olds using parent report of their children's EF. Higher levels of worry were associated with increased difficulties in EF across all the different facets of EF measured. However, age acted as a moderator for some of these. For working memory, planning, and moderating there were stronger relationships between EF and worry for younger children, suggesting that as children get older, the impact of their EF on their ability and tendency to worry decreases. This fits with cognitive models of worry, where worries become over-rehearsed with time and therefore do not require as much cognitive capacity as they do when they are not familiar cognitive processes (Hirsch & Mathews, 2012).

One of the ways in which EF might impact worry is by changing how children use past information to predict the future. In a series of experiments with children aged four to ten years of age Lagattuta and colleagues have shown that not only does children's ability to predict the future from past events develop over time (see earlier discussion) but also that EF affects that relationship. Children with better EF appear to be able to use the past information, or current ambiguous information, to predict future events and emotions (Lagattuta, Sayfan, & Harvey, 2014; Lagattuta, Tashjian, & Kramer, 2018). We would therefore expect complex relationships between EF, age, and worry. In young children the ability to predict the future from past events might increase worry, particularly for those who have had difficult early lives. However, for older children EF might protect against problematic worry by allowing children more access to possible alternative futures that are not negative or catastrophic. However, the picture is likely to be even more complicated than this. As well as age, temperamental factors impact the relationship between worry and executive functions. Gramszlo and Woodruff-Borden (2015) found that children aged 7–10 who were difficult to soothe had higher levels of self-reported worry. However, this relationship was fully mediated by parent-reported attentional and emotional control aspects of EF.

Further exploration of different aspects of EF, especially attentional control, in relation to worry is warranted to further delineate the impact age and other aspects of cognitive development have on the relationships between these two. In order to determine whether certain kinds of children are especially as risk for developing worry, and whether our adult cognitive model of worry maintenance is appropriate for younger population, we need to determine whether attentional control leads to increased worry or whether increased worry decreases attentional control abilities or both.

CATASTROPHISATION

One of the key processes in pathological worry is catastrophisation (Davey, 1994a; Wilson, 2010). This is the process whereby the iterative nature of worry leads to increasingly negative potential outcomes as people ask themselves, 'What if?' (Davey, 2006; Vasey & Borkovec, 1992). Catastrophisation is one of the processes that might distinguish problematic and non-problematic worry (see Chapter 4), and several studies with adult participants have found that people with high trait worry are able to produce more steps in a catastrophising interview (Davey, 2006). The catastrophising interview involves identifying a possible worry, either by asking the participant to identify one or by giving the participant a common situation that causes worry for many people, and then asking the participant what would be so bad about the situation or example given. This answer is written down and the participant is then asked what would be so bad about that?

> The participants were given the situation of starting a new school. So each of them were asked "what would be bad about starting a new school?". Mary's first answer was "I wouldn't know anyone." The researcher then asked "what would be bad about not knowing anyone?" Mary replied "I might be lonely." The researcher asked "what would be bad about being lonely?" Mary thought "I wouldn't have any friends" she answered. The researcher asked "what would be bad about not having any friends?" "It would mean I wouldn't want to go to school" Mary said quickly. What would be so bad about not wanting to go to school was that she wouldn't go to school, this would lead to not getting good grades, getting a bad job and being poor, sad, and lonely as an adult.

In contrast Luke replied to the first question "I wouldn't know where to sit?". When the researcher asked "what would be bad about not knowing where to sit Luke replied "nothing really, I'd just ask the teacher and then I'd know."

To date several studies have used a catastrophising interview with children and adolescents. In one of the earliest studies using a catastrophising interview with children, Vasey and colleagues (Vasey, Crnic, & Carter, 1994) interviewed 76 children between five and 12 years old. In the youngest age range (five to six years) children struggled to produce a number of steps in the catastrophising interview, but by age eight to nine, they could produce about four steps. Vasey and colleagues suggest that verbal ability might impact on the ability to produce worry steps, as when they controlled for the number of words in the answer there was no longer an effect of age on the worry steps. Osleger (2012) tested this directly in 9–11 year olds. She found that both verbal ability, as measured by the similarities subtest on the Weschler Abbreviated Scale of Intelligence (WASI), and verbal fluency predicted the number of worry steps in the catastrophising interview. We replicated this finding in 7–10 and 6–11 year olds (Wilson, Bourne, & Cuddy, in prep.) except using the vocabulary subtest of the WASI. Across these studies, we also replicated Vasey's results about number of worry steps produced. The younger children produced three to four worry steps on average, but the older children produced seven to eight. This relationship with verbal ability suggests that the catastrophising interview may not necessarily tap into worry processes and may instead be a test of verbal ability. This is also supported by the findings that in two of these three studies, and also in Turner and Wilson (2010) there were no associations between worry steps produced and measures of worry and anxiety. Furthermore, Osleger found evidence that the interview may not be particularly reliable in this population; there was a very low correlation between number of steps on two consecutive catastrophising interviews.

What might be more relevant to our understanding of worry is analysis of the content of the worries produced and interviews with participants after the interview. Vasey, Crnic, and Carter (1994) found that the worries reported by children across the wide range of ages showed a predictable developmental progression with worries about physical harm decreasing in older groups and social concerns increasing across this time-frame. Other studies have tested a much narrower age range of children and therefore cannot show this same pattern; however, different studies have explored different aspects of the worry steps. Turner and Wilson (2010) explored why participants stopped and didn't stop producing worry steps in the catastrophising interview. There appeared to be three patterns in the catastrophising interview: (1) children came to a catastrophic conclusion very quickly, (2) children ended up with a repeating circle of negative outcomes that weren't so catastrophic, or (3) children ended up after several elaborations slowly getting more and more catastrophic. Typically, it is this third group that appear to be worriers as they can produce lots of iterations. However, we may also be clinically concerned about the first group. Indeed this group also reported high levels of worry. Osleger also qualitatively examined content. Using inductive thematic analysis, she coded the pattern of responses across the interview. The worries were coded into standard worries, long term worries (about long term future), circular responses and extreme responses. Exploring the characteristics of high and low worriers, she found that long term worries were more likely in a low worry group, and circular (perseverative) and extreme (catastrophic) responses were found in the high worry group.

Number of steps in a catastrophising process may be more representative of verbal ability in children, in contrast to the studies on adults, where it does appear to be reliably associated with trait worry. However, there may well be particular processes in catastrophising that are associated with trait worry, such as perseverative patterns and extreme end points. These extreme or catastrophic end points might occur relatively quickly, bring a worry bout to an end quickly, but with a high level of emotion, or might occur slowly, encouraging perseveration.

To date no studies have examined catastrophising patterns in children with anxiety disorders. It would be very interesting to see whether the patterns are indeed different to children with normal levels of anxiety and worry. It would also be very interesting to examine whether certain patterns of catastrophising are risk factors for later anxiety or mood difficulties and in particular whether certain patterns are risks for certain anxiety disorders.

CONCLUSIONS

What is clear from reviewing the developmental literature across a number of domains is that whilst some aspects of development do change dramatically at certain time points in a child's life, most complex aspects change somewhat throughout childhood, with children gaining ability to pass developmental tasks more easily, to justify their responses verbally, and to understand and work with complexity as they age. Some of these abilities are largely intact in their adult form by early adolescence, whilst others are developing into adulthood, and possibly beyond.

Worry can be seen as one of these complex phenomena and so it is perhaps unsurprising that the trajectory of the development of worry, considering factors such as the number of iterations in a worry chain, the types of things children worry about, the ability to represent worry in words and understand it as different from fear, develops similarly across childhood into adulthood. The parallels are clear. From this perhaps we should conclude that worry is a normal and somewhat inevitable aspect of human cognition. That once we are able to iterate thought, and once we are able to look into the future and think about what it might bring, it is then inevitable that we engage from time to time in worry processes. Can then developmental psychology add to our understanding of worry and its development across childhood into adulthood? At present the literature does not allow this question to be fully answered, but a number of hypotheses might be developed. Perhaps understanding how developmental psychology can inform the study of children's worry will allow us to look for anomalies of development that might lead to certain children being at risk for developing problematic worry. It might also lead to a greater understanding of different presentations of worry.

At present our definition of worry is adapted from adult definitions. Exploring development, especially when certain aspects of it are delayed or enhanced, may help us develop a definition of worry that encompasses different presentations of worry, such as what worry looks like if someone is non-verbal, and what it looks like when following a train of thought (iterative thought) is hard.

Finally, understanding that the presentation and experience of worry is likely affected by our developmental stage may lead to different and new interventions for those whose worry interferes with their daily life. This may be especially true for children but may also be true for other populations whose development is atypical, such as those with specific learning disabilities or more global intellectual disabilities, neuro-developmental conditions, or those with acquired brain injury or cognitive degenerative conditions.

BIBLIOGRAPHY

Angelino, H., & Shedd, C. L. (1953). Shifts in the content of fears and worries relative to chronological age. *Proceedings of the Oklahoma Academy of Science, 34*, 180–186.

Astington, J., & Hughes, C. (2013). Theory of mind: Self-reflection and social understanding. In P. D. Zelazo (Ed.), *The Oxford handbook of developmental psychology, Vol. 2: Self and other* (pp. 398–423). Oxford, UK: Oxford University Press.

Atance, C. M., & Meltzoff, A. N. (2005). My future self: Young children's ability to anticipate and explain future states. *Cognitive Development, 20*(3), 341–361. https://doi.org/10.1016/j.cogdev.2005.05.001

Atance, C. M., & Meltzoff, A. N. (2006). Preschoolers' current desires warp their choices for the future. *Psychological Science, 17*(7), 583–587. https://doi.org/10.1111/j.1467-9280.2006.01748.x

Atance, C. M., & O'Neill, D. K. (2005a). Preschoolers' talk about future situations. *First Language, 25*(1), 5–18. https://doi.org/10.1177/0142723705045678

Atance, C. M., & O'Neill, D. K. (2005b). The emergence of episodic future thinking in humans. *Learning and Motivation, 36*(2), 126–144. https://doi.org/10.1016/j.lmot.2005.02.003

Bandura, A. (1969). Social-learning theory of identificatory processes. In D. A. Goslin (Ed.), *Handbook of socialization theory and research* (pp. 213–262). Chicago: Rand McNally.

Bandura, A. (2001). Social cognitive theory: An agentic perspective. *Annual Review of Psychology, 52*, 1–26. https://doi.org/10.1146/annurev.psych.52.1.1

Barahmand, U. (2008). Age and gender differences in adolescent worry. *Personality and Individual Differences, 45*(8), 778–783. https://doi.org/10.1016/j.paid.2008.08.006

Bar-Haim, Y., Lamy, D., Pergamin, L., Bakermans-Kranenburg, M. J., & van IJzendoorn, M. H. (2007). Threat-related attentional bias in anxious and nonanxious individuals: A meta-analytic study. *Psychological Bulletin, 133*(1), 1–24. https://doi.org/10.1037/0033-2909.133.1.1

Barrett, H., & Wilson, C. (2019). *The development of episodic foresight in 4–6 year olds: Methodological issues and the role of verbal and cognitive ability.* Psychological Society of Ireland Annual Conference, Kilkenny.

Beck, A. T., Brown, G., & Steer, R. T. A. (1988). An inventory for measuring clinical anxiety: Psychometric properties. *Journal of Consulting and Clinical Psychology, 56*, 893–897. https://doi: 10.1037//0022-006x.56.6.893

Beck, S. R., Weisberg, D. P., Burns, P., & Riggs, K. J. (2014). Conditional reasoning and emotional experience: A review of the development of counterfactual thinking. *Studia Logica, 102*(4), 673–689. https://doi.org/10.1007/s11225-013-9508-1

Belsky, J., Steinberg, L., & Draper, P. (1991). Childhood experience, interpersonal development, and reproductive strategy: An evolutionary theory of socialization. *Child Development, 62*(4), 647–670. https://doi: 10.1111/j.1467-8624.1991. tb01558.x

Blakemore, S.-J. (2018). *Inventing ourselves: The secret life of the teenage brain.* London: Penguin, Random House.

Brown, S. L., Teufel, J. A., Birch, D. A., & Kancherla, V. (2006). Gender, age, and behavior differences in early adolescent worry. *Journal of School Health, 76*(8), 430–437. https://doi.org/10.1111/j.1746-1561.2006.00137.x

Caes, L., Fisher, E., Clinch, J., Tobias, J. H., & Eccleston, C. (2016). The development of worry throughout childhood: Avon longitudinal study of parents and children data. *British Journal of Health Psychology, 21*(2), 389–406. https://doi.org/10.1111/bjhp.12174

Cartwright-Hatton, S. (2006). Worry in childhood and adolescence. In G. C. L. Davey, & A. Wells (Eds.), *Worry and its psychological disorders: Theory, assessment and treatment* (pp. 81–97). Chichester: John Wiley & Sons Ltd. https://doi.org/10.1002/9780470713143.ch6

Chorpita, B. F., Tracey, S. A., Brown, T. A., Collica, T. J., & Barlow, D. H. (1997). Assessment of worry in children and adolescents: An adaptation of the Penn State Worry Questionnaire. *Behaviour Research and Therapy, 35*(6), 569–581. https://doi.org/10.1016/S0005-7967(96)00116-7

Davey, G. C. L. (1994a). Pathological worrying as exacerbated problem-solving. In G. C. L. Davey, & F. Tallis (Eds.), *Worrying: Perspectives on theory, assessment and treatment* (pp. 35–59). New York: John Wiley & Sons.

Davey, G. C. L. (2006). The catastrophising interview procedure. In G. C. L. Davey, & A. Wells (Eds.), *Worry and its psychological disorders: Theory, assessment and treatment* (pp. 157–176). Chichester: John Wiley & Sons Ltd. https://doi.org/10.1002/9780470713143.ch10

Diamond, A. (2013). Executive functions. *Annual Review of Psychology, 64*(1), 135–168. https://doi.org/10.1146/annurev-psych-113011-143750

Dudeney, J., Sharpe, L., & Hunt, C. (2015). Attentional bias towards threatening stimuli in children with anxiety: A meta-analysis. *Clinical Psychology Review, 40*, 66–75. https://doi.org/10.1016/j.cpr.2015.05.007

Dumontheil, I. (2014). Development of abstract thinking during childhood and adolescence: The role of rostrolateral prefrontal cortex. *Developmental Cognitive Neuroscience, 10*, 57–76. https://doi.org/10.1016/j.dcn.2014.07.009

Dunn, J. (1988). *The beginnings of social understanding.* Cambridge, MA: Harvard University Press.

Dunn, L. M., & Dunn, D. M. (2009). *The British picture vocabulary scale.* London: GL Assessment Limited

Emde, R. N. (1992). Social referencing research. In S. Feinman (Ed.), *Social referencing and the social construction of reality in infancy* (pp. 79–94). New York: Springer US. https://doi.org/10.1007/978-1-4899-2462-9_4

Essau, C. A., Sakano, Y., Ishikawa, S., & Sasagawa, S. (2004). Anxiety symptoms in Japanese and in German children. *Behaviour Research and Therapy, 42*(5), 601–612. https://doi.org/10.1016/S0005-7967(03)00164-5

Eysenck, M. W., Derakshan, N., Santos, R., & Calvo, M. G. (2007). Anxiety and cognitive performance: Attentional control theory. *Emotion, 7*(2), 336–353. https://doi.org/10.1037/1528-3542.7.2.336

Feng, Y.-C., Krahé, C., Sumich, A., Meeten, F., Lau, J. Y. F., & Hirsch, C. R. (2019). Using event-related potential and behavioural evidence to understand interpretation bias in relation to worry. *Biological Psychology, 148*, 107746. https://doi.org/10.1016/j.biopsycho.2019.107746

Goodwin, H., Yiend, J., & Hirsch, C. R. (2017). Generalized anxiety disorder, worry and attention to threat: A systematic review. *Clinical Psychology Review, 54*, 107–122. https://doi.org/10.1016/j.cpr.2017.03.006

Goossen, B., van der Starre, J., & van der Heiden, C. (2019). A review of neuroimaging studies in generalized anxiety disorder: "So where do we stand?" *Journal of Neural Transmission, 126*(9), 1203–1216. https://doi.org/10.1007/s00702-019-02024-w

Gramszlo, C., & Woodruff-Borden, J. (2015). Emotional reactivity and executive control: A pathway of risk for the development of childhood worry. *Journal of Anxiety Disorders, 35*, 35–41. https://doi.org/10.1016/j.janxdis.2015.07.005

Gramszlo, C., Geronimi, E. M. C., Arellano, B., & Woodruff-Borden, J. (2018). Testing a cognitive pathway between temperament and childhood anxiety. *Journal of Child and Family Studies, 27*(2), 580–590. https://doi.org/10.1007/s10826-017-0914-2

Guajardo, N. R., McNally, L. F., & Wright, A. (2016). Children's spontaneous counterfactuals: The roles of valence, expectancy, and cognitive flexibility. *Journal of Experimental Child Psychology, 146*, 79–94. https://doi.org/10.1016/j.jecp.2016.01.009

Guerreiro, D. F., Cruz, D., Frasquilho, D., Santos, J. C., Figueira, M. L., & Sampaio, D. (2013). Association between deliberate self-harm and coping in adolescents: A critical review of the last 10 years' literature. *Archives of Suicide Research, 17*(2), 91–105. https://doi.org/10.1080/13811118.2013.776439

Harris, P. L., German, T., & Mills, P. (1996). Children's use of counterfactual think-ing in causal reasoning. *Cognition, 61*(3), 233–259. https://doi. org/10.1016/S0010-0277(96)00715-9

Hawton, K., Kingsbury, S., Steinhardt, K., James, A., & Fagg, J. (1999). Repetition of deliberate self-harm by adolescents: The role of psychological factors. *Journal of Adolescence, 22*(3), 369–378. https://doi.org/10.1006/jado.1999.0228

Henker, B., Whalen, C. K., & O'Neil, R. (1995). Worldly and workaday worries: Contemporary concerns of children and young adolescents. *Journal of Abnormal Child Psychology, 23*(6), 685–702. https://doi.org/10.1007/BF01447472

Hirsch, C. R., & Mathews, A. (2012). A cognitive model of pathological worry. *Behaviour Research and Therapy, 50*(10), 636–646. https://doi.org/10.1016/j.brat.2012.06.007

Hirsch, C., Hayes, S., & Mathews, A. (2009). Looking on the bright side: Accessing benign meanings reduces worry. *Journal of Abnormal Psychology, 118*(1), 44–54. https://doi.org/10.1037/a0013473

Hollocks, M. J., Jones, C. R. G., Pickles, A., Baird, G., Happé, F., Charman, T., & Simonoff, E. (2014). The association between social cognition and executive functioning and symptoms of anxiety and depression in adolescents with autism spectrum disorders: Neurocognitive ability, anxiety, and depression. *Autism Research, 7*(2), 216–228. https://doi.org/10.1002/aur.1361

Hughes, C., & Leekam, S. (2004). What are the links between theory of mind and social relations? Review, reflections and new directions for studies of typical and atypical development. *Social Development, 13*(4), 590–619. https://doi.org/10.1111/j.1467-9507.2004.00285.x

Keen, R. (2011). The development of problem solving in young children: A critical cognitive skill. *Annual Review of Psychology, 62*(1), 1–21. https://doi.org/10.1146/annurev.psych.031809.130730

Keltikangas-Jarvinen, L. (2002). Aggressive problem-solving strategies, aggressive behavior, and social acceptance in early and late adolescence. *Journal of Youth and Adolescence, 31*(4), 279–287. https://doi.org/10.1023/A:1015445500935

Kertz, S. J., Belden, A. C., Tillman, R., & Luby, J. (2016). Cognitive control deficits in shifting and inhibition in preschool age children are associated with increased depression and anxiety over 7.5 years of development. *Journal of Abnormal Child Psychology, 44*(6), 1185–1196. https://doi.org/10.1007/s10802-015-0101-0

Kramer, H. J., Goldfarb, D., Tashjian, S. M., & Lagattuta, K. H. (2017). "These pretzels are making me thirsty": Older children and adults struggle with induced-state episodic foresight. *Child Development, 88*(5), 1554–1562. https:// doi.org/10.1111/cdev.12700

Lagattuta, K. H. (2007). Thinking about the future because of the past: Young chil-dren's knowledge about the causes of worry and preventative decisions. *Child Devel-opment, 78*(5), 1492–1509. https://doi.org/10.1111/j.1467-8624.2007.01079.x

Lagattuta, K. H., & Sayfan, L. (2011). Developmental changes in children's under-standing of future likelihood and uncertainty. *Cognitive Development, 26*(4), 315–330. https://doi.org/10.1016/j.cogdev.2011.09.004

Lagattuta, K. H., & Sayfan, L. (2013a). Not all past events are equal: Biased attention and emerging heuristics in children's past-to-future forecasting. *Child Develop-ment, 84*(6), 2094–2111. https://doi.org/10.1111/cdev.12082

Lagattuta, K. H., & Sayfan, L. (2013b). Not all past events are equal: Biased attention and emerging heuristics in children's past-to-future forecasting. *Child Development, 84*(6), 2094–2111. https://doi.org/10.1111/cdev.12082

Lagattuta, K. H., & Wellman, H. M. (2001). Thinking about the past: Early knowledge about links between prior experience, thinking, and emotion. *Child Development, 72*(1), 82–102. https://doi.org/10.1111/1467-8624.00267

Lagattuta, K. H., Sayfan, L., & Harvey, C. (2014). Beliefs about thought probability: Evidence for persistent errors in mindreading and links to executive control. *Child Development, 85*(2), 659–674. https://doi.org/10.1111/cdev.12154

Lagattuta, K. H., Tashjian, S. M., & Kramer, H. J. (2018). Does the past shape anticipation for the future? Contributions of age and executive function to advanced theory of mind. *Zeitschrift Für Psychologie, 226*(2), 122–133. https://doi.org/10.1027/2151-2604/a000328

Lagattuta, K. H., Wellman, H. M., & Flavell, J. H. (1997). Preschoolers' understanding of the link between thinking and feeling: Cognitive cuing and emotional change. *Child Development, 68*(6), 1081–1104. https://doi.org/10.1111/j.1467-8624.1997.tb01986.x

Laing, S. V., Fernyhough, C., Turner, M., & Freeston, M. H. (2009). Fear, worry, and ritualistic behaviour in childhood: Developmental trends and interrelations. *Infant and Child Development, 18*(4), 351–366. https://doi.org/10.1002/icd.627

Leslie, A. M. (1994). ToMM, ToBy, and agency: Core architecture and domain specificity. In L.A. Hirschfeld, & S. A. Gelman (Eds). *Mapping the mind: Domain specificity in cognition and culture* (pp. 119–148). Cambridge: Cambridge University Press. https://doi.org/10.1017/CBO9780511752902.006

Lockman, J. J. (2000). A perception-action perspective on tool use development. *Child Development, 71*(1), 137–144. https://doi.org/10.1111/1467-8624.00127

Mahy, C. E. V., Grass, J., Wagner, S., & Kliegel, M. (2014). These pretzels are going to make me thirsty tomorrow: Differential development of hot and cool episodic foresight in early childhood? *British Journal of Developmental Psychology, 32*(1), 65–77. https://doi.org/10.1111/bjdp.12023

Muris, P., Meesters, C., Merckelbach, H., & Hülsenbeck, P. (2000). Worry in children is related to perceived parental rearing and attachment. *Behaviour Research and Therapy, 38*(5), 487–497. https://doi.org/ 10.1016/s0005-7967(99)00072-8

Muris, P., Merckelbach, H., & Luijten, M. (2002). The connection between cognitive development and specific fears and worries in normal children and children with below-average intellectual abilities: A preliminary study. *Behaviour Research and Therapy, 40*(1), 37–56. https://doi.org/10.1016/S0005-7967(00)00115-7

Muris, P., Merckelbach, H., Meesters, C., & van den Brand, K. (2002). Cognitive development and worry in normal children. *Cognitive Therapy and Research, 26*(6), 775–787. https://doi.org/10.1023/A:1021241517274

Nelson, E. E., Leibenluft, E., McCLURE, E. B., & Pine, D. S. (2005). The social re- orientation of adolescence: A neuroscience perspective on the process and its relation to psychopathology. *Psychological Medicine, 35*(2), 163–174. https://doi. org/10.1017/S0033291704003915

Ng-Cordell, E., Hanley, M., Kelly, A., & Riby, D. M. (2018). Anxiety in Williams syndrome: The role of social behaviour, executive functions and change over time. *Journal of Autism and Developmental Disorders, 48*(3), 796–808. https://doi.org/10.1007/s10803-017-3357-0

Osleger, C. (2012). *Can the catastrophizing interview technique be used to develop understanding of childhood worry?* Unpublished dissertation. Norwich: University of East Anglia.

Pasarelu, C. R., Dobrean, A., Balazsi, R., Podina, I. R., & Mogoase, C. (2017). Interpretation biases in the intergenerational transmission of worry: A path analysis. *Journal of Evidence-Based Psychotherapies, 17*(1), 31–49.

Qiu, L., Su, J., Ni, Y., Bai, Y., Zhang, X., Li, X., & Wan, X. (2018). The neural system of metacognition accompanying decision-making in the prefrontal cortex. *PLOS Biology, 16*(4), e2004037. https://doi.org/10.1371/journal.pbio.2004037

Rafetseder, E., & Perner, J. (2012). When the alternative would have been better: Counterfactual reasoning and the emergence of regret. *Cognition & Emotion, 26*(5), 800–819. https://doi.org/10.1080/02699931.2011.619744

Reinholdt-Dunne, M. L., Blicher, A., Nordahl, H., Normann, N., Esbjørn, B. H., & Wells, A. (2019). Modeling the relationships between metacognitive beliefs, attention control and symptoms in children with and without anxiety disorders: A test of the S-REF model. *Frontiers in Psychology, 10*, 1025. https://doi.org/10.3389/fpsyg.2019.01205

Riggs, K. J., Peterson, D. M., Robinson, E. J., & Mitchell, P. (1998). Are errors in false belief tasks symptomatic of a broader difficulty with counterfactuality? *Cognitive Development, 13*(1), 73–90. https://doi.org/10.1016/S0885-2014(98)90021-1

Robinson, E. J., & Beck, S. (2000). What is difficult about counterfactual reasoning? In P. Mitchell, & K. Riggs (Eds.), *Children's reasoning and the mind* (pp. 101–119). London: Psychology Press/Taylor & Francis.

Roebers, C. M. (2017). Executive function and metacognition: Towards a unifying framework of cognitive self-regulation. *Developmental Review, 45*, 31–51. https://doi.org/10.1016/j.dr.2017.04.001

Roese, N. J., & Olson, J. M. (1997). Counterfactual thinking: The intersection of affect and function. In M. P. Zanna (Ed.), *Advances in experimental social psychology* (Vol. 29, pp. 1–59). Academic Press. https://doi.org/10.1016/S0065-2601(08)60015-5

Segerstrom, S. C., Tsao, J. C. I., Alden, L. E., & Craske, M. G. (2000). Worry and rumination: Repetitive thought as a concomitant and predictor of negative mood. *Cognitive Therapy and Research, 24*(6), 671–688. https://doi.org/10.1023/A:1005587311498

Silverman, W. K., Greca, A. M., & Wasserstein, S. (1995). What do children worry about? Worries and their relation to anxiety. *Child Development, 66*(3), 671–686. https://doi.org/10.2307/1131942

Smetana, J. G. (1985). Preschool children's conceptions of transgressions: Effects of varying moral and conventional domain-related attributes. *Developmental Psychology, 21*(1), 18–29. https://doi.org/10.1037/0012-1649.21.1.18

Songco, A., Hudson, J. L., & Fox, E. (2020). A cognitive model of pathological worry in children and adolescents: A systematic review. *Clinical Child and Family Psychology Review, 23*(2), 229–249. https://doi.org/10.1007/s10567-020-00311-7

Spears, M., Montgomery, A. A., Gunnell, D., & Araya, R. (2014). Factors associated with the development of self-harm amongst a socio-economically deprived cohort of adolescents in Santiago, Chile. *Social Psychiatry and Psychiatric Epidemiology, 49*(4), 629–637. https://doi.org/10.1007/s00127-013-0767-y

Speckens, A. E. M., & Hawton, K. (2011). Social problem solving in adolescents with suicidal behavior: A systematic review. *Suicide and Life-Threatening Behavior, 35*(4), 365–387. https://doi.org/10.1521/suli.2005.35.4.365

Stallard, P., Spears, M., Montgomery, A. A., Phillips, R., & Sayal, K. (2013). Self-harm in young adolescents (12–16 years): Onset and short-term continuation in a community sample. *BMC Psychiatry, 13*(1), 328. https://doi.org/10.1186/1471-244X-13-328

Steinberg, L. (2005). Cognitive and affective development in adolescence. *Trends in Cognitive Sciences, 9*(2), 69–74. https://doi.org/10.1016/j.tics.2004.12.005

Stevenson-Hinde, J., & Shouldice, A. (1995). 4.5 to 7 years: Fearful behaviour, fears and worries. *Journal of Child Psychology and Psychiatry, 36*(6), 1027–1038. https://doi.org/10.1111/j.1469-7610.1995.tb01348.x

Stuijfzand, S., & Dodd, H. F. (2017). Young children have social worries too: Validation of a brief parent report measure of social worries in children aged 4–8 years. *Journal of Anxiety Disorders, 50*, 87–93. https://doi.org/10.1016/j.janxdis.2017.05.008

Suddendorf, T. (2010). Linking yesterday and tomorrow: Preschoolers ability to report temporally displaced events. *British Journal of Developmental Psychology, 258*(2), 491–498. https://doi.org/10.1016/j.cub.2014.10.058

Suddendorf, T., Nielsen, M., & von Gehlen, R. (2011). Children's capacity to remember a novel problem and to secure its future solution: Future solutions of novel problems. *Developmental Science, 14*(1), 26–33. https://doi.org/10.1111/j.1467-7687.2010.00950.x

Takahashi, F., Koseki, S., & Shimada, H. (2009). Developmental trends in children's aggression and social problem-solving. *Journal of Applied Developmental Psychology, 30*(3), 265–272. https://doi.org/10.1016/j.appdev.2008.12.007

Tsujimoto, S. (2008). The prefrontal cortex: Functional neural development during early childhood. *The Neuroscientist, 14*(4), 345–358. https://doi.org/10.1177/1073858408316002

Turner, L., & Wilson, C. (2010). Worry, Mood and Stop Rules in Young Adolescents: Does the Mood-as-Input Theory Apply? *Journal of Experimental Psychopathology, 1*(1), 34–51. https://doi.org/10.5127/jep.007810

Turner, S. M., Beidel, D. C., Roberson-Nay, R., & Tervo, K. (2003). Parenting behaviors in parents with anxiety disorders. *Behaviour Research and Therapy, 41*(5), 541–554. https://doi.org/10.1016/S0005-7967(02)00028-1

Ursache, A., & Raver, C. C. (2014). Trait and state anxiety: Relations to executive functioning in an at-risk sample. *Cognition and Emotion, 28*(5), 845–855. https://doi.org/10.1080/02699931.2013.855173

Varela, R. E., & Hensley-Maloney, L. (2009). The influence of culture on anxiety in Latino youth: A review. *Clinical Child and Family Psychology Review, 12*(3), 217–233. https://doi.org/10.1007/s10567-009-0044-5

Varela, R. E., Sanchez-Sosa, J. J., Biggs, B. K., & Luis, T. M. (2008). Anxiety symptoms and fears in Hispanic and European American Children: Cross- cultural measurement equivalence. *Journal of Psychopathology and Behavioral Assessment, 30*(2), 132–145. https://doi.org/10.1007/s10862-007-9056-y

Vasey, M. W., & Borkovec, T. D. (1992). A catastrophizing assessment of worrisome thoughts. *Cognitive Therapy and Research, 16*(5), 505–520. https:// doi.org/10.1007/BF01175138

Vasey, M. W., & Daleiden, E. L. (1994). Worry in Children. In G. C. L. Davey & F. Tallis (Eds.), *Worrying: Perspectives on theory, assessment and treatment* (pp. 185–208). Chichester: John Wiley & Sons Ltd.

Vasey, M. W., Crnic, K. A., & Carter, W. G. (1994). Worry in childhood: A developmental perspective. *Cognitive Therapy and Research, 18*(6), 529–549.

Visu-Petra, L., Miclea, M., & Visu-Petra, G. (2013). Individual differences in anxiety and executive functioning: A multidimensional view. *International Journal of Psychology, 48*(4), 649–659. https://doi.org/10.1080/00207594.2012.656132

Warden, D., & MacKinnon, S. (2003). Prosocial children, bullies and victims: An investigation of their sociometric status, empathy and social problem-solving strategies. *British Journal of Developmental Psychology, 21*(3), 367–385. https:// doi.org/10.1348/026151003322277757

Waters, A. M., Bradley, B. P., & Mogg, K. (2014). Biased attention to threat in paediatric anxiety disorders (generalized anxiety disorder, social phobia, specific phobia, separation anxiety disorder) as a function of "distress" versus "fear" diagnostic categorization. *Psychological Medicine, 44*(3), 607–616. https:// doi.org/10.1017/S0033291713000779

Weil, L. G., Fleming, S. M., Dumontheil, I., Kilford, E. J., Weil, R. S., Rees, G., Dolan, R. J., & Blakemore, S.-J. (2013). The development of metacognitive ability in adolescence. *Consciousness and Cognition, 22*(1), 264–271. https://doi.org/10.1016/j.concog.2013.01.004

Werner, N. E., & Crick, N. R. (2004). Maladaptive peer relationships and the development of relational and physical aggression during middle childhood. *Social Development, 13*(4), 495–514. https://doi.org/10.1111/j.1467-9507.2004.00280.x

Wilson, C. (2010). Pathological worry in children: What is currently known? *Journal of Experimental Psychopathology, 1*(1), 6–33. https://doi.org/10.5127/jep.008110

Wilson, T. D., & Gilbert, D. T. (2005). Affective forecasting: Knowing what to want. *Current Directions in Psychological Science, 14*(3), 131–134. https://doi.org/10.1111/j.0963-7214.2005.00355.x

Wright, M., Banerjee, R., Hoek, W., Rieffe, C., & Novin, S. (2010). Depression and social anxiety in children: Differential links with coping strategies. *Journal of Abnormal Child Psychology, 38*(3), 405–419. https://doi.org/10.1007/s10802-009-9375-4

2

STRESS AND PARENTING

Keith A. Crnic and Shayna S. Coburn

Introduction

Across decades of parenting research, much of it captured in this very *Handbook*, one enduring message that can be derived is that parenting is a complex and challenging experience. Without question, it can be joyous, uplifting, and fulfilling in ways few other human experiences can match. But it can also be demanding, stressful, and frustrating as parents sometimes struggle with the developmental and behavioral twists and turns that often accompany the many exigencies of childrearing. Whether under conditions of high risk or the most facilitative developmental contexts available, the stresses of parenting are apparent, and they are important features of developmental models that seek to explicate the complexity that is parenting.

This chapter specifically addresses the multidimensional and complex connections between stress and parenting. Although the predominant focus will fall on stresses associated with the experience of parenting, the connection between stress and parenting is considered more globally, as parents can be stressed by events that are external to childrearing processes and these stresses can influence the ways parents behave within the family system. Distinguishing between "stressed parenting" and "parenting stress" is important in differentiating determinants and consequences of stresses, as well as identifying potential mechanisms that explain processes that underlie such connections and their implications for child and family development.

It has been noted previously (Crnic and Low, 2002) that parenting stress is a ubiquitous experience, and others have likewise added to that perspective (Deater-Deckard, 2004; Deater-Deckard and Panneton, 2017). Not surprisingly then, research has begun to more reflect the fact that stress is common to parenting experience, and attention to such concerns has increased. In fact, a simple keyword search of PsycINFO shows that as of this writing in the late fall of 2017, there have been 570 published reports for which the words parenting stress were in the title, and nearly 5,000 published reports in which parenting stress appears anywhere in the paper. These substantial numbers indicate that the interest in creating a better understanding of parenting processes often involves attending to the stresses that parents experience. Certainly, since Belsky's (1984) seminal determinants of parenting paper promoted stress as one of a set of key conceptually critical determinants of parenting, some index of stress has been included in thousands of studies of parenting. The salience of stress as a determinant of parenting remains an important contributor (Bornstein, 2016).

The popularity of stress research in the parenting context is belied by the challenges inherent in defining stress as a construct. Although multiple perspectives exist on how best to conceptualize stress (Crum, Salovey, and Achor, 2013), some consensus has emerged. Stress response is multi-domain in that it includes behavioral, emotional, and physiological reactions (Crum et al., 2013), and arises when environmental demands exceed an individual's available resources to address those demands. This is especially true when the situation involved is appraised to be particularly meaning-ful (Aldwin, 2011). Parenting stress, in turn, reflects processes associated with aversive psychologi-cal and physiological reactions that occur specifically in adaptation to the demands of parenthood (Deater-Deckard, 2004), although again, there is no single consensus on how parenting stress can be best understood. These conceptual issues and the measurement challenges they present are addressed in greater depth in later sections of this chapter.

Despite the ubiquity of research studies that include measures of parenting stress, the field is far from fully understanding the developmental implications of this construct for parents, for children, and especially for family systems. Indeed, the preponderance of studies that have appeared have focused on rather simple main effect models confirming and reconfirming that parenting stress is associated with adverse child and parent outcomes or emerges from a wide variety of high-risk conditions. These reports align with very well worn lines of research that have clearly articulated the notion that stress is harmful to physical, psychological, and developmental well-being (Aldwin, 2011). But there remains a vast array of important process questions in which the complex mecha-nisms of effect need to be better understood. Research is now beginning to turn to these more complicated issues, with sophisticated longitudinal designs and analyses that are beginning to provide deeper answers to the ways in which stress operates to influence parenting processes and children's development.

Furthermore, research efforts have begun to recognize that parenting stress is not unidimensional in nature or effect, nor can it be assumed to be invariant across child age and parent gender. The number of children in a family seems to matter (Crnic and Greenberg, 1990; Deater-Deckard, 2004; Östberg and Hagekull, 2013), but research to date rarely considers how parenting stress may differ as a function of child age or the developmental periods represented. Although more studies have begun to explore fathers' perceptions of parenting stress), and the way they contrast with maternal experi-ence (Skreden et al., 2012), the preponderance of work still addresses mother report as the standard for identifying parenting stress. The work on fathers has shown similarities and differences with the findings on maternal parenting stress, but such efforts are just beginning to explore the complexity of stress operations within the family system (Kerig, 2019). Indeed, systems perspectives have been few and far between in studies of parenting stress despite the fact that there are very compelling systemic issues that are likely involved in understanding the potential implications of parenting stress for family well-being. Crossover effects, in which one partner's status or functioning affects the status or functioning of the other, are a prime example.

It is certainly the case that the knowledge base with respect to stress and parenting has grown dramatically. In some respects, the rise in parenting stress research is tied to the vast array of risk conditions that face children and families, and attempts to understand the ways in which risks influ-ence and are affected by parents' stressful experiences. Chronic illnesses, developmental disabilities and disorders, pre- and perinatal birth complications, behavior problems, poverty, marital conflict, single parenthood, parental psychopathology, and other conditions have created a wealth of research explicating the connection between risk and parenting stress (Deater-Deckard and Panneton, 2017). Although risk conditions and the stresses inherent in them offer important perspectives on patho-logical mechanisms, it remains the case that stress is not solely related to the presence of risk, and families with low to no ongoing risks experience normative stresses that are associated with the everyday experience of parenting.

Newer to the literature have been attempts to explore the underlying physiological mechanisms of stress in parents, creating broader biopsychosocial perspectives on the nature of the parental stress experience. Although only a few studies in this area (Merwyn, Smith, and Dougherty, 2015;

Sturge-Apple, Skibo, Rogosch, and Ignjatovic, 2011) tie biological mechanisms to behavioral stress responses in parenting, they forge new pathways for understanding the nature of stress in families within and across generations. Likewise, there has been a growing attention to culture and the experience of minority families with respect to parenting stress (Nomaguchi and House, 2013). Models of developmental process for minority children and families (Garcia Coll et al., 1996) describe critical attributes that can differentiate developmental processes for these families and children. Parenting stress is likely to be among those constructs that can be differentially understood by cultural context (Bornstein, 1995).

Whether parents are stressed by extrafamilial events and concerns, or by those processes specific to parenting itself, it seems apparent that stress creates some degree of adversity within families. When the consequences of stressful experience involve within-family or child attributes, parenting stress seems to have a somewhat stronger effect than does stress that emanates from sources external to the family (Crnic and Greenberg, 1990). That is sensible, but it remains critical to differentiate the effects of external sources of stress from those endogenous to the family. That said, it is also time now to look beyond those models that explore single-factor determinants of parenting stress or seek to connect parenting stress to some new adverse outcome. The field needs to build more complex and nuanced models of the ways in which parenting stress operates within the family system, exploring those moderating and mediating influences that create challenge that is sometimes met and sometimes not. There is a growing attention to such processes and systemic issues, and this chapter attempts to highlight these more complex approaches to the study of parenting stress.

Historical Considerations in Parenting Stress

Stress research has a long and prolific history in psychological and developmental science (Aldwin, 2011) and has been instrumental in addressing issues of human adaptation and maladaptation for decades ranging back to the mid-20th century. The efforts in previous editions of this *Handbook* have briefly documented the history that is most relevant to the emergence of parenting stress. Here, we touch again on this history but focus more extensively on research that created the context for the emergence of parenting as a critical context for stress modeling.

Early models of stress considered the experience of major life changes to be congruent with the experience of stress. That is, if one experienced life change, one experienced some degree of stress. Initially, it was just the fact of change itself that mattered. If a life change event took place, then a person was considered to experience stress and a linear relation was assumed between the number of events experienced and the degree of adverse outcome (Holmes and Rahe, 1967). Life events were broadly conceived to incorporate those general life experiences that any adult (or child to some extent) might be expected to have. Some major events would be considered relatively typical (e.g., marriage), and some less typical (e.g., incarceration), but predominantly had little to do with parenting. The events identified by Holmes and Rahe in their Social Readjustment Rating Scale, however, included pregnancy and gaining a new family member (although that did not necessarily imply the addition of a child to the family). Across many studies, life event change proved to be a reasonably strong predictor of psychological distress, but fared less well at prediction of physical illness (Rabkin and Struening, 1976).

Using a life event stress framework, a number of studies began to explore risks to parenting and child psychological well-being as a consequence of the presence of greater life stress. Coddington (1972) explored child-reported life event stress, noting that the numbers of events increased as children aged, but no gender or socioeconomic status (SES) differences were apparent. Coddington also suggested likely positive relations between numbers of life events and behavior disorders in children, although these relations were not directly assessed. Nonetheless, such predictions were borne out in later research, including work by Gersten, Langner, Eisenberg, and Orzeck (1974), Sandler and Block

(1979), and Webster-Stratton and Hammond (1988). Furthermore, reported life stress had been linked to challenges in the transition to parenthood (Cutrona, 1984; Ryan and Padilla, 2019) as well as aspects of problematic parenting, including physical child abuse (Straus, 1980; Sturge-Apple, Toth, Suor, and Adams, 2019).

Attention to the context of stress and its potential influence on families and child development grew dramatically in the 1980s as a function of a number of critical conceptual and methodological advances. Conceptually, the study of stress and resilience as critical contexts for child and family development (Garmezy and Rutter, 1983; Garmezy, Masten, and Tellegen, 1984) was growing in support of the emerging developmental psychopathology framework for understanding risk and child and family behavior problems (Cicchetti, 1984). A study by Weinberg and Richardson (1981) turned attention specifically to the notion that parenting can be a stressful experience in its own right. Using multidimensional scaling, they created a 14-item measure addressing dimensions of stress in parenting. This measure not only identified 14 salient parental experiences, but asked parents to rate these events for the degree to which they were considered unpleasant. Four dimensions of stressful parent experience emerged: (1) major versus minor child problems, (2) immediate versus long-range problem experiences, (3) child welfare versus parent welfare, and (4) restriction of self or adult activities. Each dimension was associated with the parent's experience of unpleasantness, with child behavior problems (dimension 1) having the strongest association. Restriction of self was least associated with parents' assessments of unpleasant emotion. Mothers and fathers also differed on each dimension, with the exception of restriction of self.

In some ways, the (Weinberg and Richardson (1981) effort might be considered the beginning of the specific study of stresses associated with parenting. It was not long, however, before Abidin introduced the first iteration of the Parenting Stress Index (PSI; Abidin, 1983), a measure that has since become a standard for research on parenting stress. The full version of the PSI involves 101 items that align with issues in either Parent or Child domains to which parents respond on 5-point scales that range from strongly agree to strongly disagree. The long-form measure also includes 19 items that address life stressors that are meant to provide some context for the degree of parenting stress reported. A PSI short form (36 items) became available in 1996 and has a three-scale structure (parent distress, difficult child, and dysfunctional parent-child interaction). The PSI has been a stalwart in research models that have focused on understanding the stress inherent in parenting contexts (it is currently in its 4th edition; Abidin, 2012), and although it is not without flaws, the knowledge base that has accrued on parenting stress is largely due to the formidable contribution of the PSI and its various iterations. The PSI also spurred the development of like measures for parenting stress associated with adolescents (Sheras, Abidin, and Konold, 1998) as well as for parenting in families outside the United States, such as the Swedish Parenthood Stress Questionnaire (Östberg, Hagekull, and Wettergren, 1997).

Although the PSI has been a standard for research in the field, another approach to assessing parenting stress emerged in the early 1990s based on more normative everyday aspects of childrearing. Borrowing from the daily hassles stress paradigm of Kanner, Coyne, Schaefer, and Lazarus (1981), and sharing some perspectives from the Bother Scale for parents (Easterbrooks and Goldberg, 1984), Crnic and Greenberg (1990) promoted a model of parenting daily hassles (PDH) to examine parents' responses to 20 typical parenting events or activities to which parents indicated the frequency with which the event occurred and the degree to which they found it a hassle. Both ratings were 5-point scales from low to high and attempted to reflect an objective indicator of how often the event happened (Frequency Scale) and a subjective appraisal of the degree to which it was considered stressful (Intensity Scale).

The two basic approaches to parenting stress (the PSI and the PDH), including their adaptations and variants, have dominated the way that parenting stress has been measured, and therefore understood. To date, however, the two approaches have not been included within the same study so it is not actually clear how they may be related. Regardless, the stresses associated with parenting do not exclusively capture the full nature of stress and parenting. There has been continued research on extrafamilial stressors that influence the nature and quality of parenting, parent-child relationships, and children's well-being. The disparate approaches reflect not only a number of basic theoretical differences in the approach to understanding stress contexts, but help to highlight a number of important issues that are critical for fully explicating the nature of stress and its effects on families, parenting, and children.

Background Theory in Parenting Stress

Stress is one of the most studied aspects of human experience, yet there has long been controversy about how best to define and conceptualize it. Multiple theoretical perspectives have been brought to bear, attempting to define the construct as well as conceptualize how and why stress operates to influence human experience and behavior. However, these various conceptual approaches have rarely taken an expressly developmental or lifespan frame of reference. An exception is Aldwin (2011), who described stress processes within a transactional lifespan framework that offers particular insight for current models of stress and parenting. Stress arises, she noted, when environmental demands exceed an individual's available resources to address those demands, especially when the individual appraises the situation involved as particularly meaningful. This perspective draws heavily from the Lazarus and colleagues' (Folkman, 1984; Lazarus, Delongis, Folkman, and Gruen, 1985) stress framework (discussed in previous editions of this chapter; Crnic and Low, 2002). While acknowledging perspectives that take more objective environmental event-based approaches to defining stress, Aldwin (2011) noted that the transactional perspective involving individual appraisal of environmental events is the most dominant stress model. Thus, it is an individual's appraisal of the salience and meaning of an event, and its effect, that determines the degree to which the event reflects a stressor. Most parenting stress models adopt this perspective and seek parents' perceptions of the nature of the parenting role and the quality of parent-child relationships.

Several early models of stress and parenting emerged to have substantial influences on the direction of the field (see Garmezy and Rutter, 1983), although not each of these models explicitly included current notions of parenting stress. Here, attention must be drawn to the importance of stress context, wherein stressed parenting can be differentiated from parenting stress. Extrafamilial stressors can be separated from intrafamilial factors to influence the nature of ongoing family relationships. Such considerations are exemplified by Webster-Stratton's (1990) model of stress as a disruptor of family process, as well as Abidin's (1992) more directly intrafamilial parenting stress framework. Especially salient to the daily hassle perspective was Patterson's (1983) effort to describe stress as a potential change agent within families, focusing on cumulative microsocial interactions within the family (such as coercive parent-child exchanges) that serve to escalate stress, affect subsequent interactions, and eventually lead to adverse behavioral outcomes for children. These early conceptualizations, including the work of Weinberg and Richardson (1981), formed the bedrock of the research that would follow.

Although consensus regarding a definition of stress has been difficult to reach, the approach to parenting stress has been somewhat more uniform. Parenting stress has generally been accepted to involve "a set of processes that lead to aversive psychological and physiological reactions arising from attempts to adapt to the demands of parenthood" (Deater-Deckard, 2004, p. 6). Although different methods have emerged to assess parenting stress, the field largely shares this basic understanding of the construct. Whereas the underlying premise of parenting stress may be shared, varying conceptualizations of how this stress might be represented within developmental, contextual, and risk frameworks have emerged. Both Deater-Deckard (2004) and Crnic and Ross (2017) touched on these previously, and we reiterate them briefly here. Two basic conceptual approaches are somewhat tied to the measurement processes that were developed to address them. One is the more problem-oriented

Parent-Child-Relationship framework (P-C-R) that is reflected in Abidin's (1992) parenting stress model. The other is represented by the parenting daily hassles model (Crnic and Greenberg, 1990), which attempts to capture the typical everyday frustrations that may be perceived in parenting role demands and challenging child behavior.

The basic difference between these two predominant perspectives is whether the focus is on existing problematic issues in the family context or more normative functioning (Crnic and Ross, 2017). The P-C-R framework tends to focus on conditions in which some problem may be apparent (parental distress, child behavior problems, parent-child conflict), whereas the parenting daily hassles model attempts to draw attention to everyday parent experiences and normative child behaviors that may be frustrating or irritating for parents despite their typicality. As Crnic and Ross (2017) noted, these models of parenting stress are not necessarily competing, but instead are complementary in what they attempt to explain about parenting stress. Conventional wisdom suggests that parenting is difficult and can be challenging regardless of whether problems exist within the family system. When problems do exist, stress may operate in different ways or to different degrees. Certainly, a wealth of evidence supports both models as salient to within-family functioning, and this chapter details relevant research.

Initial efforts to conceptualize parenting stress provided the base for the emergence of a substantial empirical literature that examines the nature of stressful experiences for parents, their determinants, and their consequences. The research to date has done much to substantiate the important influence of stress within parenting processes and on children's development. The effects on children have proved to be both direct and indirect, although the mechanisms and pathways for the indirect effects have not always been entirely clear. Nonetheless, the wealth of knowledge that has accrued has been instrumental in helping to understand the complexities of risk and normative familial contexts and their effects on parent and child well-being. As is often the case, however, the more knowledge that is gained, the more questions arise. Issues that had not been fully appreciated previously come into focus. In the next section, we address the central issues that have driven the field of stress and parenting, reviewing relevant research but likewise focusing attention on issues that challenge current parenting stress perspectives.

Central Issues in Stress and Parenting

It is not surprising that the wealth of research on stress and parenting has raised a host of interesting and challenging issues that have been addressed by the field. These issues focus on the nature of stressful experience, the salience of risk contexts, individual and family characteristics, developmental and systemic processes, biological mechanisms, culture, complex pathways of influence, and preventive interventions. Below we highlight some of the most salient research that touches on these issues and raise questions that are meant to encourage the next generation of research on stress and parenting processes.

Stressed Parenting Versus Parenting Stress

The relation between stress and parenting has a rich history. That history, however, sometimes tangles two specific sources from which we have come to understand this linkage: whether the source of stress is outside the family context impinging inward or within the parenting context itself and affecting family functioning and children's development. These sources of influence should be differentiated with respect to family processes.

Stressed Parenting

The differentiation between what might be termed stressed parenting where the source of the stress is extrafamilial (e.g., loss of job, legal trouble, conflicts with friends or neighbors), and parenting stress, where the source reflects parenting-specific processes, is potentially critical. There are both conceptual and empirical reasons to believe that these two sources of stress may operate differentially to influence parental well-being, parenting behavior, family system functioning, and children's development. In some research contexts, these two sources have become conflated, creating a single conceptualization of stress and parenting. They are, however, important separate sources of stress that deserve attention in their own right (Crnic and Ross, 2017; Deater-Deckard, 2004; Östberg and Hagekull, 2013). Parenting stress requires that a child or the parenting role serve as the cause of the stress the parent experiences (Deater-Deckard, 1998). Stressed parenting is a function of experience external to family context or even within the family (e.g., marital conflict) but not caused by the child or childrearing. These differing sources of stress should be conceptualized and explored as independent processes affecting parenting and child development. Indeed, there is evidence to suggest that they operate differently across domains of effect (Crnic, Gaze, and Hoffman, 2005; Östberg and Hagekull, 2013).

Concerns about stressed parenting and its implications began well before models of specific parenting stress emerged. Some of this work was touched on earlier in this chapter in the section on historical issues, where we noted that the predominant approach to exploring the nature of stressed parenting and its effects involved assessing parents' life stress. Life events, and parents' (mostly mothers) appraisals of the significance or stressfulness of those events, were used to indicate the degree of stress under which parents operated, and either the determinants of that stress or the consequences of that stress was studied (Garmezy et al., 1984). Webster-Stratton (1990) identified a number of major stressors that had been studied with parents, including negative life events, social isolation, unemployment, and daily hassles of adult life, and this information was utilized to create a conceptual model wherein extrafamilial stress created conditions for disrupted parenting through a variety of mediators that include poor social support systems, community isolation, and parent psychopathology. Extrafamilial stressors also served to amplify other parental concerns, such as low self-efficacy (Crnic and Ross, 2017).

Like most stress research, studies addressing the effects of negative life events on parental well-being and parenting processes did not produce uniform results. For certain, life stresses were generally associated with adverse outcomes for children (Sandler and Block, 1979; Webster-Stratton and Hammond, 1988) and for parents (Crnic, Greenberg, Ragozin, Robinson, and Basham, 1983; Elder, Liker, and Cross, 1984). Other research from the life stress perspective shows a lack of uniformity (Crnic et al., 2005; Emmen et al., 2013; Östberg and Hagekull, 2013; Riley, Scaramella, and McGoron, 2014) such that extrafamilial stressors help to account for adverse outcomes across both parent and child functional domains, but the specific stress associations to these attributes tend to vary within and across studies. Several longitudinal studies that explored maternal prenatal stress influences on children's behavior problems across childhood, however, showed relatively consistent predictions to children's early regulatory capacities (Lin, Crnic, Luecken, and Gonzales, 2014) and children's behavior problems, even controlling for postnatal stress experiences (Robinson et al., 2011). Although some degree of variability exists in the findings, it is apparent that stressed parenting is salient to some elements of parent and child well-being.

Economic Context

Although multiple contexts may create stressed parenting, none has been more studied than poverty or economic strain. The Family Stress Model (FSM; Masarik and Conger, 2017) offers a compelling conceptualization of the way in which economic hardship creates adverse conditions for parents and children. The FSM perspective suggests a complex pathway of influence in which perceived economic strain leads to parental distress and disrupted family relationships, which in turn lead to increased risk for child behavior problems. A wealth of research supports this model (Cassells and

Evans, 2017; Newland, Crnic, Cox, and Mills-Koonce, 2013; Scaramella, Sohr-Preston, Callahan, and Mirabile, 2008; Shelleby, Votruba-Drzal, Shaw, Dishion, Wilson, and Gardner, 2014), and other research has shown that economic strain may lead to parenting stress, which can mediate relations of economic stress to children's behavioral well-being. The FSM has been a powerful model driving research that links the stress of economic strain and poverty to parental difficulties and developmental challenges for children, but Cassells and Evans (2017) noted concerns about shared method bias in the assessment of economic strain, the limited role of children in the family processes that serve as mediators, and the need to better account for cultural frames of reference in the model. Regardless, economic stresses, which are extrafamilial in origin, have important implications for parent well-being, parenting processes, family system functions, and children's developmental well-being.

Contrasts Between Stressed Parenting and Parenting Stress

In drawing the distinction between stressed parenting and parenting stress, studies that compare these sources of stress directly are particularly useful. Yet, only a few studies have drawn specific contrasts between life event stress and stresses associated specifically with parenting. Crnic and Greenberg (1990) assessed mother-reported life stress and parenting daily hassles in families of 5-year-olds and found that both indices predicted reported child social competence, but only daily hassles accounted for reported behavior problems. The same was true for reported family system functioning. Neither stress factor predicted maternal behavior during observed interactions with the child, but parenting daily hassles were associated with less child responsiveness and more attempts to control the interaction.

In a later longitudinal study that assessed mothers and children ages across child ages 3 to 5, Crnic et al. (2005) found that both life stress and parenting daily hassles were relatively stable, although hassles seemed somewhat more so. Similar to their previous study, the parenting daily hassles and life stress measurements created differential prediction to mother and child outcomes. Neither cumulative life stress nor parenting hassles predicted observed maternal negativity at child age 5, but both independently contributed to observed maternal positivity. In contrast, hassles predicted less dyadic pleasure in mother-child interaction, whereas life stress accounted for more dyadic conflict. Both stress factors accounted for greater observed child negativity at age 5 as well as more reported child behavior problems. Of interest, the hassles factors predicted greater proportions of the variance in these outcomes than did life stress, even after parenting hassles were entered secondary to the life stress factor in hierarchical regression analyses.

Östberg and Hagekull (2013) also attempted to disentangle the effects of extrafamilial stresses from parenting stress in a sample of 436 Swedish mothers and their school-age children (mean age was nearly 7.5 years). Contrasting negative life events with parenting stress, they found that extrafamilial stressors contributed to the explained variance in children's behavior problems, but not to indices of social competence or social inhibition. Parenting stress was associated with all of the child factors and fully mediated relations between negative life events and children's externalizing behavior, internalizing behavior, and social competence.

Across these studies, it seems apparent that extrafamilial stressors at times operate in ways that are similar to parenting stress, but also in ways that differ. Parenting stress seems to be a more potent stressor than is extrafamilial stress in affecting within-family processes that involve children directly (parenting processes, parent-child relationships, and children's socioemotional functioning), a conclusion that seems coherent on its face. In contrast, relations to individual parental well-being and quality of close social relationships seem to be more susceptible to the influence of extrafamilial stressors. Marital relationships appear tied to both sources of stress, which likely reflects its place as an adult relationship within a specific family system. Much however remains to be explored with respect to sources of stress. In particular, there may be mother-father differences in the ways that different sources operate, or it may be that the salient stressors for well-being depend on the contexts in which a parent devotes more effort. If a parent spends significant effort in childrearing, parenting stress may be the more salient influence. If the parent spends more time working outside the home, extrafamilial stresses may predominate. These issues have yet to be addressed. Still, it remains important to differentiate stressed parenting from parenting stress with respect to the influence these factors exert on parents, parenting, and children's well-being.

Family Demography

The family demography of parenting stress has also been too little studied. Factors such as single- versus two-parent households (Berryhill and Durtschi, 2017) and number of children in the family (Crnic et al., 1983) appear especially salient to stress processes, but have not been fully or well explicated. Likewise, the influence of gender within parenting stress research is only beginning to be explored, as differences between male and female children are not typically studied, but are likely to be meaningful in understanding the predictions and outcomes associated with parenting stress (Crnic and Greenberg, 1990). Contrasts between fathers' and mothers' experience of parenting stress have been more frequent, but are not common. Research findings generally indicate that mothers tend to report somewhat higher parenting stress than do fathers, and different moderators and mediators operate in determining some outcomes, but there are also many similarities in stress reports and processes between mothers and fathers (Crnic, Pedersen-Arbona, Baker, and Blacher, 2009; Fagan and Lee, 2014; Gerstein et al., 2009; Halpern-Meekin and Turney, 2016; Nelson, O'Brien, Blankson, Calkins, and Keane, 2009; Nomaguchi, Brown, and Leyman, 2017; Nomaguchi and Johnson, 2016).

With respect to developmental period, the vast majority of research effort to date has focused on families of young children. The transition to parenthood has been a particular interest (Schoppe-Sullivan, Settle, Lee, and Kamp Dush, 2016), with a focus on changes that are associated with adding children to the family context. To some extent, research on parent stress with adolescents has also been of interest, given the salience of developmental challenges associated with this period (Putnick et al., 2008, 2010). Research on parent stress in middle childhood is emerging and creating a better sense of the developmental salience of parenting stress with school-age children (Nelson et al., 2009; Williford, Calkins, and Keane, 2007). Although studies exist within each developmental period, studies of parenting stress processes that cross and contrast periods are lacking.

It is likely that many existing studies have pertinent information about family demographics that might have been better explored to help illuminate some of the issues described, especially with respect to age and gender considerations. Future research should better incorporate these considerations, which can add important depth to the sophisticated conceptual parenting stress models being tested.

Developmental Perspectives on Parenting Stress

Age or Developmental Period

In the main, parenting stress has been treated as a construct that is a-developmental. That is, models of parenting stress rarely consider child age as a critical factor in the process despite the fact that the nature of stresses experienced by parents are likely to differ across developmental periods. In truth, that is acknowledged tacitly by the development of the SIPS (Sheras, Abidin, and Konold, 1998), which extended to the PSI to adolescents. Differences in parenting stress as a function of child age, or having multiple children at various ages, are likely to be quite complex. Data support change in the types of stress that parents experience over time. Östberg, Hagekull, and Hagelin (2007) showed that parental perceptions of stress related to role restriction decreases over time (infancy to early school age), whereas other sources of parenting stress (social isolation, spousal issues) remained more consistent. Families with multiple children that vary across ages likely address even broader ranges of parenting stresses, as the variety of issues they are presented extends across developmental periods.

Parenting stress may be affected by the developmental stages of the children in the family and by parents' age, parenting experiences, and parent characteristics (Rantanen, Tillemann, Metsäpelto, Kokko, and Pulkkinen, 2015). These influences may seem self-evident in some respects, but few data have been collected to demonstrate the effect. In the Rantanen et al. (2015) study, personality traits of mothers and fathers were linked longitudinally to parenting stress in a cross-lagged analysis across three age points: 33 years, 42 years, and 50 years. Reciprocal relations were found for both neuroticism and extraversion with parenting stress at the 33- and 42-year assessments in expected directions, but only high parenting stress was linked to low neuroticism from 42 to 50 years. This finding suggests that early in middle adulthood, parenting stress may operate somewhat differently than it does in later middle adulthood, at least in relation to personality. Such change may reflect increased parenting experience, changes in family size, or any number of other potential developmental characteristics. Further exploring such processes will illuminate current perspectives on the role of developmental period on the commensurate stress risks and relations to parenting that emerge. Relatively little is known at this point with respect to ways in which parenting stress may differ as a function of child age, parent age, or the interaction between the two. Furthermore, no studies were found on the nature of parenting stress associated with grown children who no longer live at home despite the fact that parenting doesn't end when children become adults.

Continuity and Stability

Only a few studies have explored parenting stress over time, expressly attending to the stability and continuity of parenting stress in families. Of those that have explored parenting stress over time, the approach has generally been to explore the stability (relative rank of individuals) of the construct more so than its continuity or change over time. Crnic et al. (2005) found high stability for parenting daily hassles measured consecutively at 6-month intervals across child ages 36 to 60 months. Furthermore, relevant to differences between stressed parenting and parenting stress, stability coefficients were notably lower for reports of extrafamilial stress across the same period, even though those coefficients demonstrated significant stability as well. Addressing both stability continuity across a similar developmental period, Williford, Calkins, and Keane (2007) reported moderate stability for parenting stress across child ages 2 to 5 years, but also found that parenting stress decreased meaningfully (discontinuity) across this same period. These relations, however, were complex as parenting stress across early childhood depended somewhat on child gender and emotion dysregulation.

In a study that explored parenting stress within the context of a parenting intervention, Östberg et al. (2007) found that parenting stress was moderately stable across a 7-year period from infancy to early school age, although those relations were somewhat dependent on the aspects of parenting stress measured as indicated above. There was a relatively large range of child age at the second measurement period (children were between 5 and 10 years old; mean of 7.5 years), but still this study assessed parenting stress into the less explored school-age period providing longer developmental windows through which to assess the stability and continuity of parenting stress. Similar to Williford's findings with parents of younger children, parenting stress decreased from infancy to the school-age period, and the intervention group was predominantly similar to the non-intervention group in the amount of change over time. The evidence continues to suggest that parenting stress during early and later childhood is fairly stable, but continuity is less apparent. There are likely moderators at play that change the nature of the parent's stress experience, and child age may be especially salient in this respect. The degree to which parenting stress shows stability and continuity during childhood may also depend on the way it is measured, as daily hassles and general parenting stress may be tapping somewhat different attributes of the stress experience.

Despite the salience of adolescence as a challenging developmental period, there has been much more limited attention to parenting stress associated with this age. Too, the research that does exist addresses the connections between parenting stress and adolescence from two perspectives: one that explores the stresses that parents of adolescents experience (Soenens, Vanteenkiste, and Beyers, 2019) and one that addresses the stresses associated with the experience of adolescents as parents themselves (Easterbrooks, Katz, and Menon, 2019). Both suggest the salience of parenting stress to the well-being of parents and offspring.

The popular conception that adolescence is a challenging time for parents maps on well to the available data. Indeed, several longitudinal studies suggest that higher parenting stress is associated with adolescent competencies in predictable ways (higher stress related to more problematic adolescent functioning). Differentiating it from earlier childhood, parenting stress with adolescents seems to be predominantly related to dysfunctional parent-child interactions, and less with parent distress and child problems (Gordon and Hinshaw, 2017a; Putnick et al., 2008, 2010). Also notable is the suggestion that parenting stress may actually increase somewhat from early to middle adolescence, which contrasts with the decreasing trajectories of parenting stress seen from early to middle childhood. Regardless, the evidence indicates that adolescence is a stressful period for both mothers and fathers (Putnick et al., 2010; Wiener, Biondic, Grimbos, and Herbert, 2016), and creates a pathway of influence in which parenting stress influences specific parenting attributes, which in turn adversely influence adolescent competence (Steeger, Gondoli, and Morrissey, 2013; Putnick et al., 2008). These stress processes are associated with adolescent biological functioning, including diurnal cortisol levels (Martin, Kim, and Fisher, 2016).

To date, an articulated and coherent developmental perspective on parenting stress has not emerged. Although stability is apparent, continuity in the experience of parenting stress is less so. Evidence suggests that differences in the perception, frequency, intensity, and function of parenting stress may exist from infancy to emerging adulthood periods and beyond. Most of our knowledge comes from early childhood periods, and middle childhood and adolescence significantly lags despite a few notable efforts. Continued longitudinal efforts will help to clarify the full developmental nature of the construct.

Current Research Perspectives in Parenting Stress

Risk Contexts

Much of our current knowledge about stress and parenting has been based on research that has focused on the presence of risk in the family. These risk contexts range across environmental (Scaramella, Sohr-Preston, Callahan, and Mirabile, 2008), socioeconomic (Cassel and Evans, 2017; Conger, Conger, and Martin 2011), parental psychopathology (Thomason, Volling, Flynn, McDonough, Marcus, Lopez, and Vazquez, 2014), and child health, behavior, and disability (Cousino and Hazen, 2013; Mackler, Kelleher, Shanahan, Calkins, Keane, and O'Brien, 2015; Neece and Chan, 2017) concerns. Although the findings tend to uniformly indicate that risk is associated with more problematic functioning for families and children, the mechanisms and parameters of such connections show some nuance. Many risk conditions have connections with parenting stress that are bidirectional or reciprocal; that is, parenting stress can be a determinant or an outcome from the risk condition or context. Given that socioeconomic risk as a stressor was previously addressed, the focus below will more specifically address risks associated with child and parent characteristics.

Behavior Problems

The presence of behavior problems in children is perhaps the most common of all risk contexts in which parenting stress has been explored, and it is difficult to find a study in which the connection between parenting stress and child behavior problems is not strongly established when both are measured. Indeed, difficult child behavior presents perhaps the most salient of parental challenges, and the often chronic nature of behavior problems allows for the accumulation of stresses over time for parents.

The reciprocal, bidirectional nature of the connections between parenting stress and behavior problems is well established. Studies in which child behavior problems predict subsequent parenting stress are plentiful (Neece and Baker, 2008; Solem, Christophersen, and Martinussen, 2011; Williford et al., 2007), as are studies in which parenting stress is conceptualized as a precursor to behavior problems (Crnic et al., 2005; Newland and Crnic, 2017; Östberg and Hagekull, 2013; Puff and Renk, 2014). But the true bidirectional nature of this relationship has been established across a number of recent studies that suggest that parent stress and child behavior problems transact over time, each influencing the other in ways that can accentuate the cumulative risk (Mackler, Kelleher, Shanahan, Calkins, Keane, and Obrien, 2015; Stone, Mares, Otten, Engels, and Janssens, 2016; Tharner, Luijk, van IJzendoorn et al., 2012). There is even evidence to suggest that maternal prenatal stress can initiate this transactional process (Lin et al., 2014; Robinson et al., 2011).

Although the linkage between parenting stress and behavior problems is really no longer at issue, whether the connection is direct or indirect remains undetermined. Evidence exists for both direct and indirect associations. It has often been suggested that the relation between parents' experience of stress and children's behavior problems is indirect, mediated by parents' behavior in interaction with their child. Parents who are stressed tend to behave less optimally with their children (Berryhill, 2016; Crnic et al., 2005; Gordon and Hinshaw, 2017b; Paulussen-Hoogeboom, Stams, Hermanns, and Peetsma, 2008), and this less optimal parenting behavior is thought to account for the connection between parenting stress and children's behavior problems. Although intuitively and conceptually appealing, empirical support for that specific stress pathway has proven elusive (see later section on Complexity and Pathways of Influence).

One final issue to raise with respect to the connection between behavior problems and parenting stress is that there is very little specificity with respect to the type of behavior problems that are addressed. Predominantly, studies assess broadband externalizing or internalizing behavior, and few studies include populations that reach clinically significant levels of these bands or address specific narrow-band problems, such as withdrawn/depressed or aggressive behavior. One exception is attention-deficit/hyperactivity disorder (ADHD), which has garnered some focused attention for its substantive relation to parenting stress (Gordon and Hinshaw, 2017a; Theule, Wiener, Tannock, and Jenkins, 2013), although it is unclear whether the associations are stronger than for other specific child diagnoses (Theule et al., 2013).

In sum, the ties between parenting stress and children's behavior problems are well established, and the transactional nature of these relations is beginning to more clearly emerge. Still, specificity of children's behavioral problems and the ways in which behavior problems and parenting stress transact across developmental periods remain to be more fully explicated.

Chronic Childhood Illness

Much the same as the literature on behavior problems, children with chronic illnesses present an understandable risk for higher levels of parenting stress. The specter of a child who must face serious ongoing health problems is certainly a context that threatens parental well-being and magnifies the nature of everyday experiences in parenting. Childhood cancer (Pai, Greenley, Lewandowski, Drotar,

Youngstrom, and Peterson, 2007), diabetes (Maas-van Schaaijk, Roeleveld-Versteegh, and van Baar, 2013), asthma (Yamamoto, 2015), cystic fibrosis (Moola, 2012), sickle cell (Yarboi, Compas, Brody, White, Patterson et al., 2017), and multiple other illnesses have been studied with documented findings that parents of children with chronic illnesses report more parenting stress.

Although the association between chronic illness and parenting stress is consistent across studies, the nature of the relations that emerge are nuanced. Two meta-analyses (Cousino and Hazen, 2013; Pinquart, 2017) detail a number of these nuanced issues. One important distinction both analyses draw is between illness—specific parenting stress and more general parenting stress. Not surprisingly, parents report higher levels of illness-specific parenting stress than general parenting stress, but general parenting stress is still greater than that reported by parents of healthy children. This analysis suggests that the stress experienced by parents of chronically ill children is not simply stress related to the nature of the disease that is present, but the typical processes associated with childrearing are also seen as more stressful when a chronic condition is present.

Some variability has been found between individual chronic illnesses and parents' stress experience, with some illnesses producing higher stress responses than others (e.g., childhood cancer), and more severe illnesses predicting higher parenting stress (Pinquart, 2017). Child age, family characteristics, and other developmental and contextual factors also seem to affect the nature of the connection between childhood chronic illness and parenting stress, but the degree to which findings can be uniformly applied across illness categories is limited by the vast diversity of childhood chronic illness and relatively small number of studies to date. The unique risk context of chronic childhood illness should encourage further research scrutiny with respect to its associations with parenting stress.

Developmental Disorders

Developmental disorders are similar in many ways to chronic illnesses in childhood, and yet there are important distinctions to be drawn with respect to socioemotional and stress processes (Crnic and Neece, 2015). The similarities center on the clear association between the presence of the developmental risk condition and reports of greater stress by parents (Neece and Chan, 2017). There is similarity as well in the differentiations between disability-specific stresses and general parenting stresses in these families. Disability-specific stresses can be high, whereas parenting daily hassles may be similar between families with and without a child with disabilities (Baker et al., 2003; Crnic et al., 2009). But research has well established that there is not uniformity in parental responses to child disability, and levels of stress can vary widely among families (Blacher and Baker, 2007; Pedersen, Crnic, Baker, and Blacher, 2015), and between the type of developmental disorder involved. Parents of children with autism spectrum disorder (ASD) appear to experience greater parenting stresses than do parents of children with other developmental disabilities (Dabrowska and Pisula, 2010).

For families of children with identified developmental disorders or intellectual disabilities (ID), parental stress tends to peak during the preschool period and decrease over time as a function of reductions in child behavior problems (Crnic et al., 2009; Neece, Green, and Baker, 2012), although evidence suggests that non-child related stresses may actually increase over time for these families (Neece and Chan, 2017). Parenting stresses related to children with ID may also recur across development, and new stressors may emerge that maintain or increase stress levels as children face new developmental challenges at key points of transition (school entry, puberty).

Another distinction specific to parenting stress and the risks associated with developmental disabilities is that the connections between the child disabilities and parenting stress appear to be mediated by the presence of behavior problems in the children. Dual diagnosis (the presence of ID and a concurrent mental health condition) is common in children with ID (Crnic and Neece, 2015), and research suggests that many social and emotional challenges, including parenting stress, that families and children face are more related to the presence of behavior problems than the cognitive and other developmental delays that are endemic to the presence of ID (Baker, Neece, Fleming, Crnic, and Blacher, 2010). In the absence of behavior problems, parenting stresses in families of children with ID appear to be more similar to non-risk families.

There seem to be clear indications that the presence of some specific high-risk condition in children is associated with greater levels of parenting stress, although there is wide variability in such parental response regardless of which risk condition is present. The developmental pathways through which stress response is moderated need to be better understood, but the extent to which behavior problems are present seem to be a key to parent stress.

Parental Psychopathology

Although child characteristics are important risk contexts for parenting stress, so too are parent characteristics. These have been addressed in depth previously (see Crnic and Low, 2002; Crnic and Ross, 2017), and the evidence in support of a connection between parental psychological well-being and parenting stress is compelling. Predominantly, studies assess parents' reports of depressed or anxious symptoms, but rarely do studies focus exclusively on parents with diagnosed clinical conditions. Consequently, the vast majority of existing knowledge represents information on the linear relation between number of symptoms and degree of stress experienced by parents. This certainly does not minimize the importance of the phenomenon. In fact, it is possible that the cumulative effect of parenting stress over time could potentially contribute to emerging clinical conditions in parents, although this direction of effect would be less likely than finding that existing parent psychopathology is likely to contribute to the degree of perceived stresses in the parenting role.

Whether or not actual clinical conditions may be present in the parent, the attributes associated with greater numbers of symptoms are likely to be important to parent-child stress processes. For example, regulatory failures (Sheppes, Suri, and Gross, 2015) and emotion dysregulation (Havighurst and Kehoe, 2017) are often judged to be major components of psychopathologies, and to affect parenting processes. Havighurst and Kehoe (2017) have specifically tied dysregulated emotion processes to parenting stress, and Platt, Williams, and Ginsburg (2016) demonstrated that a complex set of factors that included parental dysregulated emotion and parenting stress mediated relations between extrafamilial family stress and children's anxiety.

The evidence is clear that parent psychopathology, symptoms, or dysregulated emotional functioning are tied importantly to the experience of parenting stress in predictable ways. Higher stress is associated with less parental well-being regardless of whether stress leads to symptoms of depression or symptoms of depression may lead to the experience of more stress. Of course, there are important moderators and mediators of such relations (Crnic and Ross, 2017), and much work is left to do with respect to differentiation of specific parental symptoms (depression, anxiety, other dysregulated behavior) and the pathways through which parental well-being and parenting stress operate to affect child and family functioning.

Culture

Like most developmental processes, neither stressed parenting nor parenting stress can be understood from a single cultural perspective. Stress seems to be a universal experience, and parenting stress likewise crosses cultural frames of reference (Garcia Coll et al., 1996). Cultural perspectives have become much more prominent in developmental research, and the same is true for parenting stress research in particular. Nomaguchi and Milke (2017) provided a succinct review of the multiple issues involved with cultural perspectives on parenting stress, addressing the important structural components and cultural values that help to dictate the stresses experienced by parents from varied sociocultural backgrounds both within and outside the United States.

Ethnicity and the sociocultural context in the United States are both important correlates of the experience of parenting stress, but nativity is also an important consideration. The importance of nativity is especially true for Latin American families, which represent the fastest growing minority population in the United States. A number of studies have addressed parenting stress of Latin American families, and not surprising, the results are complex and depend to some extent on factors of acculturation, enculturation, generation, economic status, and living contexts. Several studies have noted that Latin American families do not differ from either African American or European American families in absolute levels of parenting stress (Cardoso, Padilla, and Sampson, 2010; Joshi and Gutierrez, 2006), but do differ in factors that moderate the effects of parenting stress such as social support and parental distress. Cardoso et al. (2010) found that social support, but not intimate partner support, was associated with less parenting stress for Latin American mothers, whereas Mortensen and Barnett (2015) reported that better romantic relationship quality for Latin American mothers was associated with less parenting stress, and parenting stress accounted for the connections found between harsh parenting and lower romantic relationship quality.

Other comparative studies have been conducted to address whether parenting stress, like other parenting attributes, might differ between different ethnic groups in the United States. It is likely the case that parenting stress is ubiquitous, but the factors that influence it vary as a function of structural and cultural factors (Nomaguchi and Milke, 2017), as well as community and neighborhood contexts (Franco, Pottick, and Huang, 2010). As noted above, parent and child country of birth determine some of the influence on parenting stress, and group differences in parenting stress more clearly emerge when nativity or immigration status is included as a study factor. For example, using data from the 2003 National Survey of Children's Health, Yu and Singh (2012) found that foreign-born parents report more parenting aggravation (a factor that was considered to be akin to parenting stress) than do native parents, with Latin American households reporting the highest levels regardless of where the children were born. They suggested that the higher level of parenting stress represented the unique challenges and risks these families face in comparison to native families. Nomaguchi and House (2013), using the Early Childhood Longitudinal Study data, found both similarities and differences between ethnic groups on parenting stress, and the degree to which differences emerged appeared were a function of nativity and its influence on cultural values, as well as contextual issues and developmental factors such as child age.

As yet, it is not entirely clear how different ethnicities experience parenting stress and what factors may serve to exacerbate or mitigate the effect of these stressors on parents and children in the United States. There remains much to be done in this regard. Studies of non-U.S. populations offer some additional insight into the role of culture and parenting stress, although it seems clear that parenting stress is an experience salient to nearly every culture (Chung et al., 2013; Dardas and Ahmad, 2014; Mejia, Calam, and Sanders, 2015; Östberg and Hagekull, 2013; Tharner et al., 2012; Yaman, Mesman, van IJzendoorn, and Bakermans-Kranenburg, 2010), and the determinants and consequences of parenting stress share similarities as well as culturally specific relations (Emmen et al., 2013). As research with more culturally diverse samples continues to emerge, these important processes involving parenting stress will clarify.

The Psychobiology of Parenting Stress

Psychobiological frameworks are predominant in current models of stress and its influence on human functioning. Yet, research on the specific psychobiology of parenting stress lags despite some work by Repetti and colleagues (Repetti, Robles, and Reynolds, 2011; Repetti and Robles, 2016) and Sturge-Apple et al. (2011). This lag is surprising given that allostatic frameworks have been suggested as potentially explanatory in understanding the ways in which physiological response systems may connect parental psychosocial stressors experienced in one context with subsequent stressful parent-child interactive behaviors (Repetti et al., 2011; Sturge-Apple et al., 2011). Indeed, Sturge-Apple et al. suggested that, as various stresses from multiple sources accumulate and magnify, allostatic systems struggle to regulate stresses associated with the typical challenges associated with parenting. These accumulating stresses over time may lead to increasing physiological dysregulation, and parents are then less likely to be able to competently regulate their behavior when faced with stressful interactions with their children.

Physiological stress can be understood as allostatic load, which refers to the physical wear and tear that results from continued attempts to adapt to challenges of chronic stressful circumstances. For our purposes, the notion of stressed parenting in combination with parenting stress can create problematic allostatic load. The attendant compromise in physiological regulation is likely to diminish parents' ability to engage effective parenting behaviors and strategies (Sturge-Apple et al., 2011).

There is some research that explores these potential physiological mechanisms and sheds light on the psychobiological mechanism involved in parenting stress. One area of interest has been maternal prenatal stress and related fetal programming hypotheses. Neuenschwander and Oberlander (2017) noted that "the period of intrauterine life represents one of the most sensitive windows during which the effects may be transmitted inter-generationally from a mother to her as yet unborn child" (p. 127). Risk can be conferred prenatally through changes in maternal mood-related physiology that then influence fetal neurobehavioral development, later maternal depression, and negative parenting during infancy (Belsky, Ruttle, Boyce, Armstrong, and Essex, 2015). The HPA axis plays a critical role in mediating the effects of maternal prenatal stress on child functioning, and fetal programming represents a potential mechanism of effect through which maternal stress experience and physiology affect children's development. Findings regarding fetal programming have been variable to date, but indications suggest that maternal prenatal stress is associated with increased reactivity in cortisol during infancy and middle childhood (Neuenschwander and Oberlander, 2017) as well as with regulatory development in early infancy (Lin et al., 2014). There is also evidence to support a connection between maternal prenatal stress and child prefrontal cortex development and executive function in middle school years (Buss, Davis, Hobel, and Sandman, 2011).

Although connections to infant and child development are of interest from the fetal programming perspective, it is also critical to know whether maternal prenatal stress has implications for later postnatal stress processes for mothers. Few studies prospectively assess parent stress from prenatal to postnatal periods, although as noted previously, parenting stress tends to be moderately stable postnatally through middle childhood. Evidence for stability between maternal prenatal distress and postnatal distress exists (Belsky et al., 2015; Coburn et al., 2016; Kingston, McDonald, Austin, and Tough, 2015) with suggestions that prenatal stress and its physiological concomitants are important to later postnatal maternal well-being and parenting.

Beyond HPA functions, a handful of genetic studies has emerged to address key processes in parenting stress. Evidence now suggests that DNA methylation can be affected by maternal stress experience, and stressed parenting can affect the epigenetic profile of the developing child in a detrimental way (Mulder et al., 2017). In maltreated children, Romens, McDonald, Svaren, and Pollak (2015) noted increased methylation in a gene that functionally depletes the formation of stress receptors, which then compromises the development of a healthy stress response system. This finding has meaning in light of the strong evidence for links between parenting stress and child maltreatment (Nair, Schuler, Black, Kettinger, and Harrington, 2003; Sprang, Clark, and Bass, 2005).

The psychobiology of parenting stress is a nascent area of study, but one that holds great promise for understanding the mechanisms through which parenting stress maintains itself over time, influences parental behavioral and emotional responsivity to children, and affects children's developmental well-being.

Systems and Complex Models in Parenting Stress

Family System Perspectives

Parenting stress is rarely conceptualized from a systems perspective, despite the fact that it occurs within families and requires at least a dyadic parent-child context to exist. Typically, families involve more than a single dyadic relationship, and have multiple subsystems that compose a notably complex whole. Stress in the parenting context is unlikely to be limited to just one parent, or to just one child when multiple children are present in the home. In two-parent families, both mothers and fathers share a marital relationship while they also have their own perceptions of the parenting role. Their shared relationship is likely to affect each other's experience of parenting stress, implicating coparenting and parent to parent crossover effects in the process. Furthermore, in all families with multiple children, parenting stress is likely to reflect the complex interplay of those children's ages, characteristics, and relationships with each other as well as with each parent. Thus, parenting stress is best conceptualized as a dynamic family systems construct that represents the cumulative and simultaneous integrative influences of all children in the home, regardless of variations in age, behavior, or risk (Crnic and Ross, 2017). Yet, almost every study of parenting stress focuses on a specific child at a specific age of interest for that study (see Deater-Deckard, Smith, Ivy, and Petril, 2005, for an exception), and the potential contribution of other children in the family are rarely considered. In contrast, research has begun to explore coparenting and crossover effects in two-parent families, and to some extent has attempted to differentiate mother and father parenting stress perceptions.

Coparenting

Coparenting involves the various ways in which mothers and fathers (or care providers) coordinate their parenting efforts, engage in supportive or undermining actions toward each other, and manage the inevitable childrearing conflicts that arise in families (Feinberg and Kan, 2008; Minuchin, Rosman, and Baker, 1978). Coparenting has been consistently linked to parent adjustment, parenting behaviors, and child competencies (Feinberg, Kan, and Hetherington, 2007) and to the ways in which parenting stress operates in families.

There is a direct link between coparenting effectiveness and parenting stress, such that in families for which parenting stress is low, coparenting is typically more effective (Feinberg, Jones, Kan, and Goslin, 2010; Riina and McHale, 2012). But much of the effort to link coparenting and parenting stress has explored more complex meditational and moderating processes, often with longitudinal methods, to understand the possible pathways through which coparenting and parenting stress affect family relationships. Several studies suggest that coparenting quality mediates relations between problematic circumstances and parenting stress in theoretically consistent directions (Delvecchio, Sciandra, Finos, Mazzeschi, and De Riso, 2015; Fagan and Lee, 2014; Schoppe-Sullivan, Settle, Lee, and Kamp Dush, 2016). In a longitudinal study, using the Fragile Families and Child Well Being Study data set, Durtschi, Soloski, and Kimmes (2017) showed that supportive coparenting from fathers buffered the adverse effects of maternal parenting stress on reported couple relationship quality. Multiple mediating and moderating pathways involving coparenting are likely to exist.

Coparenting processes are often linked with marital relationship quality (Holland and McElwain, 2013), but it is surprising to find that few studies directly assess marital relationship quality and parenting stress. Chester and Blandon (2016) reported that for mothers of toddlers marital intimacy was negatively related to parenting stress, and Gerstein, Crnic, Blacher, and Baker (2009) showed that the quality of the marital relationship can buffer the effects of parenting stress on parent well-being. Relationship transitions between parents have also been explored. Osborne, Berger, and Magnuson

(2012) found that transitioning out of relationships was associated with higher parenting stress than was transitioning into relationships, and relationship churning (repeatedly separating and getting back together) was associated with greater parenting stress than was a stably engaged or stably disengaged situation (Halpern-Meekin and Turney, 2016).

Although not a direct index of the marital relationship, but certainly a relevant marker, intimate partner violence (IPV) has been explored for its connection to parenting stress. Not surprisingly, IPV is associated with greater parenting stress as well as more behavior problems in children. Some studies found only direct associations between parenting stress and child behavior problems in the context of IPV (Huth-Bocks and Hughes, 2008), but others found pathways in which parenting stress mediated the connection between IPV and child behavioral problems. Regardless, extreme risk conditions such as IPV are stressful in any respect. In all, the quality of the couple relationship and the ways in which couples coparent are complexly related to the degree to which one or both partners experience parenting stress.

Crossover

Given the relative dearth of studies on parenting stress that include both mothers and fathers, it is not surprising that that only a handful of studies report on crossover effects. Crossover represents partner effects in a relationship, such that an individual's functioning in one domain affects the behavior of functioning of their partner in one or more relevant domains. With respect to parenting stress, one individual's stress or behavior may affect their partner's stress or behavior in one or another context.

Findings from studies that assess crossover effects with respect to parenting stress suggest that crossover is salient in some domains, or but not others. Nelson et al. (2009) tested potential crossover effects of family stress on parenting behaviors in a study of 101 parents of school-age children. They found crossover effects related to parent job dissatisfaction, such that both mothers' and fathers' job dissatisfactions decreased their spouses' supportive responses to children's negative emotions, but did not affect the degree of unsupportive responses. Other tested factors (for example, marital dissatisfaction, home chaos) did not create crossover effects. In a study of children at developmental risk, Gerstein et al. (2009) found that for both mothers and fathers, levels of distress and positive marital adjustment predicted less increasing parenting stress in the partner, supporting notions of emotion transmission in families (Larson and Almeida, 1999). Similarly, in a like sample of children at developmental risks, Mitchell, Szczerepa, and Hauser-Cram (2016) found that higher levels of partner stress predicted reports of lower family cohesion for both mothers and fathers, although marital satisfaction suppressed the associations.

Crossover and coparenting processes are just two systemic processes that merit further attention in parenting stress research. Sibling relationships, triadic interactions among parents and children, simultaneously competing child demands, and multigenerational caregiving contexts among multiple other issues remain to be explored in understanding systemic stress processes within families. But whether direct or indirect in effect, research findings to date demonstrate the importance of focusing more on systemic aspects of family functioning.

Complexity and Pathways of Influence

Related to system perspectives are notions about the mechanisms that help to explain the emerging complexity of relations between stress and parenting processes. As noted, the field of parenting stress has moved well beyond the main effect models that sought to identify straightforward connections between risk and stress, and then between stress and some adverse parent or child outcome. That was important work to be sure, and much was learned from identifying the many determinants of parenting stress and its meaningful consequences.

Now, however, complex developmental modeling has begun to be applied to parenting stress processes, helping the field to move beyond the relatively simplistic perspectives that stress leads to poor outcomes and/or is predicted by adverse circumstances. Complexity now comes from studies that employ thoughtful longitudinal designs and integrate conceptually meaningful mediating and moderating processes that help to explicate the various pathways through which parenting stress operates. These efforts are critical in helping to explain the rich variability in parenting stress processes both within and across families.

The explosive growth of this literature precludes an exhaustive review, but a number of studies that address complex, potentially bidirectional pathways among risk, parenting stress, parenting behaviors, and children's behavior and emotional problems are illustrative. The ability to examine direct and indirect influences of parenting stress on the emergence of child behavior and emotion problems has been an issue of some conceptual interest, as the connection between parental stress and child behavior problems has been thought to be more indirect and mediated by parent behavior, than directly influential. Multiple longitudinal studies have established connections between parenting stress and children's behavior problems in the context of a variety of family situations (Östberg and Hagekull, 2013; Puff and Renk, 2014; Robinson et al., 2011), establishing pathways of direct effects from infancy through adolescence. Both Crnic et al. (2005) and Mackler et al. (2015) tested mediated pathways by which parenting behavior would either fully or partially account for connections between parenting stress and later child behavior problems either in early or middle childhood. Neither study, however, found evidence for mediation, despite connections between parenting stress and maternal parenting behaviors or attributes.

Mackler et al. (2015) offered a specific example of the rich complexity inherent in exploring transactional processes in parenting stress research. In a longitudinal paradigm that stretched across four measurement periods from age 4 to 10, the authors explored the transactional relations between parenting stress, parents' perceived negative reactions to children's emotion, and children's externalizing behavior. Despite the absence of mediating effects for parental reactions to child emotion, Mackler et al. found that a transactional model that allowed for both direct and indirect relations among all study variables across time best fit the data. This pattern suggested that both parent-effect pathways and child-effect pathways were operative across time. Exploring each pathway specifically, both parent- and child-effect paths were equally operative when children were younger (ages 4–7), but child-effect pathways were stronger when children were older such that child externalizing behavior was more predictive of parenting stress than parenting stress was of child externalizing behavior.

Other studies have examined pathways that explore parent and family contributions to change in parenting stress over time (Williford et al., 2007), cultural influences on the connection between parenting stress and behavior problems over time (Yaman et al., 2010), and the moderating roles of parenting stress in understanding associations between coparenting and parental self-efficacy (Schoppe-Sullivan et al., 2016), among others. In all, studies that integrate multidimensional and multimodal perspectives on parenting stress for developmental processes across time represent a significant step forward for conceptualizations of parenting stress processes, and illuminate the risk and resilience mechanisms that operate within families.

Intervention for Parenting Stress

It is apparent that parenting stress is an important component of family risk processes that can lead to adverse outcomes for parents, children, and families. Given this risk status, developmentalists and clinicians alike have suggested the need to incorporate a parenting stress focus into early interventions that are aimed at supporting high-risk families and children. A handful of interventions has been developed, and evaluation results suggest that interventions can successfully ameliorate parenting stress or the links between parents' experiences of stress and child and family well-being.

Interventions vary in the models they employ, ranging from those that focus on parent training approaches (Hodes et al., 2017: Moreland et al., 2016; Strauss et al., 2012), and support system facilitation (Castel et al., 2016) to mindfulness interventions (Dykens, Fisher, Taylor, Lambert, and Miodrag, 2014; Neece, 2014). Although parenting stress might sometimes be an explicit target of the intervention (Neece, 2014), it is also included in intervention research as an indirect effect of treatments that focus more on parent skill building (Misri, Reebye, Milis, and Shah, 2006; Moreland et al., 2016). Whether the intervention addresses parenting stress directly or indirectly, the evidence suggests that most parent interventions, regardless of modality, find corresponding reductions in parenting stress. These reductions tend to be stronger in the short term than the long term (Golfenshtein, Srulovici, and Deatrick, 2016; Singer, Ethridge, and Aldana, 2007), suggesting that maintaining parenting stress reduction in the face of ongoing challenge is difficult.

Even if longer-term effects have proven elusive in some cases, the focused treatment of parenting stress appears to facilitate therapeutic change for child behavior problems (Kazdin and Whitley, 2003). Parenting stress interventions have provided positive effects on parent and child well-being across risk conditions that include developmental disabilities (Neece, 2014; Singer et al., 2007), autism spectrum disorder (Bluth, Roberson, Billen, and Sams, 2013), preterm birth (Castel et al., 2016), childhood illness (Golfenshtein et al., 2016), and child abuse risk (Shenk et al., 2017).

The complexity of indirect intervention effects can be seen in the study by Shenk et al. (2017), in which a home visiting intervention for high-risk new mothers assessed the impact of a history of child maltreatment on the parenting outcomes in the study. Mothers with a history of child maltreatment, in addition to the high-risk criteria to enter the home visiting program, reported worsening parenting stress at 18 months postpartum, and these relations were mediated by levels of social support when the mothers enrolled in the intervention, and the persistence of depressive symptoms across the intervention period.

Timing of intervention for parenting stress may be an important consideration, and indications are that the transition to parenthood for couples and their relationship may be a prime opportunity to intervene to influence parenting and coparenting processes (Petch, Halford, Creedy, and Gamble, 2012). Coparenting interventions targeting the transition to parenthood have addressed parenting stress as an important factor associated with successful intervention outcome. Feinberg and colleagues' Family Foundations program is a specific example in which expectant cohabitating couples are provided eight skill building intervention sessions that aim to enhance the coparenting relationship (Feinberg, Jones, Kan, and Goslin, 2010). Results from this intervention program have shown lower rates of parenting stress across the infancy and early preschool periods for parents in the intervention group, suggesting that better coparenting relationships can facilitate less stressful circumstances in the context of parenting. Other home visiting programs in the transition to parenthood period that focus on parenting more broadly show similar positive effects on parenting stress (Jacobs et al., 2016), indicating the promise of such interventions for ameliorating the developmental risks associated with parenting stress experience.

In sum, a variety of interventions that either directly or indirectly target parenting stress have proven effective in the short term for stress reduction even though maintaining effects over time has been a challenge. It may be that changes in the nature and function of parenting stress over time, and the contexts in which it emerges, make it difficult for intervention programs to be sufficiently adaptive. Regardless, the successes are encouraging and efforts to promote maintenance effects should be the next steps in intervention programs for parenting stress.

Conclusion

It is hard not be impressed by the sheer volume of work that has explored parenting stress and the ways it is associated with parent, child, and family well-being. It is apparent that parenting stress is common, multidimensional, and determined by an extensive array of risk conditions and normative circumstances. Stressed parenting is associated with a cadre of potentially adverse outcomes, and it operates through multiple mechanisms involving mediated and moderated pathways that illustrate its developmental complexity.

Although conceptual and empirical approaches have come a long way in explicating the nature of parenting stress, there remain areas of confusion and issues that have been poorly represented in the work to date. This chapter has attempted to detail many of these issues. Now, more explicit attention to the developmental nature of parenting stress is needed, as there is simply too little known about the ways in which parenting stress may change or operate across developmental periods and parental lifespans. The systemic nature of parenting stress needs further recognition and research as well. Although contrasts between mothers' and fathers' experiences are helpful, and marital and coparenting processes are illustrative, much more needs to be done to explore the effects of multiple child families, triadic (or greater!) relationships, and multigenerational contexts. Finally, research needs to further pursue transactional mechanisms that operate over time and tie factors of risk, family relationships, developmental psychobiology, and stress contexts together in ways that create coherent pathways of influence through which parent, child, and family well-being can be better understood.

References

Abidin, R.R. (1983). *Parenting stress index*. Charlottesville, VA: Pediatric Psychology Press.

Abidin, R.R. (1992). The determinants of parenting behavior. *Journal of Clinical Child Psychology, 21*(4), 407–412. https://doi.org/10.1207/s15374424jccp2104_12

Abidin, R.R. (2012). *Parenting stress index* (4th ed.). Lutz, FL: PAR.

Aldwin, C. (2011). Stress and coping across the lifespan. In S. Folkman (Ed.), *The Oxford handbook of stress, health, and coping: The Oxford handbook of stress, health, and coping* (pp. 15–34). New York: Oxford University Press.

Baker, B.L., McIntyre, L.L., Blacher, J.B., Crnic, K., Edelbrock, C., and Low, C. (2003). Preschool children with and without developmental delay: Behavior problems and parenting stress over time. *Journal of Intellectual Disability Research, 47*, 217–230. doi.10.1046/j.1365-2788.2003.00484.x

Baker, B.L., Neece, C.L., Fleming, R.M., Crnic, K.A., and Blacher, J. (2010). Mental disorders in five-year old children with or without developmental delay: Focus on ADHD. *Journal of Clinical Child and Adolescent Psychology, 39*, 492–505.

Belsky, J. (1984). The determinants of parenting: A process model. *Child Development, 55*(1), 83–96. https://doi.org/10.2307/1129836

Belsky, J., Ruttle, P.L., Boyce, W.T., Armstrong, J.M., and Essex, M.J. (2015). Early adversity, elevated stress physiology, accelerated sexual maturation, and poor health in females. *Developmental Psychology, 51*(6), 816–822. https://doi.org/10.1037/dev0000017

Berryhill, M.B. (2016). Mothers' parenting stress and engagement: Mediating role of parental competence. *Marriage and Family Review, 52*(5), 461–480. https://doi.org/1080/01494929.2015.1113600

Berryhill, M.B., and Durtschi, J.A. (2017). Understanding single mothers' parenting stress trajectories. *Marriage and Family Review, 53*(3), 227–245. https://doi.org/10.1080/01494929.2016.1204406

Blacher, J., and Baker, B.L. (2007). Positive impact of intellectual disability on families. *American Journal on Mental Retardation, 112*, 330–348.

Bluth, K., Roberson, P.N.E., Billen, R.M., and Sams, J.M. (2013). A stress model for couples parenting children with autism spectrum disorders and the introduction of a mindfulness intervention. *Journal of Family Theory and Review, 5*(3), 194–213. doi.10.1111/jftr.12015

Bornstein, M.H. (1995). Form and function: Implications for studies of culture and human development. *Culture and Psychology, 1*, 123–137. https://doi.org/10.1177/1354067X9511009

Bornstein, M.H. (2016). Determinants of parenting. In D. Cicchetti (Ed.), *Developmental psychopathology: Risk, resilience, and intervention* (Vol. 4, 3rd ed., pp. 180–270, Chapter xiii, 1137 Pages). Hoboken, NJ: John Wiley & Sons.

Buss, C., Davis, E.P., Hobel, C.J., and Sandman, C.A. (2011). Maternal pregnancy-specific anxiety is associated with child executive function at 6–9 years. *The International Journal on the Biology of Stress, 14*(6), 665–676. https://doi.org/10.3109/10253890.2011.623250

Cardoso, J.B., Padilla, Y.C., and Sampson, M. (2010). Racial and ethnic variation in the predictors of maternal parenting stress. *Journal of Social Service Research, 36*(5), 429–444. https://doi.org/10.1080/01488376.2010.51094

Cassells, R.C., and Evans, G.W. (2017). Ethnic variation in poverty and parenting stress. In K. Deater-Deckard and R. Panneton (Eds.), *Parental stress and early child development: Adaptive and maladaptive outcomes* (pp. 15–46). Cham, Switzerland: Springer.

Castel, S., Creveuil, C., Beunard, A., Blaizot, X., Proia, N., and Guillois, B. (2016). Effects of an intervention program on maternal and paternal parenting stress after preterm birth: A randomized trial. *Early Human Development, 103*, 17–25. https://doi.org/10.1016/j.earlhumdev.2016.05.007

Chester, C.E., and Blandon, A.Y. (2016). Dual trajectories of maternal parenting stress and marital intimacy during toddlerhood. *Personal Relationships, 23*(2), 265–279. https://doi.org/10.1111/pere.12122

Chung, K., Ebesutani, C., Bang, H.M., Kim, J., Chorpita, B.F., Weisz, J.R., . . . Byun, H. (2013). Parenting stress and child behavior problems among clinic-referred youth: Cross-cultural differences across the US and Korea. *Child Psychiatry and Human Development, 44*(3), 460–468. https://doi.org/10.1007/s10578-012-0340-z

Cicchetti, D. (1984). The emergence of developmental psychopathology. *Child Development, 55*(1), 1–7. https://doi.org/10.2307/1129830

Coburn, S.S., Gonzales, N.A., Luecken, L.J., and Crnic, K.A. (2016). Multiple domains of stress predict postpartum depressive symptoms in low-income Mexican American women: the moderating effect of social support. *Archives of Women's Mental Health*, 1–10. DOI: 10.1007/s00737-016-0649-x

Coddington, R.D. (1972). The significance of life events as etiologic factors in the diseases of children: II. A study of a normal population. *Journal of Psychosomatic Research, 16*(3), 205–213. https://doi.org/10.1016/0022-3999(72)90045-1

Conger, R.D., Conger, K.J., and Martin, M.J. (2011). Socioeconomic status, family processes, and individual development. *Journal of Marriage and the Family, 72*, 685–704. https://doi.org/10.1111/j.1741-3737.2010.00725.x. socioeconomic

Cousino, M.K., and Hazen, R.A. (2013). Parenting stress among caregivers of children with chronic illness: A systematic review. *Journal of Pediatric Psychology, 38*(8), 809–828. https://doi.org/10.1093/jpepsy/jst049

Crnic, K.A., Gaze, C., and Hoffman, C. (2005). Cumulative parenting stress across the preschool period: Relations to maternal parenting and child behavior at age five. *Infant and Child Development, 14*, 117–132.

Crnic, K.A., and Greenberg, M.T. (1990). Minor parenting stresses with young children. *Child Development, 61*, 1628–1637.

Crnic, K.A., Greenberg, M.T., Ragozin, A.S., Robinson, N.M., and Basham, R.B. (1983). Effects of stress and social support on mothers and preterm and full-term infants. *Child Development, 54*, 209–217.

Crnic, K.A., and Low, C. (2002). Everyday stresses and parenting. In M. Bornstein (Ed.), *Handbook of parenting* (Vol. 4, 2nd ed., pp. 243–268). Hillsdale, NJ: Lawrence Erlbaum Associates.

Crnic, K.A., and Neece, C.L. (2015). Socioemotional consequences of illness and disability. In M.E. Lamb (Ed.), *Social, emotional, and personality development: Handbook of child psychology and developmental science* (Vol. 3, 7th ed., pp. 287–323). New York, NY: Wiley-Blackwell.

Crnic, K.A., Pedersen y Arbona, A., Baker, B., and Blacher, J. (2009). Mothers and fathers together: Contrasts in parenting across preschool to early school age in children with developmental delay. In L. Glidden and M. Seltzer (Eds.), *International Review of Research in Mental Retardation, IRRMR* (Vol. 37, pp. 3–30). Oxford: Elsevier.

Crnic, K.A., and Ross, E. (2017). Parenting stress and parental self-efficacy. In K. Deater-Deckard and R. Panneton (Eds.), *Parental stress and early child development: Adaptive and maladaptive outcomes* (pp. 263–284). Cham, Switzerland: Springer.

Crum, A.J., Salovey, P., and Achor, S. (2013). Rethinking stress: The role of mindsets in determining the stress response. *Journal of Personality and Social Psychology, 104*(4), 716–733. https://doi.org/10.1037/a0031201

Cutrona, C.E. (1984). Social support and stress in the transition to parenthood. *Journal of Abnormal Psychology, 93*(4), 378–390. https://doi.org/10.1037/0021-843X.93.4.378

Dabrowska, A., and Pisula, E. (2010). Parenting stress and coping styles in mothers and fathers of pre-school children with autism and down syndrome. *Journal of Intellectual Disability Research, 54*, 266–280.

Dardas, L.A., and Ahmad, M.M. (2014). Quality of life among parents of children with autistic disorder: A sample from the Arab world. *Research in Developmental Disabilities, 35*(2), 278–287. https://doi.org/10.1016/j.ridd.2013.10.029

Deater-Deckard, K. (1998). Parenting stress and child adjustment: Some old hypotheses and new questions. *Clinical Psychology: Science and Practice, 5*(3), 314–332. doi.10.1111/j.1468-2850.1998.tb00152.x

Deater-Deckard, K. (2004). *Parenting stress*. New Haven, CT: Yale University Press. https://doi.org/10.12987/yale/9780300103939.001.000

Deater-Deckard, K., and Panneton, R. (2017). *Parental stress and early child development*. Cham, Switzerland: Springer.

Deater-Deckard, K., Smith, J., Ivy, L., and Petril, S.A. (2005). Differential perceptions of and feelings about sibling children: Implications for research on parenting stress. *Infant and Child Development, 14*(2), 211–225. https://doi.org/10.1002/icd.389

Delvecchio, E., Sciandra, A., Finos, L., Mazzeschi, C., and Di Riso, D. (2015). The role of co-parenting alliance as a mediator between trait anxiety, family system maladjustment, and parenting stress in a sample of non-clinical Italian parents. *Frontiers in Psychology*, *6*, 8.

Durtschi, J.A., Soloski, K.L., and Kimmes, J. (2017). The dyadic effects of supportive coparenting and parental stress on relationship quality across the transition to parenthood. *Journal of Marital and Family Therapy*, *43*(2), 308–321. https://doi.org/10.1111/jmft.12194

Dykens, E.M., Fisher, M.H., Taylor, J.L., Lambert, W., and Miodrag, N. (2014). Reducing distress in mothers of children with autism and other disabilities: A randomized trial. *Pediatrics*, *134*(2), e454–e463. https://doi.org/10.1542/peds.2013-3164

Easterbrooks, M.A., and Goldberg, W.A. (1984). Toddler development in the family: Impact of father involvement and parenting characteristics. *Child Development*, *55*(3), 740–752. https://doi.org/10.2307/1130126

Easterbrooks, M.A., Katz, R.C., and Menon, M. (2019). Adolescent parenting. In M.H. Bornstein (Ed.), *Handbook of parenting Vol. 3: Being and becoming a parent* (3rd ed., pp. 199–231). New York, NY: Routledge.

Elder, G.H., Liker, J., and Cross, C. (1984). Parent-child behavior in the great depression: Life course and intergenerational influences. In P. Baltes and O. Brim (Eds.), *Life span development and behavior* (Vol. 6, pp. 109–158). Orlando, FL: Academic Press.

Emmen, R.A.G., Malda, M., Mesman, J., van IJzendoorn, M.H., Prevoo, M.J.L., and Yeniad, N. (2013). Socioeconomic status and parenting in ethnic minority families: Testing a minority family stress model. *Journal of Family Psychology*, *27*(6), 896–904. https://doi.org/10.1037/a0034693

Fagan, J., and Lee, Y. (2014). Longitudinal associations among fathers' perception of coparenting, partner relationship quality, and paternal stress during early childhood. *Family Process*, *53*(1), 80–96. https://doi.org/10.1111/famp.12055

Feinberg, M.E., Jones, D.E., Kan, M.L., and Goslin, M.C. (2010). Effects of family foundations on parents and children: 3.5 years after baseline. *Journal of Family Psychology*, *24*(5), 532–542. https://doi.org/10.1037/a0020837

Feinberg, M.E., and Kan, M.L. (2008). Establishing family foundations: Intervention effects on coparenting, parent/infant well-being, and parent-child relations. *Journal of Family Psychology*, *22*(2), 253–263. https://doi.org/10.1037/0893-3200.22.2.253

Feinberg, M.E., Kan, M.L., and Hetherington, E.M. (2007). The longitudinal influence of coparenting conflict on parental negativity and adolescent maladjustment. *Journal of Marriage and Family*, *69*(3), 687–702. doi.10.1111/j.1741-3737.2007.00400.x

Folkman, S. (1984). Personal control and stress and coping processes: A theoretical analysis. *Journal of Personality and Social Psychology*, *46*(4), 839–852. https://doi.org/10.1037/0022-3514.46.4.839

Franco, L.M., Pottick, K.J., and Huang, C. (2010). Early parenthood in a community context: Neighborhood conditions, race-ethnicity, and parenting stress. *Journal of Community Psychology*, *38*(5), 574–590. https://doi.org/10.1002/jcop.20382

Garcia Coll, C.G., Lamberty, G., Jenkins, R., McAdoo, H.P., Crnic, K., Wasik, B.H., and Garcia, H.V. (1996). An integrative model for the study of developmental competencies in minority children. *Child Development*, *67*(5), 1891–1914. https://doi.org/10.2307/1131600

Garmezy, N., Masten, A.S., and Tellegen, A. (1984). The study of stress and competence in children: A building block for developmental psychopathology. *Child Development*, *55*(1), 97–111. https://doi.org/10.2307/1129837

Garmezy, N., and Rutter, M. (1983). *Stress, coping, and development in children*. New York, NY: McGraw-Hill.

Gerstein, E., Crnic, K., Blacher, J., and Baker, B. (2009). Resilience and the course of daily parenting stress in families of young children with intellectual disabilities. *Journal of Intellectual Disabilities Research*, *53*, 981–997.

Gersten, J.C., Langner, T.S., Eisenberg, J.G., and Orzeck, L. (1974). Child behavior and life events: Undesirable change or change per se? In B.S. Dohrenwend and B.P. Dohrenwend (Eds.), *Stressful life events: Their nature and effects; stressful life events: Their nature and effects* (p. 340, Chapter xi, 340 Pages). Oxford: John Wiley & Sons.

Golfenshtein, N., Srulovici, E., and Deatrick, J.A. (2016). Interventions for reducing parenting stress in families with pediatric conditions: An integrative review. *Journal of Family Nursing*, *22*(4), 460–492. https://doi.org/10.1177/1074840716676083

Gordon, C.T., and Hinshaw, S.P. (2017a). Parenting stress and youth symptoms among girls with and without attention-deficit/hyperactivity disorder. *Parenting: Science and Practice*, *17*(1), 11–29. https://doi.org/10.1080/15295192.2016.1262178

Gordon, C.T., and Hinshaw, S.P. (2017b). Parenting stress as a mediator between childhood ADHD and early adult female outcomes. *Journal of Clinical Child and Adolescent Psychology*, *46*(4), 588–599. https://doi.org/10.1080/15374416.2015.1041595

Halpern Meekin, S., and Turney, K. (2016). Relationship churning and parenting stress among mothers and fathers. *Journal of Marriage and Family*, 78(3), 715–729. https://doi.org/10.1111/jomf.12297

Havighurst, S., and Kehoe, C. (2017). The role of parental emotion regulation in parent emotion socialization: Implications for intervention. In K. Deater Deckard and R. Panneton (Eds.), *Parental stress and early child development: Adaptive and maladaptive outcomes* (pp. 285–308). Cham, Switzerland: Springer.

Hodes, M.W., Meppelder, M., de Moor, M., Kef, S., and Schuengel, C. (2017). Alleviating parenting stress in parents with intellectual disabilities: A randomized controlled trial of a video feedback intervention to promote positive parenting. *Journal of Applied Research in Intellectual Disabilities*, 30(3), 423–432. https://doi.org/10.1111/jar.12302

Holland, A.S., and McElwain, N.L. (2013). Maternal and paternal perceptions of coparenting as a link between marital quality and the parent-toddler relationship. *Journal of Family Psychology*, 27(1), 117–126. https://doi.org/10.1037/a003142

Holmes, T.H., and Rahe, R.H. (1967). The social readjustment rating scale. *Journal of Psychosomatic Research*, 11(2), 213–218. doi.10.1016/0022-3999(67)90010-4

Huth-bocks, A., and Hughes, H.M. (2008). Parenting stress, parenting behavior, and children's adjustment in families experiencing intimate partner violence. *Journal of Family Violence*, 23(4), 243–251. https://doi.org/10.1007/s10896-007-9148-1

Jacobs, F., Easterbrooks, M.A., Goldberg, J., Mistry, J., Bumgarner, E., Raskin, M., . . . Fauth, R. (2016). Improving adolescent parenting: Results from a randomized controlled trial of a home visiting program for young families. *American Journal of Public Health*, 106(2), 342–349. https://doi.org/10.2105/AJPH.2015.302919

Joshi, A., and Gutierrez, B.J. (2006). Parenting stress in parents of Hispanic adolescents. *North American Journal of Psychology*, 8(2), 209–216.

Kanner, A.D., Coyne, J.C., Schaefer, C., and Lazarus, R.S. (1981). Comparison of two modes of stress measurement: Daily hassles and uplifts versus major life events. *Journal of Behavioral Medicine*, 4(1), 1–39. https://doi.org/10.1007/BF00844845

Kazdin, A.E., and Whitley, M.K. (2003). Treatment of parental stress to enhance therapeutic change among children referred for aggressive and antisocial behavior. *Journal of Consulting and Clinical Psychology*, 71(3), 504–515. https://doi.org.ezproxy1.lib.asu.edu/10.1037/0022-006X.71.3.504

Kerig, P. (2019). Parenting and family systems. In M.H. Bornstein (Ed.), *Handbook of parenting Vol. 3: Being and becoming a parent* (3rd ed., pp. 3–35). New York, NY: Routledge.

Kingston, D., McDonald, S., Austin, M., and Tough, S. (2015). Association between prenatal and postnatal psychological distress and toddler cognitive development: A systematic review: E0126929. *PLoS ONE*, 10(5) https://doi.org/10.1371/journal.pone.0126929

Larson, R.W., and Almeida, D.M. (1999). Emotional transmission in the daily lives of families: A new paradigm for studying family process. *Journal of Marriage and the Family*, 61(1), 5–20. https://doi.org/10.2307/353879

Lazarus, R.S., DeLongis, A., Folkman, S., and Gruen, R. (1985). Stress and adaptational outcomes: The problem of confounded measures. *American Psychologist*, 40(7), 770–779. https://doi.org/10.1037/0003-066X.40.7.770

Lin, B.L., Crnic, K.A., Luecken, L.J., and Gonzales, N.A. (2014). Maternal prenatal stress and infant regulatory capacity in Mexican Americans. *Infant Behavior and Development*, 37, 571–582.

Maas-van Schaaijk, N.M., Roeleveld-Versteegh, A., and van Baar, A.L. (2013). The interrelationships among paternal and maternal parenting stress, metabolic control, and depressive symptoms in adolescents with type 1 diabetes mellitus. *Journal of Pediatric Psychology*, 38(1), 30–40. https://doi.org/10.1093/jpepsy/jss096

Mackler, J.S., Kelleher, R.T., Shanahan, L., Calkins, S.D., Keane, S.P., and O'Brien, M. (2015). Parenting stress, parental reactions, and externalizing behavior from ages 4 to 10. *Journal of Marriage and Family*, 77(2), 388–406. https://doi.org/10.1111/jomf.12163

Martin, C.G., Kim, H.K., and Fisher, P.A. (2016). Differential sensitization of parenting on early adolescent cortisol: Moderation by profiles of maternal stress. *Psychoneuroendocrinology*, 67, 18–26. https://doi.org/10.1016/j.psyneuen.2016.01.025

Masarik, A.S., and Conger, R.D. (2017). Stress and child development: A review of the family stress model. *Current Opinion in Psychology*, 13, 85–90. https://doi.org/10.1016/j.copsyc.2016.05.008

Mejia, A., Calam, R., and Sanders, M.R. (2015). Examining delivery preferences and cultural relevance of an evidence-based parenting program in a low-resource setting of Central America: Approaching parents as consumers. *Journal of Child and Family Studies*, 24(4), 1004–1015. https://doi.org/10.1007/s10826-014-9911-x

Merwyn, S.M., Smith, V.C., and Dougherty, L.R. (2015). It takes two: The interaction between parenting and child temperament on parents' stress physiology. *Developmental Psychobiology*, 57, 336–348. https://doi.org/10.1002/dev.21301

Minuchin, S., Rosman, B.L., and Baker, L. (1978). *Psychosomatic families: Anorexia nervosa in context*. Cambridge, MA: Harvard University Press.

Misri, S., Reebye, P., Milis, L., and Shah, S. (2006). The impact of treatment intervention on parenting stress in postpartum depressed mothers: A prospective study. *American Journal of Orthopsychiatry, 76*(1), 115–119. https://doi.org.ezproxy1.lib.asu.edu/10.1037/0002-9432.76.1.115

Mitchell, D.B., Szczerepa, A., and Hauser-Cram, P. (2016). Spilling over: Partner parenting stress as a predictor of family cohesion in parents of adolescents with developmental disabilities. *Research in Developmental Disabilities, 49–50*, 258–267. https://doi.org/10.1016/j.ridd.2015.12.007

Moola, F.J. (2012). "This is the best fatal illness that you can have": Contrasting and comparing the experiences of parenting youth with cystic fibrosis and congenital heart disease. *Qualitative Health Research, 22*(2), 212–225. https://doi.org/10.1177/104973231142148

Moreland, A.D., Felton, J.W., Hanson, R.F., Jackson, C., and Dumas, J.E. (2016). The relation between parenting stress, locus of control and child outcomes: Predictors of change in a parenting intervention. *Journal of Child and Family Studies, 25*(6), 2046–2054. https://doi.org/10.1007/s10826-016-0370-4

Mortensen, J.A., and Barnett, M.A. (2015). Risk and protective factors, parenting stress, and harsh parenting in Mexican origin mothers with toddlers. *Marriage and Family Review, 51*(1), 1–21. https://doi.org/10.1080/01494929.2014.955937

Mulder, R.H., Rijlaarsdam, J., Luijk, M.P.C.M., Verhulst, F.C., Felix, J.F., Tiemeier, H., . . . Van IJzendoorn, M.H. (2017). Methylation matters: FK506 Binding Protein 51 (FKBP5) methylation moderates the associations of FKBP5 genotype and resistant attachment with stress regulation. *Development and Psychopathology, 29*(2), 491–503. https://doi.org/10.1017/S095457941700013X

Nair, P., Schuler, M.E., Black, M.M., Kettinger, L., and Harrington, D. (2003). Cumulative environmental risk in substance abusing women: Early intervention, parenting stress, child abuse potential, and child development. *Child Abuse and Neglect, 27*, 997–1017. https://doi.org/10.1016/S01452134(03)00169-8

Neece, C.L. (2014). Mindfulness based stress reduction for parents of young children with developmental delays: Implications for parental mental health and child behavior problems. *Journal of Applied Research in Intellectual Disabilities, 27*(2), 174–186. https://doi.org/10.1111/jar.12064

Neece, C., and Baker, B. (2008). Predicting maternal parenting stress in middle childhood: The roles of child intellectual status, behaviour problems and social skills. *Journal of Intellectual Disability Research, 52*, 1114–1128. https://doi.org/10.1111/j.1365-2788.2008.01071.x

Neece, C.L., and Chan, N. (2017). The stress of parenting children with developmental disabilities. In K. Deater Deckard and R. Panneton (Eds.), *Parental stress and early child development: Adaptive and maladaptive outcomes* (pp. 263–284). Cham, Switzerland: Springer.

Neece, C.L., Green, S.A., and Baker, B.L. (2012). Parenting stress and child behavior problems: A transactional relationship across time. *American Journal on Intellectual and Developmental Disabilities, 117*(1), 48–66. https://doi.org.ezproxy1.lib.asu.edu/10.1352/1944-7558-117.1.48

Nelson, J.A., O'Brien, M., Blankson, A.N., Calkins, S.D., and Keane, S.P. (2009). Family stress and parental responses to children's negative emotions: Tests of the spillover, crossover, and compensatory hypotheses. *Journal of Family Psychology, 23*(5), 671–679. https://doi.org/10.1037/a0015977

Neuenschwander, R., and Oberlander, T.F. (2017). Developmental origins of self-regulation: Prenatal maternal stress and psychobiological development during childhood. In K. Deater Deckard and R. Panneton (Eds.), *Parental stress and early child development: Adaptive and maladaptive outcomes* (pp. 263–284). Cham, Switzerland: Springer.

Newland, R.P., and Crnic, K.A. (2017). Developmental risk and goodness of fit in the mother-child relationship: Links to parenting stress and children's behaviour problems. *Infant and Child Development, 26*(2). https://doi.org/10.1002/icd.1980

Newland, R.P., Crnic, K.A., Cox, M.J., and Mills-Koonce, W. (2013). The family model stress and maternal psychological symptoms: Mediated pathways from economic hardship to parenting. *Journal of Family Psychology, 27*(1), 96–105. https://doi.org/10.1037/a0031112

Nomaguchi, K., Brown, S., and Leyman, T.M. (2017). Fathers' participation in parenting and maternal parenting stress: Variation by relationship status. *Journal of Family Issues, 38*(8), 1132–1156. https://doi.org/10.1177/0192513X15623586

Nomaguchi, K., and House, A.N. (2013). Racial-ethnic disparities in maternal parenting stress: The role of structural disadvantages and parenting values. *Journal of Health and Social Behavior, 54*(3), 386–404. https://doi.org/10.1177/0022146513498511

Nomaguchi, K., and Johnson, W. (2016). Parenting stress among low-income and working-class fathers: The role of employment. *Journal of Family Issues, 37*(11), 1535–1557. https://doi.org/10.1177/0192513X14560642

Nomaguchi, K., and Milke, M.A. (2017). Sociological perspectives on parenting stress: How social structure and culture shape parental strain and the well being of parents and children. In K. Deater Deckard and R. Panneton (Eds.), *Parental stress and early child development: Adaptive and maladaptive outcomes* (pp. 263–284). Cham, Switzerland: Springer.

Osborne, C., Berger, L.M., and Magnuson, K. (2012). Family structure transitions and changes in maternal resources and well-being. *Demography, 49,* 23–47. https://doi.org/10.1007/s13524-011-0080-x

Östberg, M., and Hagekull, B. (2013). Parenting stress and external stressors as predictors of maternal ratings of child adjustment. *Scandinavian Journal of Psychology, 54*(3), 213–221. https://doi.org/10.1111/sjop.12045

Östberg, M., Hagekull, B., and Hagelin, E. (2007). Stability and prediction of parenting stress. *Infant and Child Development, 16*(2), 207–223. https://doi.org/10.1002/icd.516

Östberg, M., Hagekull, B., and Wettergren, S. (1997). A measure of parental stress in mothers with small children: Dimensionality, stability and validity. *Scandinavian Journal of Psychology, 38,* 199–208.

Pai, A., Greenley, R., Lewandowski, A., Drotar, D., Youngstrom, E., and Peterson, C. (2007). A meta-analytic review of the influence of pediatric cancer on parent and family functioning. *Journal of Family Psychology, 21,* 407–415. https://doi.org/10.1037/0893-3200.21.3.407

Patterson, C.R. (1983). Stress: A change agent for family process. In N. Garmezy and M. Rutter (Eds.), *Stress, coping, and development in children* (pp. 235–264). New York, NY: McGraw-Hill.

Paulussen-Hoogeboom, M., Stams, G.J.J.M., Hermanns, J.M.A., and Peetsma, T.T.D. (2008). Relations among child negative emotionality, parenting stress, and maternal sensitive responsiveness in early childhood. *Parenting: Science and Practice, 8*(1), 1–16. https://doi.org/10.1080/15295190701830656

Pedersen, A.L., Crnic, K.A., Baker, B.L., and Blacher, J. (2015). Reconceptualizing family adaptation to developmental delay. *American Journal on Intellectual and Developmental Disabilities, 120*(4), 346–370. https://doi.org.ezproxy1.lib.asu.edu/10.1352/1944-7558-120.4.346

Petch, J.F., Halford, W.K., Creedy, D.K., and Gamble, J. (2012). A randomized controlled trial of a couple relationship and coparenting program (couple CARE for parents) for high- and low-risk new parents. *Journal of Consulting and Clinical Psychology, 80*(4), 662–673. https://doi.org/10.1037/a0028781

Pinquart, M. (2017). Parenting stress in caregivers of children with chronic physical condition—a meta-analysis. *Stress and Health: Journal of the International Society for the Investigation of Stress.* https://doi.org/10.1002/smi.2780

Platt, R., Williams, S.R., and Ginsburg, G.S. (2016). Stressful life events and child anxiety: Examining parent and child mediators. *Child Psychiatry and Human Development, 47,* 23–34. https://doi.org/10.1007/s10578-015-0540-4

Puff, J., and Renk, K. (2014). Relationships among parents' economic stress, parenting, and young children's behavior problems. *Child Psychiatry and Human Development, 45*(6), 712–27. https://doi.org/10.1007/s10578-014-0440-z

Putnick, D.L., Bornstein, M.H., Hendricks, C., Painter, K.M., Suwalsky, J.T.D., and Collins, W.A. (2008). Parenting stress, perceived parenting behaviors, and adolescent self-concept in European American families. *Journal of Family Psychology, 22*(5), 752–762. https://doi.org/10.1037/a0013177

Putnick, D.L., Bornstein, M.H., Hendricks, C., Painter, K.M., Suwalsky, J.T.D., and Collins, W.A. (2010). Stability, continuity, and similarity of parenting stress in European American mothers and fathers across their child's transition to adolescence. *Parenting: Science and Practice, 10*(1), 60–77. https://doi.org/10.1080/15295190903014638

Rabkin, J.G., and Struening, E.L. (1976). Life events, stress, and illness. *Science, 194*(4269), 1013–1020. https://doi.org.ezproxy1.lib.asu.edu/10.1126/science.7905

Rantanen, J., Tillemann, K., Metsäpelto, R., Kokko, K., and Pulkkinen, L. (2015). Longitudinal study on reciprocity between personality traits and parenting stress. *International Journal of Behavioral Development, 39*(1), 65–76. https://doi.org/10.1177/0165025414548776

Repetti, R.L., and Robles, T.F. (2016). Nontoxic family stress: Potential benefits and underlying biology. *Family Relations: An Interdisciplinary Journal of Applied Family Studies, 65*(1), 163–175. https://doi.org/10.1111/fare.12180

Repetti, R.L., Robles, T.F., and Reynolds, B. (2011). Allostatic processes in the family. *Development and Psychopathology, 23,* 921–938. https://doi.org/10.1017/S095457941100040X

Riina, E.M., and McHale, S.M. (2012). The trajectory of coparenting satisfaction in African American families: The impact of sociocultural stressors and supports. *Journal of Family Psychology, 26*(6), 896–905. https://doi.org/10.1037/a0030055

Riley, M.R., Scaramella, L.V., and McGoron, L. (2014). Disentangling the associations between contextual stress, sensitive parenting, and children's social development. *Family Relations, 63*(2), 287–299. https://doi.org/10.1111/fare.12063

Robinson, M., Mattes, E., Oddy, W.H., Pennell, C.E., van Eekelen, A., McLean, N.J., . . . Newnham, J.P. (2011). Prenatal stress and risk of behavioral morbidity from age 2 to 14 years: The influence of the number, type, and timing of stressful life events. *Development and Psychopathology, 23*(2), 507–20. https://doi.org/10.1017/S0954579411000241

Romens, S.E., McDonald, J., Svaren, J., and Pollak, S.D. (2015). Associations between early life stress and gene methylation in children. *Child Development, 86*(1), 303–309. https://doi.org/10.1111/cdev.12270

Ryan, R.M., and Padilla, C.M. (2019). Transition to parenthood. In M.H. Bornstein (Ed.), *Handbook of parenting Vol. 3: Being and becoming a parent* (3rd ed., pp. 513–555). New York, NY: Routledge.

Sandler, I.N., and Block, M. (1979). Life stress and maladaptation of children. *American Journal of Community Psychology, 7*(4), 425–440. https://doi.org/10.1007/BF00894384

Scaramella, L.V., Sohr-Preston, S., Callahan, K.L., and Mirabile, S.P. (2008). A test of the family stress model on toddler-aged children's adjustment among hurricane Katrina impacted and nonimpacted low-income families. *Journal of Clinical Child and Adolescent Psychology, 37*(3), 530–541. https://doi.org/10.1080/15374 410802148202

Schoppe-Sullivan, S., Settle, T., Lee, J., and Kamp Dush, C.M. (2016). Supportive coparenting relationships as a haven of psychological safety at the transition to parenthood. *Research in Human Development, 13*(1), 32–48. https://doi.org/10.1080/15427609.2016.1141281

Shelleby, E.C., Votruba-Drzal, E., Shaw, D.S., Dishion, T.J., Wilson, M.N., and Gardner, F. (2014). Income and children's behavioral functioning: A sequential mediation analysis. *Journal of Family Psychology, 28*(6), 936–946. https://doi.org/10.1037/fam0000035

Shenk, C.E., Ammerman, R.T., Teeters, A.R., Bensman, H.E., Allen, E.K., Putnam, F.W., and Van Ginkel, J.B. (2017). History of maltreatment in childhood and subsequent parenting stress in at-risk, first-time mothers: Identifying points of intervention during home visiting. *Prevention Science, 18*(3), 361–370. https://doi. org/10.1007/s11121-017-0758-4

Sheppes, G., Suri, G., and Gross, J.J. (2015). Emotion regulation and psychopathology. *Annual Review of Clinical Psychology, 11*, 379–405.

Sheras, P.L., Abidin, R.R., and Konold, T.R. (1998). *Stress index for parents of adolescents: Professional manual.* Odessa, FL: Psychological Assessment Resources.

Singer, G.H.S., Ethridge, B.L., and Aldana, S.I. (2007). Primary and secondary effects of parenting and stress management interventions for parents of children with developmental disabilities: A meta-analysis. *Mental Retardation and Developmental Disabilities Research Reviews, 13*(4), 357–369. https://doi.org/10.1002/mrdd.20175

Skreden, M., Skari, H., Malt, U.F., Pripp, A.H., Björk, M.D., Faugli, A., and Emblem, R. (2012). Parenting stress and emotional wellbeing in mothers and fathers of preschool children. *Scandinavian Journal of Public Health, 40*(7), 596–604. https://doi.org/10.1177/1403494812460347

Soenens, B., Vanteenkiste, M., and Beyers, W. (2019). Parenting adolescents. In M.H. Bornstein (Ed.), *Handbook of parenting Vol. 1: Children and parenting* (3rd ed., pp. 111–167). New York, NY: Routledge.

Solem, M., Christophersen, K., and Martinussen, M. (2011). Predicting parenting stress: Children's behavioural problems and parents' coping. *Infant and Child Development, 20*(2), 162–180. https://doi.org/10.1002/icd.681

Sprang, G., Clark, J.J., and Bass, S. (2005). Factors that contribute to child maltreatment severity: A multi-method and multidimensional investigation. *Child Abuse and Neglect, 29*(4), 335–350. https://doi.org.ezproxy1.lib. asu.edu/10.1016/j.chiabu.2004.08.008

Steeger, C.M., Gondoli, D.M., and Morrissey, R.A. (2013). Maternal avoidant coping mediates the effect of parenting stress on depressive symptoms during early adolescence. *Journal of Child and Family Studies, 22*(7), 952–961. https://doi.org/10.1007/s10826-012-9657-2

Stone, L.L., Mares, S.H.W., Otten, R., Engels, R.C.M.E., and Janssens, J.M.A.M. (2016). The co-development of parenting stress and childhood internalizing and externalizing problems. *Journal of Psychopathology and Behavioral Assessment, 38*(1), 76–86. https://doi.org/10.1007/s10862-015-9500-3

Straus, M.A. (1980). Stress and physical child abuse. *Child Abuse and Neglect, 4*(2), 75–88.

Strauss, K., Vicari, S., Valeri, G., D'Elia, L., Arima, S., and Fava, L. (2012). Parent inclusion in early intensive behavioral intervention: The influence of parental stress, parent treatment fidelity, and parent mediated generalization of behavior targets on child outcomes. *Research in Developmental Disabilities, 33*, 688–703. doi:10.1016/j.ridd.2011.11.008

Sturge-Apple, M., Skibo, M.A., Rogosch, F.A., Ignjatovic, Z., and Heinzelman, W. (2011). The impact of allostatic load on maternal sympathovagal functioning in stressful child contexts: Implications for problematic parenting. *Development and Psychopathology, 23*(3), 831–844. https://doi.org/10.1017/S0954579411000332

Sturge-Apple, M.A., Toth, S.L., Suor, J.H., and Adams, T.R. (2019). Parental maltreatment. In M.H. Bornstein (Ed.), *Handbook of parenting Vol. 4: Social conditions and applied parenting* (3rd ed., pp. 556–589). New York, NY: Routledge.

Tharner, A., Luijk, M.P.C.M., van IJzendoorn, M.H., Bakermans-Kranenburg, M., Jaddoe, V.W.V., Hofman, A., . . . Tiemeier, H. (2012). Infant attachment, parenting stress, and child emotional and behavioral problems at age 3 years. *Parenting: Science and Practice, 12*(4), 261–281. https://doi.org/10.1080/15295192.2012. 709150

Theule, J., Wiener, J., Tannock, R., and Jenkins, J.M. (2013). Parenting stress in families of children with ADHD: A meta-analysis. *Journal of Emotional and Behavioral Disorders, 21*(1), 3–17.

Thomason, E., Volling, B.L., Flynn, H.A., McDonough, S.C., Marcus, S.M., Lopez, J.F., and Vazquez, D.M. (2014). Parenting stress and depressive symptoms in postpartum mothers: Bidirectional or unidirectional effects? *Infant Behavior and Development, 37*(3), 406–415. https://doi.org/10.1016/j.infbeh.2014.05.009

Webster-Stratton, C. (1990). Stress: A potential disruptor of parent perceptions and family interactions. *Journal of Clinical Child Psychology, 19*(4), 302–312. https://doi.org/10.1207/s15374424jccp1904_2

Webster-Stratton, C., and Hammond, M. (1988). Maternal depression and its relationship to life stress, perceptions of child behavior problems, parenting behaviors, and child conduct problems. *Journal of Abnormal Child Psychology, 16*(3), 299–315. https://doi.org/10.1007/BF00913802

Weinberg, S.L., and Richardson, M.S. (1981). Dimensions of stress in early parenting. *Journal of Consulting and Clinical Psychology, 49*(5), 686–693. https://doi.org/10.1037/0022-006X.49.5.686

Wiener, J., Biondic, D., Grimbos, T., and Herbert, M. (2016). Parenting stress of parents of adolescents with attention-deficit hyperactivity disorder. *Journal of Abnormal Child Psychology, 44*(3), 561–574. https://doi.org/10.1007/s10802-015-0050-7

Williford, A.P., Calkins, S.D., and Keane, S.P. (2007). Predicting change in parenting stress across early childhood: Child and maternal factors. *Journal of Abnormal Child Psychology, 35*(2), 251–263. https://doi.org/10.1007/s10802-006-9082-3

Yamamoto, N., and Nagano, J. (2015). Parental stress and the onset and course of childhood asthma. *BioPsychoSocial Medicine, 9*, 8. https://doi.org/10.1186/s13030-015-0034-4

Yaman, A., Mesman, J., van IJzendoorn, M.H., and Bakermans-Kranenburg, M. (2010). Perceived family stress, parenting efficacy, and child externalizing behaviors in second-generation immigrant mothers. *Social Psychiatry and Psychiatric Epidemiology, 45*(4), 505–512. https://doi.org/10.1007/s00127-009-0097-2

Yarboi, J., Compas, B.E., Brody, G.H., White, D., Patterson, J.R., Ziara, K., and King, A. (2017). Association of social-environmental factors with cognitive function in children with sickle cell disease. *Child Neuropsychology, 23*(3), 343–360. https://doi.org/10.1080/09297049.2015.1111318

Yu, S.M., and Singh, G.K. (2012). High parenting aggravation among US immigrant families. *American Journal of Public Health, 102*(11), 2102–2108. https://doi.org/10.2105/AJPH.2012.300698

3

YOUTH–ADULT RELATIONSHIPS AS ASSETS FOR YOUTH

Promoting Positive Development in Stressful Times

Stephen F. Hamilton, Mary Agnes Hamilton, David L. DuBois , M. Loreto Martínez, Patricio Cumsille, Bernadine Brady, Pat Dolan, Susana Núñez Rodriguez, and Deborah E. Sellers

In this chapter we examine relationships between youth and adults outside their families as sources of strength that can help young people thrive even in the face of stressful economic and social change. Such relationships are counted among the assets that promote positive youth development (Eccles & Gootman, 2002). Our treatment of the topic will emphasize the needs of low-income and otherwise marginalized youth. While acknowledging the primacy of family relationships for nearly all youth, we focus primarily on relationships with adults who are not family members, addressing the value of these relationships, what forms they take, which adults are most likely to be involved, and finally how such relationships can be fostered so that more of the youth who need them have access to, and benefit from, them.

The metaphor, social capital, is useful for our purpose. In a seminal article, Coleman (1988) wrote about "social capital in the creation of human capital," calling attention to the link between people's capacity to earn a living and the nature of their social networks. Lin (2001, p. 29) defined social capital as, "resources embedded in a social structure that are accessed and/or mobilized in purposive actions." In simpler language, social capital inheres in a person's ability to achieve her or his goals with the aid of people she or he knows. A person whose family, friends, neighbors, and other acquaintances can be called upon to help out has more social capital than one who is either more isolated – having a sparser social network – or whose acquaintances are less able to help.

A classic example is finding a job through "contacts," acquaintances who know about openings and perhaps can offer a recommendation. Three refinements of social capital theory are especially useful in the present context. The first is from Granovetter (1983), whose phrase, "the strength of weak ties," captures his discovery that the best sources for job prospects are people the job-seeker knows only slightly, such as a friend of a friend. The reason is that people with whom a person is closely associated tend to have the same sources of information and access. As a result, they add little to the job-seeker's search. People on the periphery of the job-seeker's network are most likely to know about new prospects and to be acquainted with people the job-seeker does not know. Hence it is through "weak ties" that a job search is most likely to succeed. More generally, this example illustrates how expanding one's network beyond close acquaintances can provide access to new resources that can prove important in achieving a goal.

The strong vs. weak tie distinction is related to a second refinement, the distinction Putnam (2000) made between "bonding" and "bridging" social capital. Bonding social capital exists among people who share many characteristics. Families, for example, share a common culture, traditions, language, often religion, and political preferences as well. Neighbors, members of religious congregations, and voluntary associations are also high in bonding social capital, which gives them a sense of identity with the group, of belonging, of being part of something larger than themselves. Bridging social capital, as the metaphor suggests, reaches across these kinds of group boundaries, making connections between people who belong to different groups. These connections enable people to encounter others who are different and to make connections and be stimulated in ways that may not happen within their more closely bonded communities. A low-income youth of color who attends an elite university not only gains a good education but builds bridging social capital as well.

The third refinement to social capital theory, related to bridging social capital, is the designation of some social network members as "institutional agents" (Stanton-Salazar, 2001, 2011), that is, as representatives of important social institutions who by virtue of their position and knowledge are able to aid outsiders, young people among them, in gaining entrée to those institutions and access to their resources.[1] College admissions officers are exemplars of institutional agents, as are people with authority to make or influence hiring decisions.

This conceptual orientation strongly suggests that family connections (i.e., bonding) are necessary but not sufficient as sources of social capital for youth from families and communities with limited resources. The job recommendation from such a family member might help a youth find a position in a beauty parlor or a corner grocery store but not a business office or large factory. That person might accurately urge the youth to study hard to get into college but have no knowledge of financial aid or of the difference between enrolling in a nearby college that is a local institution and another whose alumni move on to top graduate and professional schools.

The studies cited and reported in this chapter further elaborate evidence of the social class-based differentiation of young people's opportunities to form relationships with adults. Young people from low-income families whose parents have little education need assistance in building bridging social capital, in the form of relationships with people who have more resources, to aid their acquisition of greater human capital. A second topic is the contribution of youth organizations and schools to young people's opportunities to form development-enhancing relationships with adults. While these relationships arise in the course of youth program activities as a kind of second-order effect (Hirsch, Deutsch, & DuBois, 2011), growing appreciation of the importance of young people's relationships with adults outside their families has contributed to a movement to make mentors available to vulnerable youth (Rhodes, 2002), not only in the US, but in other countries as well. Data from a study of the Irish version of Big Brothers Big Sisters illuminates the different kinds of support mentors can provide. However, there are never enough volunteers and program staff to meet the needs of youth who could benefit from a mentor (Stukas, Clary, & Snyder, 2014). Moreover, most mentoring-type relationships occur naturally or informally, outside of mentoring programs. Hence, it is useful to examine how mentoring occurs naturally, both to deepen our understanding of who mentors are and what they do, and to gain leverage to foster such relationships intentionally, among other ways by designing programs in which mentoring occurs without formal one-to-one matching of youth with mentors.

The four studies reported in this chapter, from Brazil, Chile, Ireland, and the US, will be described serially. Themes tying the studies together will be identified as well and discussed in the conclusion section.

The Importance of Social Class: Differences in Brazilian Youths' Perceived Autonomy

In times of economic distress, those who are already in distress inevitably suffer the most. A dramatic illustration of this fact of life is found in a study of "informal mentors" in US high schools by Erickson, McDonald, and Elder (2009). Drawing on the National Longitudinal Study of Adolescent Health, the investigators found that students from families with lower parent education and family income who nonetheless had someone at school they could talk to – a teacher mentor – were nearly twice as likely to enroll in college as comparable students without such an adult relationship (65% compared to 35%), and nearly as likely to enroll as students whose parents had more education and more money but no teacher mentor (67%). Those students with more family resources, who had a teacher mentor as well were even more likely to enroll in college (75%) but the difference attributable to having a teacher mentor was not nearly so great. This study, employing a representative sample of the US student population and controls for other likely influences on the dependent variable such as grades and test scores, indicates that youth whose families have the least resources benefit the most from relationships with adults outside the family.

Susana Núñez Rodriguez studied autonomy and relatedness in Brazilian youth. At the time of this study, Brazil was experiencing strong economic growth combined with modest declines in income inequality and dramatically rising secondary school completion rates. Autonomy, competence, and relatedness are the three basic psychological needs identified in self-determination theory (Deci & Ryan, 1985, 2000). According to this theory, human behavior is driven by the quest for their fulfillment. The need for autonomy refers to the individual's will and desire to organize experiences and carry out activities coherently within an integrated sense of self (Deci & Ryan, 2000). According to Chirkov (2007), individuals may choose experiences that allow them to fulfill their need for autonomy within a collectivist environment as well as an individualistic one. The need for relatedness is met when a person has satisfying relations with friends and family, feels accepted by and is accepting of others for who they truly are, and is able to establish and maintain close and committed intimate relationships (Kasser, Cohn, Kanner, & Ryan, 2007).

Brazilian Study Design

Núñez's study included 970 participants, ages 18–30 years ($M = 22.8$; $SD = 3.4$) recruited from universities and schools in different regions of the country. In addition to a sociodemographic questionnaire, participants filled out, online or on paper, a Portuguese version of the Basic Psychological Needs Scale (BPNS, Gagné, 2003) and the Satisfaction with Life Scale (SWLS, Diener, Emmons, Larsen, & Griffin, 1985). Exploratory and confirmatory factor analyses were performed on the BPNS results. Multidimensional scaling was used to test for differences in autonomy related to participants' socioeconomic status (SES). Being predominately university and graduate students (90%), most participants were classified as coming from middle (54%) or high (32%) income families.

Brazilian Study Findings

Two findings are of particular interest for this chapter. One is that social class conditioned the association between relatedness and autonomy. For participants classified as lower SES, a stronger association was evident between autonomy and relatedness than those classified as higher SES. There was a statistically significant difference in need for autonomy according to SES (H(3, 970) = 10.274, p = .001), with high SES showing an average level of 516.58 and lower SES showing an average of 416.25. The investigators linked this finding to other research in Brazil indicating differences in the appraisal of autonomy and its association with SES (Vieira et al., 2010; Seidl-de-Moura et al., 2008; Barbosa & Wagner, 2013). These results suggest that, at least for lower-class Brazilian youth, autonomy is not necessarily a matter of gaining independence by leaving behind close ties but is a need that also can be fulfilled on the foundation of relationships.

The second finding is that the three-factor solution to the model of basic psychological needs that has been validated in the US and several other countries did not fit the Brazilian data, another indication of cultural differences in the meaning of autonomy to Brazilian youth. Rather than forming three distinct factors representing autonomy, relatedness, and competence, the responses of the Brazilian sample loaded on two factors that were best understood as representing competence and relatedness (see Table 10.1). While some items from the autonomy sub-scale could be joined with one of the other sub-scales, the most satisfactory solution dropped autonomy completely, in recognition that the BPNS did not adequately capture the meaning of autonomy for Brazilian youth. The resulting two-factor version demonstrated good internal consistency (alphas of .76 and .73 for relatedness and competence, respectively) and the subscales correlated well (.45, .54, p < .01) with the Satisfaction with Life Scale, demonstrating evidence of construct validity.

TABLE 10.1   Fit Indexes of the 3 and 2 Factor Models obtained in the Factorial Analysis

Factor Analysis	X^2	*df*	*WRMR/ SRMR[1]*	*RMSEA[2]*	*CFI[3]*	*TLI[4]*
CFA[5] (3 factors) (N = 294)	1558.797*	186	2.057	.112	.799	.773
EFA[6] (2 factors**) (N = 294)	905.771*	169	.060	.086	.892	.866
CFA (2 factors) (N = 301)	126.375*	43	.081	.087	.938	.921

(* p < .001; **Common shared variance = 64.96%)

1 Weighted Root Mean Square Residual/Standardized Root Mean Square Residual
2 Root Mean Square Error of Approximation
3 Comparative Fit Index
4 Tucker Lewis Index
5 Confirmatory Factor Analysis
6 Exploratory Factor Analysis

Brazilian Study Implications

The findings of this study suggest that relatedness and autonomy, even if they are fundamental human needs, along with competence, have different meanings depending on young people's social class and on their cultural background. Perceptions of relatedness and competence were differentiated among Brazilian youth, as captured in the factorial model. However, the items did not capture the perception of autonomy for Brazilian youth from different social class backgrounds, as they did in other countries, despite a very careful translation process. In Brazil, especially among lower-SES youth, the sense of self is associated with their relationships with others (e.g., family) and associations with their environment (e.g., school). In addition to pursuing the measurement issues raised by these findings, it would be intriguing to explore the behavioral implications, especially to learn what relatedness and autonomy mean for lower-class Brazilian youth and how both can be enhanced. (See also comparable findings from Chile by Martínez, Pérez, & Cumsille, 2014.)

Contexts for Adult Relationships: Youth Organizations in Chile

Participation in youth organizations can cultivate values (e.g., tolerance, social responsibility; Flanagan & Faison, 2001) and promote skills (Kirshner, 2008) that advance youth civic development when they provide opportunities for interaction and learning that match youths' developmental needs, abilities, and interests (Zeldin, 2004). Young people are most likely to benefit when organizations foster their active participation and when the quality of relationships that adults establish with young participants is high. Adult partners in youth programs and organizations can promote positive outcomes by encouraging participation, by mentoring (Rhodes, Reddy, Roffman, & Grossman, 2005), by employing good teaching skills, and by linking youth with community resources and leaders (Camino & Zeldin, 2002; Zeldin, Petrokubi, & MacNeil, 2008). The benefits of participation in youth organizations can be expected to occur when youth hold meaningful roles, have opportunities for collaboration in decision making (Finn & Checkoway, 1998; Zeldin, Camino, & Calvert, 2003), and share power with adults (Watts, Williams, & Jaegers, 2003). One such benefit that is especially important because it has implications for a healthy civil society is a growing sense of sociopolitical control, which includes leadership competence and political efficacy (Zimmerman & Zahniser, 1991).

Chilean Study Design

M. Loreto Martínez and Patricio Cumsille examined Chilean youth organizations as contexts for youth–adult relationships, focusing specifically on how those relationships build a sense of sociopolitical control. In addition to calling attention to the importance of the quality of youth–adult relationships and the distinctive characteristics of youth organizations in their country, they explored the function of identity as a mediator.

Growing up in a country that is still recovering its democratic institutions, Chilean youth are skeptical about government and the efficacy of participation in politics. Only 34% of 18–29-year-olds [INJUV, 2012] endorsed compliance with government as essential for democracy and 40% reported that they did not think it was possible to influence political matters. On the other hand, half were favorable toward participation in civil society and 45% said they participated in social organizations; 61% said social networks are more effective channels for expressing demands than voting (INJUV, 2012).

Participants in Martínez and Cumsille's study were recruited through youth organizations, assuring a higher than average level of membership. The sample included 370 older adolescents and young adults ($M = 21.18$, $SD = 2.37$, range = 17–26 years; 50.9% males), from Santiago and the Maule region. Most were students (89.7%); the majority came from middle-SES families (56%), indexed by parental education; low- and high-SES were equally represented among the remainder (i.e., about 22% each). Participants filled out a questionnaire on their perceptions of their *relationships with adults* in the organizations in which they were involved, including *caring/support* (6 items, $\alpha = .89$), *opportunities for reflection/processing* (4 items, $\alpha = .81$), and for *active participation in decision-making* within the organization (8 items, $\alpha = .87$). Identity measures included questions about *future orientation goals* (6 items, $\alpha = .82$) and *sense of personal coherence* (3 items, $\alpha = .80$). Finally, two indicators of sense of sociopolitical control were included as dependent variables, namely *leadership* (5 items, $\alpha = .76$) and *political efficacy* (4 items, $\alpha = .76$).

Chilean Study Results

These measures allowed for a test of a hypothesized model proposing that youth gain sociopolitical control when adults provide emotional support, opportunities for reflecting on experience, and opportunities to have a voice and role and when those characteristics of youth–adult relationships positively relate to youth identity. As Figure 10.1 shows, all measured indicators loaded high on their corresponding latent variables, thus providing evidence of the measurement properties of the model. Overall, the hypothesized model had an excellent fit to the data [$\chi^2 (11, n = 370) = 11.11, p = .43$, CFI $= 1$, TLI $= 1$, RMSEA $= .005$]. As hypothesized, the quality of youth–adult relationships within organizations had a positive association with identity ($\beta = .36, p < .001$), which in turn had a positive association with sense of sociopolitical control ($\beta = .57, p < .001$). More important, the hypothesized mediational role of identity was supported by the data ($.20, p = <.001$, 95% CI [.13:31]). Unlike the bivariate association between relational context and sociopolitical control, the regression coefficient

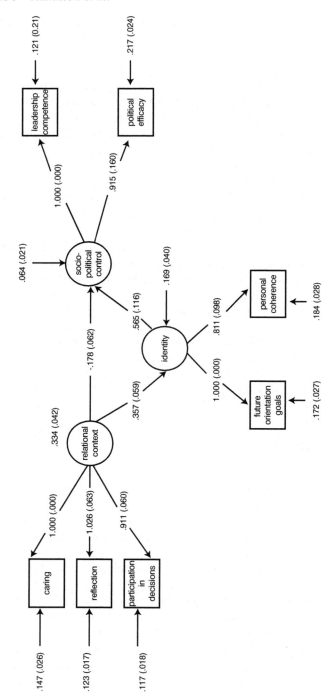

FIGURE 10.1 Hypothesized Model

linking relational context to sociopolitical control, even while controlling for the effect of identity, was significant. However, the association was, unexpectedly, negative ($\beta = -0.18$, $p < .01$), suggesting that identity acts as a suppressor in the relation between relational context and sociopolitical control.

Chilean Study Implications

This study offers support for the idea that the interpersonal context provided by supportive and caring adults in youth organizations allows adolescents and young adults to explore and consolidate their identity (Eccles, 2005; Kirshner, 2009; Larson, 2006; Larson & Angus, 2011). In turn, identity consolidation is reflected in youths' beliefs about their capacity to exert influence on sociopolitical issues. The findings also suggest that the quality of the relationships that youth establish with adults are relevant to identity across a range of organizational contexts. However, the unexpected negative direct association between relational context and sociopolitical control, after accounting for contributions of identity, suggests that whatever positive effects the relational context has on sociopolitical control goes through identity and, further, that the remaining variability in sociopolitical control that is not associated with identity is negatively associated to relational context. This latter possible process remains obscure, requiring further research. Perhaps when the relational context does not promote an autonomous self (identity), it is not conducive to an enhanced sense of sociopolitical efficacy but may be useful in other ways, such as for mental health or personal well-being. Both replication and triangulation using observational methods would help illuminate this issue. However, the capacity of youth organizations to give youth access to close relationships with adults who matter to them is clearly supported.

Forms of Support Adults Give to Youth: Findings from an Irish Mentoring Program

The creation of mentoring programs is the most direct response to the perception that youth benefit from close, caring, and enduring relationships with adults who are not family members. Resilience (Rutter, 1985; Werner & Smith, 1982) is one of multiple strands of theory and research that has contributed to the rationale for and design of mentoring programs. Previous research has revealed much about how youth mentoring programs work, including the contexts in which they are most likely to be successful, and their limitations (see DuBois & Karcher, 2013 for a comprehensive treatment of mentoring programs). Positive outcomes have been demonstrated in an array of areas, including emotional well-being, educational achievement, risky behavior, and relationships with parents and peers (Blinn-Pike 2007; DuBois, Portillo, Rhodes, Silverthorn, & Valentine,

2011; Tierney, Grossman, & Resch, 1995). Qualitative studies have explored some of the processes underpinning mentoring relationships. For example, studies by Spencer illustrated relational processes of authenticity, empathy, collaboration, and companionship in mentoring relationships (Spencer, 2006), reasons behind the termination of relationships (Spencer et al., 2014), and ways families are involved in mentoring programs (Spencer & Basualdo-Delmonico, 2014).

One of the primary purposes of mentoring programs is to strengthen the social support that young people receive (Barrera & Bonds, 2005). We know that the presence of at least one caring adult in a young person's life can help reduce stress and improve mental well-being (Dooley & Fitzgerald, 2012). However, the mentoring literature provides little guidance on the nature of the support provided by adults in youth mentoring relationships. By drawing on an in-depth study of nine successful mentoring pairs in the Irish Big Brothers Big Sisters (BBBS) program, Bernadine Brady and Patrick Dolan sought to identify distinctive types of support and highlight perceived improvements in the young person's welfare, particularly in terms of their emotional and behavioral well-being, that may have occurred as a result of this support.

Irish Study Design

The qualitative data reported here were collected as part of a larger mixed methods investigation that include a longitudinal quantitative study using a randomized controlled design ($n = 164$) (see Dolan et al., 2011a & b). At the time of recruitment to the qualitative strand, approximately 50 young people had been matched with mentors as part of the longitudinal quantitative strand of the study. BBBS project staff asked these participants (young people and parents) if they would also be willing to participate in a series of interviews with the research team. Twenty-one youth–parent pairs agreed and a purposive sample of 10 was selected to represent a balance across age, gender, location, family situation, and reason for referral. Two interviews were conducted with the mentor and youth as well as with the parent and caseworker on two occasions – at the early stages of the relationship and approximately six months later. One youth declined to participate after the first interview, leaving a sample of nine. At both the first and second round, five interviews could not be conducted (yielding 35 interviews in round one and 31 in round two).

After reading interview notes and transcripts several times to get a sense of the development of each match, and to note whether and how outcomes were reported in each case, the researcher identified themes and coded the data according to them, using NVivo software. Initial themes were then grouped into higher order categories. After coding all interviews, the researcher re-read transcripts and interview notes in full and made some revisions to the codes. Having four perspectives (mentee, mentor, parent, and caseworker) on each mentoring relationship enabled triangulation among different viewpoints regarding outcomes and processes.

Five male and four female mentees took part in the study. Their average age at the time of referral was 12 years. Only three of the youth lived with both parents at the time of the study intake. All the young people were Irish and all lived in rural areas or towns in the West of Ireland. The young people were dealing with a range of family and personal issues, including break-up of their parents' relationship, bereavement, incarceration of family members, behavioral problems, and low literacy. The average age of the mentor was 33 years on recruitment to the program; most mentors were single and had some higher education. Mentors and youth were matched by gender.

Irish Study Findings

Previous studies of social support in interpersonal relationships (Cutrona & Russell, 1990; Wills, 1991) have identified five types of social support: concrete (also called tangible, instrumental, or practical), companionship, emotional, esteem, and advice. These categories served well to group the kinds of support described in the interviews.

Concrete support is defined as the provision of practical acts of assistance (Cutrona, 2000; Dolan & Brady, 2012), whereas *companionship support* is defined as giving people a sense of social belonging (Wills, 1991). It enhances the pleasure of everyday life and contributes to emotional well-being (Rook & Underwood, 2000; Spencer, 2006). In mentoring relationships these two types of support are often intertwined. Many parents commented that their child "did not get out much," mostly because they as parents did not have time, money, or resources to make that possible and, in some cases, because the young person was shy and unwilling to engage in social events with peers. One of the most obvious forms of support offered by mentors was the companionship support of taking the young person out of the house to do something different for a few hours every week. The weekly activities involved companionship, including one-to-one activities such as going to cafes, cinema, and cooking, but also group events such as sports or youth clubs.[2] Parents and mentors who described this type of support also tied it to desirable outcomes, including increased confidence and new relationships with others in the community.

Concrete and companionship support was evident at initial interviews. Based on the analysis of interview data, it can be argued that this support can be provided before a close bond has been formed, helping to create a context and structure from which a friendship and discovery of shared interests can emerge, and from which emotional, esteem, and advice support can more readily be offered and accepted (see Keller, 2005, for a related discussion of the interplay of more relational and instrumental forms of activity, including the potential for instrumental activities to serve as important contexts for relationship development in a reciprocal manner).

Cobb (1976) defined *emotional support* as actions that lead a person to believe he or she is cared for. Emotional support took many forms in the mentoring relationships studied, including the mentor listening to and empathizing with the young person and acting as a "sounding board," and listening to accounts of daily events and challenges. Theoretically, emotional support can and should be provided in different ways to match the needs and coping styles of the youth. Illustrations in line with this idea were found in the interviews, for example, of girls who appreciated having someone to talk to about the stresses they were feeling. In comparison, the mentors' emotional support for boys was often less direct. One boy, for example, did not confide to his mentor for several months that his parents had broken up, yet seemed to gain emotional strength from the consistency of his relationship with the mentor.

> Myself and his father broke up in the last year, so there has been an awful lot of changes for Brendan. But I just think that Alan gives him that stability whereas I didn't, and his father didn't, you know? He still has a continuum with Alan; Alan was still here on the dot every week, once a week, sometimes twice a week. So it's certainly helped … He's had consistency as far as Brendan goes.
>
> (parent)

Esteem support results from one person expressing love and concern for another (Cutrona, 2000). Youth inferred their mentors' concern for them from the time they spent with them, while mentors' encouragement and praise for their mentees added to this feeling. There were also examples in the research of a mentee showing a mentor how to play or improve their skills in particular activities (such as music, swimming, or handball) and enjoying the positive feedback or esteem of the mentor for doing so.

Advice support is the fourth type identified. Mentors offered information and guidance. The feedback from research participants is that the ability to offer advice was something that came more easily when the relationship was better established, and where advice could be given in the course of a normal conversation, rather than more didactically. For example, one mentor, Liam, described how his mentee, Dylan, asked his advice regarding school and education.

> With regard to school I suppose he has not been asking me advice but we have kind of ended up talking about school and what he was going to do … so yes, I suppose he would have asked me advice on that or I'd have given my advice, I'm not sure which.
>
> (Liam, mentor)

Irish Study Implications

Inferences about the effects of these types of social support are all based on the testimony of those interviewed, not on formal measures. Yet, that testimony tended to converge around some of the same changes in emotional well-being and behavior control. Mentees were described as happier and calmer, more involved with other people, and more confident. Among their conclusions, the researchers found that their data and interpretation support the findings of other studies that if they are to flourish, mentoring relationships need frequent, consistent, and enduring meetings – and space – openness, and responsiveness to the needs of the youth.

Functional Roles of Natural Mentors in the US

Mentoring programs exist because, as Erickson et al. (2009) reported, those who most need mentors are least likely to have them. Most adult mentors of youth are not part of mentoring programs, and those programs face a chronic shortage of appropriate volunteers (MENTOR, 2005). Another concern is that mentoring programs can have iatrogenic effects (i.e., harm resulting from treatment). A young person whose assigned mentor does not work out for some reason can suffer from that failure, looking worse than a control group participant who never had a match (Grossman & Rhodes, 2002). The magnitude of the estimated effect found by Erickson et al. of having a natural mentor is noteworthy. The near doubling of college enrollment among low-resource students with a school-related natural mentor is far greater than effect sizes reported from mentoring program evaluations (DuBois et al., 2011). Although they applied multiple controls, Erickson and his colleagues reported a correlational finding, meaning that other factors may be at play. Still, their findings are certainly notable enough to warrant further research.

Natural mentors are non-parental adults who act as mentors without being assigned to do so through a program designed for that purpose (Hamilton & Hamilton, 2004; Zimmerman, Bingenheimer, & Behrendt, 2005). Young people find natural mentors in schools (Greenberger, Chen & Beam, 1998), workplaces (Mortimer, 2003), youth development organizations (Hirsch, Deutsch, & DuBois, 2011), other organizations, and in their communities. In addition to looking at natural mentors, this study asked youth about more than the provision of social support by mentors. While Brady and Dolan's focus on social support is prominent and appropriate in studies of mentoring, especially for younger youth, developmental theory and research tell us that older youth also need a goal orientation (Clausen, 1993; Schneider & Stevenson, 1999). Karcher and Nakkula (2010; see also Nakkula & Harris, 2014) helpfully treat the goal orientation (or instrumental) and socioemotional emphases of mentoring relationships as compatible.

US Study Design

These considerations motivated Mary Agnes Hamilton, Stephen F. Hamilton, David L. DuBois, and Deborah E. Sellers to investigate natural (or informal) mentors. The study employed the concept of functional roles (Darling, Hamilton, Toyokawa, & Matsuda, 2002; Hamilton & Darling, 1989), which adds depth and detail to the broad distinction between socioemotional and instrumental mentoring. The research drew both on the research just cited, which was done with middle school students and college students, and on retrospective interviews with two groups of young adults from low-income and minority communities on promising paths (Hamilton & Hamilton, 2012). Interview respondents talked about adults who taught them useful lessons and supported or encouraged them, who inspired and challenged them, who linked them with other people and resources, and who helped them acquire a sense of direction or purpose. We designated these functional roles: *Teacher, Supporter, Role Model, Challenger, Connector,* and *Compass.*

The study was conducted in two small southern California high schools that are part of a charter school organization. Students are accepted by lottery, to represent the income and ethnicity/racial diversity of their district. The mean age of students in both schools was 15.7 years (SD = 1.2). Young women were slightly over-represented in each school. A majority (70%) of Site 1 students self-identified as Hispanic/Latino(a), whereas this was true of 38% of students at Site 2. These percentages are close to the overall percent Hispanic/Latino(a) reported by each school. The response rate at Site 1 was 59% (n = 355 of 598); at Site 2 it was 54% (n = 313 of 583).

Following basic demographic questions, the survey asked students to identify their primary caregivers (i.e., parents or up to two other adults who were most responsible for raising them), then up to one additional important relative, and, finally, up to three important adults outside their family. For each of these adults, youth were asked to respond to the same set of 21 functional role items on a five-point response scale: not at all, a little, some, quite a bit, a lot. Students accessed the web-based survey on a computer, tablet, or smartphone. Exploratory factor analysis was used to investigate the factor structure of the items as rated for students' relationships with important non-familial adults. If a youth reported more than one such adult, ratings from the first (most important) adult were used. Additional analyses examined whether a similar factor structure was evident in ratings of students' experiences in their relationships with their parent/guardians and other important related adults (see Hamilton, Hamilton, DuBois, & Sellers, 2016).

US Study Findings

Surprisingly, only 22% of the students who took the survey (n = 148) reported having an important non-related adult in their lives; of those who did, 44% (n

= 66) identified just one such adult, 34% (*n* = 50) identified two, and 22% (*n* = 32) identified three. Students reported that they knew most of these adults (66%) in their school, either as teachers or in another role such as an advisor, administrator, or coach; 18% of the adults were reported to be known through involvement in other organizations (e.g., faith-based, sports, arts); the remaining 16% were described as having informal social roles in the youth's life such as an older friend, neighbor, or family friend.

Factor analyses of the functional role items for important non-related adults were conducted using an iterative process. The final solution was based on 14 of the 21 items and included four factors that accounted for 72.1% of the variance in the items. This factor solution is shown in Table 10.2.

Three of the factors consisted entirely of items intended for the *Supporter*, *Challenger*, and *Connector* roles, respectively, whereas the remaining factor included a mix of items intended for either the *Model* or *Compass* roles (the items intended for each functional role are indicated in Table 10.2). Scales based on the items that loaded most strongly on each of the factors demonstrated satisfactory internal reliability (coefficient alphas ranging from .77 to .87).

US Study Implications

This research sought to empirically differentiate the functions of mentors for youth with a higher level of detail and theoretical grounding than has been typical of prior work. Initial findings are consistent with the value of a functional roles framework for understanding natural mentoring among youth and, as such, could ultimately prove useful in the design and evaluation of initiatives to foster youth access to mentoring as one strategy to reduce inequalities (Putnam, 2015).

The survey measure that resulted from this research clearly should be regarded as preliminary and in need of further investigation, which should include examining support for the salience of the associated functional roles within larger and more demographically diverse samples of youth. Also meriting study are the associations of functional roles of familial and non-familial important adults as assessed on the instrument with expected influences on youth access to mentoring (e.g., neighborhood resources, school environment) as well as anticipated outcomes of mentoring (e.g., academic achievement, health, delinquent activity). Such research would serve the dual purposes of clarifying issues of construct validity and advancing theory (Smith, 2005).

These needs for further research notwithstanding, the four functional roles identified offer promising characterizations of the ways in which youth see their mentors. Combining the Compass and Model roles makes some sense insofar as youth may tend to look to mentors they want to emulate as sources for values. Distinguishing among mentors' functional roles opens the door to more refined studies in which the independent variable is not simply the presence

TABLE 10.2   Factor Loadings and Intercorrelations for Mentoring Functional Role Items

Item[a]	Supporter	Model/Compass	Challenger	Connector
	Rotated Factor Pattern Loadings[b]			
This person stands up for me.	.79			
This person is there when I need him/her.	.73			
This person cares about me.	.72			
This person helps me understand things about life.		.84		
This person helps me reflect on my purpose in life.[c]		.66		
I want to be like this person in some ways.[d]		.90		
I want to do things as well as this person.[d]		.65		
This person pushes me to do my best.			−.91	
This person gets me to work harder.			−.79	
This person holds me to high standards.			−.76	
This person points out where I need to improve.			−.75	
This person connected me to someone to learn what I want to know.				.86
This person connected me to someone to help me meet my goals.				.82
This person takes me to new places.				.42
Factor	*Factor Intercorrelations*			
Supporter	−			
Model/Compass	.45	−		
Challenger	−.33	−.46	−	
Connector	.25	.37	.38	−

Note. The following seven items were not included in the final factor solutions (intended functional roles are indicated in parentheses): "This person supports me in what I do" (Supporter), "This person teaches me how to do things" (Model), "I respect what this person has achieved" (Model), "I get values from this person" (Compass), "Ideas I have about right/wrong come from this person" (Compass), "This person helps me see the impact of my behavior on others" (Compass), and "I do things with this person I haven't done before" (Connector).

a For each item, the youth rated how much the statement described their relationship with this adult: Not at all, A little, Some, Quite a bit, A lot.

b Factor loadings <.35 are not included in the table.

c Item intended to assess the Compass functional role.

d Item intended to assess the Model functional role.

of a mentor but the profile of mentoring functions a youth is receiving. It also makes possible examination of different functions that might be performed by multiple mentors for one youth, simultaneously or sequentially, thus informing a social network perspective on mentoring that to date is largely lacking in the literature (Keller & Blakeslee, 2014).

A concern raised by this study is that only a minority of survey respondents reported an important unrelated adult: 21% of those at Site 1, 23% at Site 2. This aspect of our findings was discordant with previous research (e.g., Bruce & Bridgeland, 2014; DuBois & Silverthorn, 2005). In an effort to better understand what might have happened, we conducted brief focus groups and interviews with students in both schools. Seven focus groups were conducted with a total of 77 students and individual interviews were conducted with 27 additional students, five of whom had not taken the survey. These were convenience samples; they included approximately equal numbers of male and female students from all racial and ethnic groups. In stark contrast to the survey, nearly every student we asked face-to-face told us about at least one important non-family adult in his or her life. Only two of the students interviewed said they could not identify such an adult.

Although average completion time for the survey was only 12 minutes, our conversations with students revealed that several of them found the survey too long and too repetitive. They simply stopped responding before getting to the questions about non-family adults. We believe improving the survey design and recruitment would increase participation. We had both higher response rates and far more reports of important adults outside the family on a simpler paper-and-pencil survey in a pre-test. In the focus groups, students told us they would have been more likely to complete the survey if they had been asked to do it in class-time. Some suggested using Instagram or Facebook, technology more appealing than web surveys. Students also told us that talking face-to-face and hearing our explanation of why we were asking the questions and what we planned to do with the data made them more interested in participating. They also said incentives for participation were appealing. Finally, several students strongly endorsed the idea of engaging students in designing and conducting a survey.

Implications and Conclusions from the Four Studies

The four studies presented in this chapter from three continents all sound variations on the theme of young people's relationships with adults outside their families as resources in times of stressful economic and social change. The importance of those relationships is well-grounded in the research literature; these studies illuminate some of the intricacies inherent in them.

By showing that relatedness and autonomy are positively associated among low-SES Brazilian youth and that the factor structure of the widely used Basic Psychological Needs Scale works best without autonomy for their Brazilian sample (with only relatedness and competence), Nuñéz's work reminds us that neither relationships nor their impact should be expected to be uniform across social classes and cultures. This poses a warning to researchers planning to measure these constructs that instruments developed in one culture may not be valid in another and to policy makers and practitioners that mentoring and other interventions designed to meet young people's basic psychological needs are not necessarily transferable. What works for some youth in some contexts may well not work for others.

Martínez and Cumsille's study of Chilean youth is encouraging. Despite considerable skepticism among youth about conventional political engagement, Chilean youth organizations offer a space for participation, leadership, and the development and enactment of caring and supportive relationships with adults, decision making, leadership, political efficacy, and opportunities for reflection, all desirable and productive. Unexpectedly, the predicted association of the quality of youths' relationships with adults in these settings with sociopolitical control proved to be negative, raising questions to be answered in the future. But two conclusions seem warranted. One is that youth organizations can provide many constructive experiences for young people, including the chance to build relationships with adults outside the family. The other is that simply being there is not enough. Quality counts. The programs and the relationships have to be good. The adults need to be skilled. Most of all they need to be willing and able to share power with young people, to give them real responsibility, making them part of the decision-making process. Adults must create partnerships with youth (Zeldin, Camino, & Mook, 2005) and make multiple careful judgments in the moment about what young people can manage, when to push, and when to stand back (Larson, Walker, & Pearce, 2005).

Brady and Dolan help to open up the nature of high-quality youth–adult relationships, differentiating the core concept of social support into five types: concrete, companionship, emotional, esteem, and advice. This typology helps to explicate what a high-quality relationship looks like between an adult mentor and a young person, especially one whose family has limited capacity. The observation that a mentor can provide concrete and companionship support without a close and strong relationship but that such support can become a platform for the more personal types of support (emotional and esteem) offers a suggestion about the possible developmental trajectory of a close and enduring mentoring relationship that should be useful to mentors and those who work with them.

Hamilton, Hamilton, DuBois, and Sellers (2016) offer a related but somewhat different typology in which support(er) is an important function of mentoring but is joined by three more functions: challenger, connector, and model/compass, all having a more instrumental or goal-directed orientation, possibly because they studied older youth. When mentoring programs, youth organizations, schools, and communities are all considered potential sources of adult relationships for youth, the opportunities appear broader. These findings also point to different facets of mentoring relationships, both natural and program-supported, that merit further examination both in terms of processes involved and developmental outcomes to examine. We need to learn more about the nature of support exchanges and roles in mentoring, the quality of youth–adult relationships in youth programs and their association with different developmental outcomes. The Brazilian study reminds us that the influences of culture and social class should be examined in relation to all of these issues.

Social Inventions to Increase Access to Natural Mentors

If we accept the premise of this chapter that such relationships are beneficial and that they are especially important for youth facing stressful times with few resources, then the question becomes how to create more opportunities for those youth. Mentoring programs have demonstrated their value in giving youth greater access to adults. While advocating their greater use we also propose the modification of existing organizations and institutions creating social inventions (Hamilton & Hamilton, 2015) to enhance natural mentoring without necessarily matching mentors and mentees one-to-one. Some illustrations follow, drawn from or suggested by the reports above.

Advisory Groups

The small high schools studied by Hamilton et al. (2015) are examples of what Freedman (1993) called "mentor-rich environments," places where mentoring is likely to happen without formal intervention. One social invention (Whyte, 1982) in those schools, but not unique to them, is the advisory group, in which a stable cross-age set of students meets regularly with a teacher or staff member to do things together and talk about issues of mutual interest. This group is an example of the kind of invention that is needed to take full advantage of making any school experientially smaller for students even if the school's total size remains large.

Civic Engagement Projects

Martínez and Cumsille's study of Chilean youth organizations demonstrates that political attitudes and the skills needed for community involvement are formed not only in explicitly political contexts but also in civil society more broadly. Participation in decision making as well as experiences in leadership and planning in contexts such as youth organizations and school can build a sense of competence and commitment that carries over to political and non-political organizations in the larger community and nation. As they and others pointed out, adults need to make it possible for youth to take real responsibilities, wield genuine power, and have a chance to think and talk or reflect on their experiences. Service-learning is an especially powerful form of civic engagement for youth in which action to improve the community is central, but opportunities for youth learning are equally important. The convergence between mentoring and service-learning is illustrated by the Irish Big Brothers Big Sisters program's sponsorship of citizenship projects by participants (www.foroige.ie/citizenship/inspiration-your-citizenship-project).

Jobs and Internships

Work and work-like experiences can be used for career exploration, job training, or more general education. They give young people paid or unpaid work-based learning experiences in which they can engage with adults in goal-directed activity. As with civic engagement projects done in partnership with adults, these experiences are conducive to the formation of close relationships (Hamilton & Hamilton, 2004). Despite the fact that many youth jobs offer only limited contact with adults, a surprising number of young workers report that their adult supervisors are important people in their lives (Mortimer, 2003). We can hypothesize that the process of joint engagement in instrumentally meaningful activities can foster close ties, or, in functional role terms, that instrumental roles may evolve into more personal, emotional roles. This would appear to be a complementary trajectory to concrete and companionship support serving as a foundation for deeper and more personal mentoring relationships observed in the Irish study.

Community Activation

When citizens and leaders, including youth, come together and agree that it is important for youth to be incorporated into the life of their community, they can find many ways to change organizations, in addition to creating new programs, for this purpose.[3] Consider, for example, taking greater advantage of the cross-age membership of faith-based organizations. Although families may participate in some services, other activities are age-graded when young people might be intentionally integrated with adults as a way of sharing the responsibilities of nurturing children beyond the immediate family and enabling the youth to get to know a wider range of caring adults. This kind of change, like adding youth members to local government committees, takes a consensus within the community or organization that youth belong in such places, that they should have a voice, and that adults who are not their parents and teachers bear some responsibility for promoting their development. In view of the sad reality that some adults are capable of doing harm to young people, that consensus should extend to the creation of new norms, expectations, and procedures around youth–adult relationships. Youth can learn how to invite adults to become their mentors and then how to make the most of the opportunity. Adults can be encouraged to welcome such invitations, to initiate them, and be coached in how to be an effective mentor. Parents should be involved appropriately in those relationships in recognition that they retain primary responsibility for their child's welfare and that one of the benefits of having a mentor is that it can improve relations with parents (Rhodes, Grossman, & Resch, 2000).

Cultural Norms and Youth Voice

We should also acknowledge that our recommendations presume an appreciation of youth empowerment that is not universal. Some societies and certainly some segments of all societies emphasize subordination to elders and view the idea of youth–adult partnership as improper. This may mean that the relationships look different in different locations and cultures, as suggested by Núñez's study, perhaps more hierarchical than we have envisioned. Research on this topic would be welcome.

That young people facing economic and social change need education and jobs is indisputable. Far too many need food, shelter, and protection from violence and diseases as well. Their parents and other family members should remain their primary sources of support whenever possible. But as we seek to promote the positive development of all youth we need to attend to their opportunities to watch, talk with, learn from, pattern themselves after, and interact on a progressively more equal way with adults who are not family members. Access to these opportunities comes with the privilege of attending a well-resourced institution of higher education, indenture in a high-quality apprenticeship, or membership in a high-functioning community. For the vast majority of young people who do not enjoy these privileges we must be more intentional and invest more resources to make these opportunities available. The studies reported and cited in this chapter provide some guidance toward that aim.

Acknowledgments

S. F. Hamilton organized the symposium at which the studies reported in this chapter were presented and was the principal author of the chapter. M. A. Hamilton collaborated in shaping and editing the chapter. D. L. DuBois, M. L. Martínez, and P. Cumsille also contributed to improving the entire chapter. The other co-authors are listed alphabetically.

Notes

1 This construct is related to "linking social capital," which is used in public health. See, for example, Szreter and Woolcock, 2004.

2 Unlike in the USA, the Irish BBBS programme is integrated into a "parent" youth service, which gives mentors and mentees access to groups and facilities if desired.
3 The Search Institute has methods and capacity to help communities coalesce around youth development goals.

References

Barbosa, P. V., & Wagner, A. (2013). A autonomia na adolescência: Revisando conceitos, modelos e variáveis. *Estudos de Psicologia (Natal)*, *18*(4), 649–658. doi:10.1590/S1413--294X2013000400013

Barrera, M., & Bonds, D. D. (2005). Mentoring relationships and social support. In D. L. DuBois & M. J. Karcher (Eds), *The handbook of youth mentoring* (pp. 133–142). Thousand Oaks, CA: Sage.

Blinn-Pike, L. (2007). The benefits associated with youth mentoring relationships. In T. D. All, & L. T. Eby (Eds), *The Blackwell handbook of mentoring: A multiple perspectives approach* (pp. 165–188). Malden, MA: Blackwell Publishing.

Bruce, M., & Bridgeland, J. (2014). *The mentoring effect: Young people's perspectives on the outcomes and availability of mentoring.* Washington, DC: Civic Enterprises in association with Hart Research Associates for MENTOR, the National Mentoring Partnership. Retrieved from www.mentoring.org/images/uploads/Report_TheMentoringEffect.pdf (accessed 15/03/2015).

Camino, L., & Zeldin, S. (2002). From periphery to center: Pathways for youth civic engagement in the day-to-day life of communities. *Applied Developmental Science, 6*(4), 213–220.

Chirkov, V. I. (2007). Culture, personal autonomy, and individualism: Their relationships and implications for personal growth and well-being. In G. Zheng, K. Leung, & J. G. Adair (Eds), *Perspectives and progress in contemporary cross-cultural psychology* (pp. 247–263). Beijing, China: China Light Industry Press.

Clausen, J. S. (1993). *American lives: Looking back at the children of the Great Depression.* New York: Free Press.

Cobb, S. (1976). Social support as a moderator of life stress. *Psychosomatic Medicine, Vol. 38* (No. 5 September–October 1976), 300–313.

Coleman, J. S. (1988). Social capital in the creation of human capital. *American Journal of Sociology, 94* (Suppl.), S95–S120.

Cutrona, C. E. (2000). Social support principles for strengthening families. In J. Canavan, P. Dolan, & J. Pinkerton (Eds), *Family support: Direction from diversity* (pp. 103–122). London: Jessica Kingsley.

Cutrona, C. E., & Russell, D. W. (1990). Type of social support and specific stress: Toward a theory of optimal matching. In B. R. Sarason, I. G. Sarason, & G. R. Pierce (Eds), *Social support: An interactional view* (pp. 319–366). New York: John Wiley & Sons.

Darling, N., Hamilton, S. F., Toyokawa, T., & Matsuda, S. (2002). Naturally occurring mentoring in Japan and the United States: Social roles and correlates. *American Journal of Community Psychology, 30*(2), 245–270.

Deci, E. L., & Ryan, R. M. (1985). The general causality orientation scale: Self-determination in personality. *Journal of Research in Personality, 19*(2), 109–134.

Deci, E. L., & Ryan, R. M. (2000). The "what" and "why" of goal pursuits: Human needs and the self-determination of behavior. *Psychological Inquiry, 11*(4), 227–268.

Diener, E., Emmons, R. A., Larsen, R. J., & Griffin, S. (1985). The Satisfaction with Life Scale. *Journal of Personality Assessment, 49*(1), 71–75.

Dolan P., & Brady B. (2012). *A guide to youth mentoring. Providing effective social support.* London: Jessica Kingsley Publishers.

Dolan, P., Brady, B., O'Regan, C., Russell, D., Canavan, J., & Forkan, C. (2011a). Big Brothers Big Sisters of Ireland: Evaluation study. Report one: Randomised controlled trial and implementation report. Galway: Child and Family Research Centre.

Dolan, P., Brady, B., O'Regan, C., Russell, D., Canavan, J., & Forkan, C., (2011b). *Big Brothers Big Sisters of Ireland: Evaluation study. Report two: Qualitative evidence.* Galway: Child and Family Research Centre.

Dooley, B., & Fitzgerald, A. (2012). *My World survey: National study of youth mental health.* Dublin: Headstrong & UCD School of Psychology.

DuBois, D. L., & Karcher, M. J. (Eds) (2013) *Handbook of youth mentoring* (2nd ed.). Thousand Oaks, CA: Sage.

DuBois, D. L., & Silverthorn, N. (2005). Characteristics of natural mentoring relationships and adolescent adjustment: Evidence from a national study. *Journal of Primary Prevention, 26*(2), 69–92.

DuBois, D. L., Portillo, N., Rhodes, J. E., Silverthorn, N., & Valentine, J. C. (2011). How effective are mentoring programs for youth? A systematic assessment of the evidence. *Psychological Science in the Public Interest, 12*(2), 57–91.

Eccles, J. (2005). The present and future of research on activity settings. In J. Mahoney, R. Larson,, & J. Eccles (Eds) *Organized activities as contexts of development* (pp. 353–371). Mahwah, NJ: Lawrence Erlbaum Associates.

Eccles, J., & Gootman, J. A. (Eds) (2002). *Community programs to promote youth development.* Washington, DC: National Academy Press.

Erickson L. D., McDonald S., & Elder, Jr., G. H. (2009). Informal mentors and education: Complementary or compensatory resources? *Sociology of Education, 82*(4), 344–367.

Finn, J. L., & Checkoway, B. (1998). Young people as competent community builders: A challenge to social work. *Social Work, 43*(4), 335–345.

Flanagan, C., & Faison, N. (2001). Youth civic development: Implications of research for social policy and programs. *Social Policy Report, 15*(1), 3–14.

Freedman, M. (1993). *The kindness of strangers: Reflections on the mentoring movement.* San Francisco, CA: Jossey-Bass.

Gagné, M. (2003). The role of autonomy support and autonomy orientation in prosocial behavior engagement. *Motivation and Emotion, 27*(3), 199–223.

Granovetter, M. (1983). The strength of weak ties: A network theory revisited. *Sociological Theory, 1*, 201–233.

Greenberger, E., Chen, C., & Beam, M. (1998). The role of "very important" nonparental adults in adolescent development. *Journal of Youth and Adolescence, 27*(3), 321–343.

Grossman, J. B., & Rhodes, J. E. (2002). The test of time: Predictors and effects of duration in youth mentoring relationships. *American Journal of Community Psychology, 30*(2), 199–218.

Hamilton, S. F., & Darling, N. (1989). Mentors in adolescents' lives. In K. Hurrelmann & U. Engel (Eds), *The social world of adolescents: International perspectives* (pp. 121–139). Berlin: Walter deGruyter.

Hamilton, S. F., & Hamilton, M. A. (2004). Contexts for mentoring: Adolescent-adult relationships in workplaces and communities. In R. M. Lerner & L. Steinberg (Eds), *Handbook of adolescent psychology* (pp. 492–526). New York: Wiley.

Hamilton, M. A., & Hamilton, S. F. (2012, October). *Mentoring in retrospect*. Presentation at the Society for Research on Child Development Themed Conference on Transition to Adulthood. Tampa, FL.

Hamilton, M.A., & Hamilton, S.F. (2015). Seeking social inventions to improve the transition to adulthood. *Applied Developmental Science, 19*(2), 87–107.

Hamilton, M. A., Hamilton, S. F., DuBois, D. A., & Sellers, D. E. (2016). Functional roles of important nonfamily adults for youth. *Journal of Community Psychology 44*(6), 799–806. doi: 10.1002/jcop.21792

Hirsch, B. J., Deutsch, N. J., & DuBois, D. L. (2011). *After-school centers and youth development: Case studies of success and failure.* New York: Cambridge University Press.

INJUV (2012). *7a Encuesta Nacional de Juventud 2012* [7th National Survey of Youth 2012]. Retrieved from: http://www.injuv.gob.cl/portal/wp-content/files_mf/septimaencuesta nacionainjuvcorr2.pdf (accessed 31/08/2016).

Karcher, M. J., & Nakkula, M. J. (2010). Youth mentoring with a balanced focus, shared purpose, and collaborative interactions. In M. J. Karcher & M. J. Nakkula (Eds), *Play, talk, learn: Promising practices in youth mentoring. New Directions in Youth Development* (No. 126, pp. 13–32). San Francisco: Jossey-Bass.

Kasser, T., Cohn, S., Kanner, A. D., & Ryan, R. M. (2007). Some costs of American corporate capitalism: A psychological exploration of value and goal conflicts. *Psychological Inquiry, 18*(1), 1–22.

Keller, T. E. (2005). The stages of development of mentoring relationships. In D. L. DuBois & M. J. Karcher (Eds), *Handbook of youth mentoring* (pp. 82–99). Thousand Oaks, CA: Sage.

Keller, T. E., & Blakeslee, J. E. (2014). Social networks and mentoring. In D. L. DuBois & M. J. Karcher (Eds), *Handbook of youth mentoring* (2nd ed., pp. 129–142). Thousand Oaks, CA: Sage.

Kirshner, B. (2008). Guided participation in three youth activism organizations: Facilitation, apprenticeship, and joint work. *Journal of Learning Sciences, 17*(1), 60–101.

Kirshner, B. (2009). "Power in numbers": Youth organizing as a context for exploring civic identity. *Journal of Research on Adolescence, 19*(3), 414–440.

Larson, R. (2006). Positive youth development, willful adolescents, and mentoring. *Journal of Community Psychology, 34*(6), 677–689.

Larson, R. W., & Angus, R. M. (2011). Adolescents' development of skills for agency in youth programs: Learning to think strategically. *Child Development, 82*(1), 277–294.

Larson, R., Walker, K., & Pearce, N. (2005). A comparison of youth-driven and adult-driven youth programs: Balancing inputs from youth and adults. *Journal of Community Psychology, 33*(1), 57–74.

Lin, N. (2001). *Social capital: A theory of social structure and action.* Cambridge, UK: Cambridge University Press.

Martínez, M. L., Pérez, J. C., & Cumsille, P. (2014). Chilean adolescents' and parents' views on autonomy development. *Youth and Society, 46*(2), 176–200.

MENTOR (2005). *Mentoring in America 2005: A snapshot of the current state of mentoring.* Washington, DC: Author. Retrieved from www.mentoring.org/downloads/mentoring_523.pdf (accessed 03/10/2015).

Mortimer, J. T. (2003). *Working and growing up in America.* Cambridge, MA: Harvard University Press.

Nakkula, M. J., & Harris, J. T. (2014). Assessing mentoring relationships. In D. L. DuBois & M. J. Karcher (Eds), *Handbook of youth mentoring* (2nd ed., pp. 45–62). Thousand Oaks, CA: Sage.

Putnam, R. D. (2000). *Bowling alone: The collapse and revival of American community*. New York: Simon & Schuster.

Putnam, R. D. (2015). *Our kids: The American dream in crisis*. New York: Simon & Schuster.

Rhodes, J. E. (2002). *Stand by me: The risks and rewards of mentoring today's youth*. Cambridge, MA: Harvard University Press.

Rhodes, J. E., Grossman, J. B., & Resch, N. L. (2000). Agents of change: Pathways through which mentoring relationships influence adolescents' academic adjustment. *Child Development, 71*(6), 1662–1671.

Rhodes, J., Reddy, R., Roffman, J., & Grossman, J. (2005). Promoting successful youth mentoring relationships: A preliminary screening questionnaire. *Journal of Primary Prevention, 26*(2), 147–167.

Rook, K. S., & Underwood, L. G. (2000). Social support measurement and interventions: Comments and future directions. In S. Cohen, L. Underwood & B. Gottlieb (Eds), *Social support measurement and intervention: A guide for health and social scientists* (pp. 311–334). Oxford: Oxford University Press.

Rutter, M. (1985). Resilience in the face of adversity: Protective factors and resistance to psychiatric disorders. *British Journal of Psychiatry, 147*(6), 589–611.

Schneider, B., & Stevenson, D. (1999). *The ambitious generation: America's teenagers, motivated but directionless*. New Haven, CT: Yale University Press.

Seidl-de-Moura, M. L., Lordelo, E., Vieira, M. L., Piccinini, C. A., Siqueira, J. O., Magalhaes, C. M. C., Pontes, F. A. R., Salomao, N. M., & Rimoli, A. (2008). Brazilian mothers' socialization goals: Intracultural differences in seven Brazilian cities. *International Journal of Behavioral Development, 32*(6), 465–472.

Smith, G. T. (2005). On construct validity: Issues of method and measurement. *Psychological Assessment, 17*(4), 396–408.

Spencer, R. (2006) Understanding the mentoring process between adolescents and adults. *Youth & Society, 37*(3), 287–315.

Spencer, R., & Basualdo-Delmonico, A. (2014) Family involvement in the youth mentoring process: A focus group study with program staff. *Children and Youth Services Review, 41*, 75–82.

Spencer, R., Basualdo-Delmonico, A., Walsh, J., & Drew, A.L. (2014) Breaking up is hard to do: A qualitative interview study of how and why youth mentoring relationships end. *Youth & Society*, 1–23. doi: 10.1177/0044118X14535416

Stanton-Salazar, R. D. (2001). *Manufacturing hope and despair: The school and kin support networks of U.S.–Mexican youth*. New York: Teachers College Press.

Stanton-Salazar, R. D. (2011). A social capital framework for the study of institutional agents and their role in the empowerment of low-status students and youth. *Youth and Society, 43*(3), 1066–1109.

Stukas, A. A., Clary, E. G., & Snyder, G. (2014). Mentor recruitment and retention. In D. L. DuBois & M. J. Karcher (Eds), *Handbook of youth mentoring* (2nd ed., pp. 397–409). Thousand Oaks, CA: Sage.

Szreter, S., & Woolcock, M. (2004). Health by association? Social capital, social theory, and the political economy of public health. *International Journal of Epidemiology, 33*(4), 650–667.

Tierney, J., Grossman, J., & Resch, N. (1995) *Making a difference: An impact study of Big Brothers Big Sisters of America*. Philadelphia, PA: Public Private Ventures.

Vieira, M. L., Seidl-de-Moura, M. L., Macarini, S. M., Martins, G. D. F., Lordelo, E. R., Tokumaru, R. S., & Oliva, A. D. (2010). Autonomy and interdependence: Beliefs of Brazilian mothers from state capitals and small towns. *The Spanish Journal of Psychology, 13*(2), 818–826.

Watts, R.J., Williams, N. C., & Jaegers, R. J. (2003). Sociopolitical development. *American Journal of Community Psychology, 31*(1–2), 185–194.

Werner, E. E., & Smith, R. S. (1982). *Vulnerable but invincible: A study of resilient children*. New York: McGraw-Hill.

Whyte, W. F. (1982). Social inventions for solving human problems. *American Sociological Review, 47*(1), 1–13.

Wills, T. A. (1991). Social support and interpersonal relationships. In C. Margaret (Ed.), *Pro-social behavior, review of personality and social psychology* (pp. 265–289). Thousand Oaks, CA: Sage.

Zeldin, S. (2004). Youth as agents of adult and community development: Mapping the processes and outcomes of youth engaged in organizational governance. *Applied Developmental Science, 8*(2), 75–90.

Zeldin, S., Camino, L., & Calvert, M. (2003). Toward an understanding of youth in community governance: Policy priorities and research directions. *Social Policy Report, 23*(3), 3–20.

Zeldin, S., Camino, L., & Mook, C. (2005). The adoption of innovation in youth organizations. *American Journal of Community Psychology, 33*(1), 121–135.

Zeldin, S., Petrokubi, J., & MacNeil, C. (2008). Youth–adult partnerships in decision making: disseminating and implementing an innovative idea into established organizations and communities. *American Journal of Community Psychology, 41*(3–4), 262–277.

Zimmerman, M. A., & Zahniser, J. H. (1991). Refinements of sphere-specific measures of perceived control: Development of a sociopolitical scale. *Journal of Community Psychology, 19(2)*, 189–204.

Zimmerman, M. A., Bingenheimer, J. B., & Behrendt, D. E. (2005). Natural mentoring relationships. In D. L. DuBois, & M. J. Karcher (Eds), *Handbook of youth mentoring* (pp. 143–157). Thousand Oaks, CA: Sage.

4

EMPLOYMENT AND PARENTING

Wen-Jui Han, Nina Philipsen Hetzner, and Jeanne Brooks-Gunn

Introduction

In this chapter, we review the prevalence and trends in parental employment over the past decades as well as in the foreseeable coming years, how trends in parental employment situated in the current global economy may shape parenting, and how that, in turn, may shape child cognitive, socioemotional, and physical well-being. We draw on literature primarily from the United States but also globally to expand our understanding of the topic and to provide international comparisons.

A family's ability to rear happy and healthy children depends heavily on resources, including those within and outside of the family. Parental employment is a critical component shaping resources available to the family. Mothers and fathers have been engaged in labor activity throughout human history, but the intensity and extensity of work and the degree of support from family members and from society have changed over time, as have trends in parenting. Dramatic macrodemographic and economic shifts in the past half century in the United States and around the world have shaped how parents conduct their daily lives and care for their children. Since the turn of the 20th century, women's labor force participation rates have risen, and women are increasingly working throughout their adult lives. Mothers, particularly those with young children, have entered the workforce in record numbers, and the 24/7 economy has altered when, how, and where parents work. The timing, intensity, work schedules, flexibility, and job stability of parental employment have become ever more critical to children's daily lives and well-being. At the same time, we have witnessed increasing involvement of fathers in childrearing and caring tasks as both parents manage the balancing act of family and work responsibilities. These changes have triggered intense debate about the implications for children's well-being, not only short term but also long term.

Theory and empirical evidence from different disciplines have posited that parental investments, including money (to nurture physical and psychological well-being and human capital, such as purchasing childcare, cognitively stimulating materials and environments), time, human capital (e.g., parental education) and psychological capital (e.g., parental mental health) influence optimal child development, but the level and types of parental investment depend heavily on parental employment. In this chapter, we refer to *parental employment* or *work* or *labor force participation* to mean an occupation by which a parent earns a living through salary or wages.

In approaching this topic theoretically, we begin with the notion that a young child's life revolves around parents and/or caregivers—from when to wake up, when and what to eat, when and how to play, and when and where to sleep—young children rely on a sensitive and responsive caregiver to have their most basic needs met. Aspects of parental employment such as timing, intensity, schedules, job stability, and job quality might all have an effect on child well-being through mechanisms including parenting. This chapter builds on scholarship on child and family development in sociology, economics, demography, and psychology to examine how parental employment might be associated with parenting and why it is important for children's well-being.

Trends and Changes in Parental Employment

Since the 1950s, we have seen a consistent rise in labor force participation—the percentage of the population working or looking for work—among women, particularly among mothers with young children, and this rise has occurred globally (OECD Social Policy Division, 2010). Nearly all the Organisation for Economic Co-operation and Development (OECD) countries have witnessed a substantial increase in parental employment particularly among mothers with children over the past half century (see Figure 8.1 from Schildberg-Hörisch, 2016, for 2011 rates of employment of mothers whose children are under the age of 3, between ages 3 and 5, and ages 6–14 in 38 countries). As can be seen in Figure 8.1, more than 60% of mothers with children under age of 6 were working, and the employment rate varied substantially between countries for mothers with children under age of 3 due to the availability of universal parental leave; countries such as those in Scandinavian regions with universal parental leave tended to have lower employment rates among mothers than their counterparts (Schildberg-Hörisch, 2016). For example, maternal employment rates are much higher during children's first year of life in countries without universal paid family leave such as the United States. Although the employment rate among mothers with young children has increased substantially over the past several decades, fathers' employment rates have remained fairly stable at about 90% for those with children under the age of 6 (Schildberg-Hörisch, 2016). Moreover, there is an increase in the overall hours worked by parents, particularly mothers, with children aged 14 or younger, and early return to the labor market by mothers after birth.

In the following sections, data from the United States are presented on the following topics—the rise in labor force participation, the increase in maternal employment in children's early years, the uptick in long hours of work, the emergence of the 24/7 economy and the push for nonstandard work hours by the service economy, the trend for less stable jobs, the increase in unemployment or underemployment during economic shocks, and changes in time spent with children.

Rising Labor Force Participation, Early Return, and Long Work Hours

In 1950 in the United States, one-third of females (aged 16 or older) were employed. By 2000 that percentage had increased to two-thirds (Bureau of Labor Statistics, 2007; Fullerton, 1999). Such dramatic increases occurred for women both with and without children. Currently, the labor force participation rates are far higher than they were in the recent past. In 1975 (the first year with public official data), about half of mothers (47%) with children younger than 18 were in the labor force, and about a third of those with children younger than 3 years old were in the labor force. By 2000, 73% of mothers with children under age of 18 were in the labor force and two-thirds of those with children under age of 3 were in the labor force (Bureau of Labor Statistics, 2007). Labor force participation in 2016 stands at 70% among all mothers of children younger than 18; among them, mothers with children aged 6–17 had the highest labor force participation (75%), followed by mothers with children aged 1–5 (64%) and by mothers with children under 1 year (58%) (Bureau of Labor Statistics, 2016a). However, labor force participation rate and employment rates grew the most for mothers with children under age of 3.

In 2015, the United States had about 34.4 million families with children under age 18, and about 90% of these families had at least one employed parent. In two-parent families, 97% had at least one

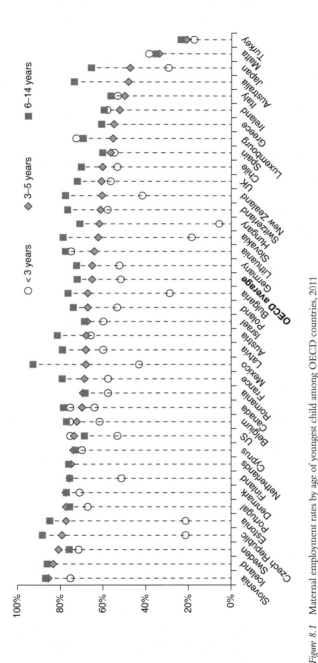

Figure 8.1 Maternal employment rates by age of youngest child among OECD countries, 2011

Source: Reprint from Schildberg-Hörisch, H. (2016). Parental employment and children's academic achievement. IZA World of Labor. Retrieved from https://wol.iza.org/articles/parental-employment-and-childrens-academic-achievement/long

employed parent, and 61% had two employed parents. Among single-parent families, 71% of the mothers in the female-headed families were employed, and 82% of the fathers in male-headed families were employed, although this last group is relatively small (Bureau of Labor Statistics, 2016b). In 2015, the labor force participation rates were 68% for married mothers and 75% for non-married mothers. The rates were 94% for married fathers and 87% for non-married fathers.

Among mothers with children younger than 18, African American mothers are the most likely to be in the labor force—about three-fourths are, followed by 70% among European American mothers. About 64% of Asian American mothers and 62% of Latin American mothers are in the labor force. Asian and Latin American mothers' relatively lower labor force involvement may have to do with the relatively high proportions of immigrants in these groups who are less likely to be working than their U.S.-born counterparts (Pew Research Center, 2015).

Work hours have also increased. The total annual parental work hours have increased by about 20% since the late 1960s, and more parents are working long hours (e.g., 50 hours or more per week; Fox, Han, Ruhm, and Waldfogel, 2013). Total annual parental work hours increased in both two- and single-parent families between 1967 and 2009; the increase was 16% from 2,663 to 3,092 hours in a two-parent family and was 35% from 938 to 1,262 hours in a single-parent family. In 2015, about three-fourths of all employed mothers with children under age of 18 were working full time. Of importance, the increase in work hours was concentrated among highly educated parents with children (Bianchi, 2011; Fox et al., 2013).

The rising educational achievements by females have also motivated women to join the labor market once they complete their schooling and stay in the labor force even on getting married and having children. For example, in the United States, in 1970, marriage and motherhood hold strong effects on women's labor force participation rates; the participation rate reached its initial peak at ages 20–24, fell at ages 25–34, and then gradually rose to another peak at ages 45–54 before tapering off. In 2006, this pattern of peaks and valleys was no longer evident, as women were more likely to work continuously throughout their lives. Now, women's labor force participation pattern by age looks like that of men, despite at a lower overall participation rate. Additionally, women now return to the labor market sooner after giving birth. Using a national birth-cohort sample born in 2001 in the United States, researchers documented the return to work within the first 9 months of a child's life—although only 7% of the mothers were working within the first month after giving birth, 26% of the mothers were working after 2 months, 41% by 3 months, and almost 60% were working by 9 months (Han, Ruhm, Waldfogel, and Washbrook, 2008). These trends were more pronounced in an urban birth cohort from the same period where almost three quarters of mothers were working by the time their children turned one year old (Berger, Brooks-Gunn, Paxson, and Waldfogel, 2008). Increasing employment by mothers with young children carries important implications for the early days of a child's life when attachment is formed to establish the foundation for healthy social relationship in a long run (Cummings and Warmuth, 2019). The recent increases in work—through maternal participation, early return after birth, and extended work hours—may have raised incomes for the two-parent family but not necessarily so for single-parent families (Fox et al., 2013).

24/7 Economy and Nonstandard Work Schedule

Together with the increase in female labor force participation, there has been an increased need for services that used to be fulfilled by mothers not in the workforce (e.g., childcare providers and health aides). In addition, jobs requiring nonstandard hours (often in the service and health sectors) have increased, given technological advances. Finally, jobs expecting rapid and continuous availability all have contributed to what is sometimes called the "24/7 economy." Nonstandard and variable work hours are more likely in service industries and continuous access to employees in more professional industries. The transformation of the market economy combining service and technology along with its deregulation of the labor and financial markets, privatization, and social spending cuts has contributed to a polarized labor market. At one end of this polarization is a significant proportion of skilled and highly skilled workers including working parents who work very long hours. At the other end is the large proportion of low- and semi-skilled workers who tend to work at non-daytime hours (or so-called nonstandard hours) and struggle to secure adequate employment or good quality jobs

Prior studies show that nonstandard work schedules are not unusual in many countries; in fact, at least one-third of the labor force in Australia, Canada, the United Kingdom, and the United States work such schedules (OECD, 2007; Presser, Gornick, and Parashar, 2008). Nonstandard work schedules are particularly prevalent among workers who have low wages (OECD, 2007). In the United States, African Americans, the less educated, and low-skilled parents are more likely than others to work nonstandard hours. Moreover, single mothers and parents with young children under age 6 are also more likely to have nonstandard work schedules (Presser, 2003).

In 1997, in the United States, one-third of married dual-earner parents with at least one child under the age of 5 had at least one parent working nonstandard hours during the week, and that figure went up to 60% if weekends were included (Presser, 2003). The prevalence of nonstandard work schedules was even higher among low-income or single-parent families. Sixty-eight percent of low-income dual-earner families with children under the age of 5 had at least one parent working at nonstandard hours, whereas 46% of single mothers with a child under the age of 5 worked at nonstandard hours (Presser, 2003).

Around a third of mothers report "childcare" as their primary reason for taking on nonstandard schedules (Presser, 2003). Working in the evenings, at nights, or on the weekend has thus become an adaptive strategy for many families to manage their childcare needs, especially when these needs are not met by formal care. The availability and cost of formal childcare during non-daytime hours is a barrier for many families who may have limited access to affordable care and informal care provided by friends and family.

Job Changes and Stability

As parental employment becomes more important, job stability also becomes more important to the well-being of the family. Job stability may be defined as changes in jobs, job loss, fluctuating job schedules, or income instability due to changes in jobs (Brand, 2015). Indeed, parental employment, including maternal employment during early years of a child's life, tends to fluctuate. For example, one study, using a national representative U.S. sample, examined maternal employment patterns within the first year of a child's life among women who were employed before childbirth, given these women would be more attached to the labor force than those who were not employed before the birth (Lu, Wang, and Han, 2017). The researchers found four distinctive patterns of maternal employment within the first year of a child's life: (1) mothers showed a high degree of labor market continuity and job stability before and after childbirth despite many mother's moves to scale back work after birth (57%); (2) mothers employed primarily part time before and after childbirth, with a small proportion of these women being self-employed (20%); (3) mothers who withdrew from the labor market over time (15%); and (4) mothers who gradually transitioned from full- to part-time employment, undergoing multiple transitions, resulting in dropping out or returning to full-time employment by the end of the first year (9%). Taken together, more than 40% of mothers within the first year of their child's life experienced transitions related to work intensity and type of work. Indeed, with a sample from an urban, predominately low-income, population of families, Pilkauskas, Waldfogel, and Brooks-Gunn (in press) documented that, over the first 5 years of a child's life, mothers were employed, on average, for 36 months out of 64 months. Great variation was observed: 20% were always (or stably) employed, 20% were employed for most of early childhood (48–59 months),

21% of mothers were employed for less than a year, and equally split percentages of the remaining 40% of mothers were employed between 1–2, 2–3, and 3–4 years.

Unemployment

Another set of issues related to parental work has to do with unemployment and underemployment. The unemployment rate is defined as being out of the labor force but looking for work. This rate includes those who have lost a job (quit or fired or laid off) as well as those who have not worked previously. It does not include those who are no longer looking for work (and thus is an underestimate of adults out of the workforce). Underemployment, which is typically not captured by labor statistics, means that individuals would like to work more hours.

Unemployed and underemployed adults fall into four groups: Those who are (1) marginally attached to the labor market (those who want a job, are available to work, and have searched for a job in the past year, but who currently are not actively looking for work—that is, they are not unemployed), (2) part-timers for economic reasons (referred to as involuntary part-time workers—those who worked 1 to 34 hours for reasons such as slack work or an inability to find full-time work), (3) unemployed (those who are without work, are available for work, and have actively searched for work in the previous 4 weeks), or (4) out of labor force (those who are neither employed nor unemployed).

In the United States, about 3% of the labor force was either unemployed or lost their jobs in 1994. These percentages climbed substantially during the Great Recession, which occurred from 2007 to 2009. The total percentage of people who fall into one of the four groups mentioned above was 9% in December 2007 and 17% by December 2009 (Brundage, 2014). At the onset of the 2007 recession, 7.6 million people were unemployed. When the recession officially ended in June 2009, the number of unemployed individuals had nearly doubled to 14.7 million, and it continued to rise well into 2010, before beginning to recover. In September 2014, the unemployment level had fallen to 9.3 million, as it continued to decline in the direction of its prerecession level. In December 2007, there were 1.3 million marginally attached workers. By June 2009, that number had increased substantially to 2.2 million, and stayed the same in September 2014. During the 2007–2009 recession, the number of people working part time for economic reasons rose to historically high levels—from 4.6 million in December 2007 to 9.2 million in March 2010. There were still 7.1 million working part time for economic reasons in September 2014. People who were unemployed or worked part time for economic reasons are two primary forces behind the finding that almost 20% of the civilian labor force is either underemployed or unemployed (Brundage, 2014). In 2012, more than one in six children, or 12.1 million, were affected by parental unemployment and underemployment, although this number was down from 13.5 million in 2010 (Isaacs, 2013).

This chapter does not focus on unemployment, but we would be remiss not to acknowledge the research on this topic. Job loss has been studied most often in relation to the Great Depression, the Iowa Farm Crisis, plant closings, and, more recently, the Great Recession. The first three unemployment events focused on fathers' job (or farm) loss. Elder (1974) and Conger and Elder (1994) studied the effects of job loss on family relationships and conflict, parental mental health, and parenting behaviors. The Family Stress Model is based on their findings as paternal job loss is associated with parental conflict, depression, and drinking, which are in turn related to harsh parenting (Conger and Elder, 1994). Similar findings are found for job loss in other periods (Brand, 2015; Coelli, 2011; Kalil, 2013).

Many studies have examined the impact of job loss and employment instability and found that both are predictive of poorer outcomes for children around the globe (Brand and Thomas, 2014; Kalil, 2013; Kalil and Ziol-Guest, 2005; Oreopoulos, Page, and Stevens, 2008; Rege, Telle, and Votruba, 2011) with particularly detrimental effects for low-income children (Gyamfi, Brooks-Gunn, and

Jackson, 2001; Hill, Morris, Castells, and Walker, 2011; Johnson, Kalil, and Dunifon, 2012). These adverse outcomes are likely explained by links between job loss and decreases in responsive parenting (Raver, 2003), poorer parental mental health (Chatterji, Markowitz, and Brooks-Gunn, 2013), lower quality of childcare, income instability, and residential instability (Kalil, 2013), and decreased quality in parent-child time together (Kalil, 2013).

Even when parents do not lose their jobs during a period of financial instability (like the Great Recession), parenting is affected by an overall loss in consumer confidence (Brooks-Gunn, Schneider, and Waldfogel, 2013; Lee et al., 2013; Schneider, Waldfogel, and Brooks-Gunn, 2017). These analyses drew upon the Fragile Families and Child Wellbeing Study which was in the field for several years since a child's birth until when they turned 9 years of age (2001 to 2010). Monthly national consumer confidence ratings as well as monthly national and local unemployment rates are available and matched to the interview month. Besides influencing parenting, national consumer confidence ratings were associated with child behavior problems (Schneider, Waldfogel, and Brooks-Gunn, 2015).

Time Spent With Children

Parental employment influences both the quality and quantity of parent-child time together. Using the 2003–2007 American Time Use Survey, Levin (2011) found that parental employment shapes the amount of time children spend with the parent. In general, for children aged under 13 in the United States, both married and unmarried mothers who were out of the labor force spent the largest amounts of time with their children (184 and 145 minutes per day on a weekday, respectively), followed by those who worked part time (140 and 101 minutes, respectively), those who were unemployed (121 and 97 minutes, respectively), and those who worked full time (90 and 76 minutes, respectively). Married fathers who were out of the labor force spent the largest amount of time with their children (111 minutes per day on a weekday), followed by those who were unemployed (98 minutes), those who were employed part time (67 minutes), and those who worked full time (54 minutes) (Levin, 2011, p. 321, Table 15.1).

At the same time, increases in parental employment do not always reduce time spent with children. Indeed, an extensive literature analyzing trends in parental time has reported that the increase in work hours by mothers has not brought about large decreases in primary childcare by parents. Literature has suggested two primary reasons for this: (1) parenting norms that have become more intensive mothering have increased the time mothers spend on childcare tasks, no matter what the employment status is (Sandberg and Hofferth, 2001), and (2) resident fathers have become increasingly involved in childcare and/or are spending more time with their children (Bianchi, Robinson, and Milkie, 2006; Sandberg and Hofferth, 2001). Specifically, research using time use surveys (Aguiar and Hurst, 2007; Bianchi et al., 2006) found that hours spent in primary childcare either somewhat declined or stayed constant from 1965 to the early 1990s, increased substantially from the mid-1990s to 2000–2003, and have leveled off since 2003. Considering changes in demographics and fertility rates over the entire period, Aguiar and Hurst (2007) found that, on average, both fathers and mothers have experienced an increase of 2 hours per week from 1965 to 2003 in time spent in childcare. Additionally, although longer work hours reduce total nonmarket time, employed mothers have at least partially protected time with children by decreasing hours spent in other activities, such as leisure (Fox et al., 2013). For some dual-earner families, non-daytime work schedules provide an alternative of managing childrearing tasks by jointly arranging employment schedules while protecting the time spent with the child (Fox et al., 2013; Presser, 1989). Fathers have spent substantially more time with children in families where mothers worked than those in families where mothers did not work between 1981 and 1997 (Sandberg and Hofferth, 2001).

For preschool and school-age children, activities outside the home (including both childcare and extracurricular activities, such as sports, music, and lessons of various kinds) have become increasingly popular and prevalent (Blau and Currie, 2006; Lareau and Weninger, 2008; Vandell, Simpkins, and Wegemer, 2019). Extracurricular activities for older children may increase parental time spent transporting and supervising children, whereas other activities such as preschool attendance may serve to level the amount of time both employed and not-employed mothers may spend with their children (Bianchi, 2000).

Time use surveys provide a detailed portrait of how much time parents spend with children, but information on the quality of that time is usually, if not always, lacking. When parents are working, child and parental well-being may suffer because of stress and time pressure, lack of sleep, and increases in multitasking (particularly if parents are taking care of tasks related to work while also caring for children), all of which may in turn compromise the parent-child relationship and the quality of parenting (e.g., less energy to attend to a child's cue). Bianchi et al. (2006) found that employment reduces the number of hours spent on housework by married mothers, reduces the number of hours for sleep and other personal care activities by single mothers, and doubled the number of hours spent multitasking for both groups.

Although it could be assumed that unemployed parents may be able to spend more time with their children, that may not necessarily to be the case, both in terms of quantity and quality. Studies examining time use during the Great Recession found that only 30% of lost market work hours are allocated to household chores and only 5% to increased childcare, and the bulk of the lost market work hours is allocated to leisure; however, women tend to allocate most of lost market work hours to household chores, whereas men tend to allocate a large fraction of the lost market work hours to watching TV and education (Aguiar, Hurst, and Karabarbounis, 2013). Such allocation of lost market work hours is not necessarily the case for all families, as some parents reduce children's extracurricular activities, which in turn saves some expenses and increases the time the parent and the child spend together (Morrill and Pabilonia, 2012). Increased time parents and children spend together due to job loss, however, may not necessarily result in quality time spent together, especially when it is the father who has lost his job (Elder, 1974). The normative gender roles endorsed by society may put greater psychological stress on unemployed fathers than on unemployed mothers. Studies have found fewer adverse effects of maternal unemployment compared to paternal unemployment on children's well-being. This was true even for families in which mothers were the primary earners (Kalil and Ziol-Guest, 2008; Rege et al., 2011).

Future Considerations on Studying Parental Employment

Dual-earner families have become the norm, and men's and women's roles have been converging, with men taking a more active role at home, doing a greater share of housework and childcare, and women spending more time in paid work (OECD Social Policy Division, 2010; Parker and Wong, 2013). Despite increases in employment among mothers, mothers still spend more time on unpaid work and less time on leisure than men. This may have in turn resulted in mothers still working and earning less than fathers. Below we highlight a few areas that warrant further research on parental employment.

1. Longitudinal data on parental employment throughout the first 17 years of a child's life. We have documented recent trends in parental employment, particularly the substantial increase in female labor force participation, especially among mothers with young children. Yet, we have not had literature documenting the pattern of parental employment over the first 17 years of a child's life and how that may shape parenting and child well-being (Pilkauskas et al., in press). Examining the pattern of parental employment, including the continuity, stability, and job characteristics (e.g., quality, intensity, schedules, and flexibility), through a longitudinal lens throughout a child's life offers invaluable insights into the pathways and trajectories of child

development being shaped and evolving, as well as the threshold and dosage of the contexts (e.g., family socioeconomic status, poverty status, family structure) helping or hurting optimal child development.

2. The link between job characteristics (e.g., variable hours, unpredictable schedules) and child well-being. More data and attention should also be paid to the importance of job characteristics to child well-being through parental mental health and parenting (Menaghan, 2005). For parents, schedule unpredictability makes it particularly difficult to arrange reliable childcare and participate in family activities and routines important to child development, such as monitoring homework and establishing bedtime routines. Involuntary part-time employment together with unpredictable work schedules may lead to economic insecurity, especially for low-wage workers.

3. Long work hours with nonstandard hours among socioeconomically advantaged families. A decent set of studies has documented the potential adverse effects of parents working at nonstandard hours on child development through compromised parenting and home environment (Li et al., 2014). This adverse effect is particularly salient for single-parent families and for families with low incomes. What the field has not paid much attention to is the other side of polarization—parents with high levels of education and professional jobs who work extremely long hours (e.g., 50 hours or more per week) including evenings and weekends. Although it is likely that children are more likely to be cushioned from the potential adverse effects of parents working extremely long hours due to rich family resources (e.g., purchasing quality care, providing an educational stimulating environment) than children of families with fewer resources, we have little empirical evidence to support the hypothesis.

4. The link between job loss/unemployment/recession on child well-being. Although increasing attention, particularly due to the most recent Great Recession, has been paid to how parental unemployment and job loss may be linked with child development, there is much we do not know (Kalil, 2013; Schneider et al., 2015, 2017). Parental employment is becoming fragile in the globalized economy and economies in which capitalism is exercised to the extreme (such as in the United States), and consequently, parental unemployment and job loss are becoming more likely than ever. The time it takes for the United States to rebound from recessions has increased since the 1980s (Bivens, 2016). As low-wage and low-skilled workers tend to be hit the earliest, the hardest, and the longest, understanding the impacts of parental unemployment and job loss has become more important than ever. The importance of parental unemployment and job loss is further underscored by the possibility that not only children whose parents experience such loss and disruption are hurting, but also children whose communities have suffered from economic downturns despite their parents still having jobs.

5. Gender roles in the 21st century. To fully understand the links between parental employment and child well-being through various mechanisms including parenting, we also need to pay attention to how gender roles may shape the impact of paternal and maternal employment and unemployment on child well-being. Increasing father involvement, particularly among married-couple families, has redefined the roles of fathers and mothers in shaping child development (Williams, Blair-Loy, and Berdahl, 2013). Although studies have documented the transformation of fatherhood between the 20th and 21st centuries from primarily providing money to the family to being both a breadwinner and a nurturing caregiver by making themselves available to be involved in the daily lives and routines of their children (Cabrera, Tamis-LeMonda, Bradley, Hofferth, and Lamb, 2000; Henwood and Procter, 2003), it is not clear if the primary breadwinner role of the father has diminished (Strazdins, Baxter, and Li, 2017; Williams et al., 2013), and mothers are still expected to do more caregiving (Sinno and Killen, 2011).

Without doubt, parental employment is linked with how mothers and fathers parent, which is tremendously important for child development. To understand how parental employment might shape child outcomes, it is critical to start with an understanding of how child development evolves and the social factors that influence it in the early years (Bornstein, 2002; Bronfenbrenner, 2005; Maccoby and Martin, 1983; Shonkoff and Phillips, 2000; Sroufe, 1979; Thompson, 2006). Below we focus on how parenting has direct influences on children's overall well-being and how one such factor, parental employment, may shape parenting.

Parental Employment, Parenting, and Child Development

Bronfenbrenner's Ecological Systems Theory informs our understanding of how child development is shaped by proximal environments and by children themselves in reaction to changing environments (Bronfenbrenner, 1979). Children's daily experiences and environments likely vary significantly by parental employment status throughout their first 17 years of life. Parents who are employed may juggle multiple demands from both the family and the workplace that may in turn lead to less positive family dynamics, including reduced time spent with children, lower quality home environment, and having less energy or time to enact parenting practices that facilitate positive development in children. Possibly, juggling multiple demands particularly when compounded with little or no support from the family or the society (e.g., lack of affordable and quality childcare, lack of flexible work arrangements, availability of sick or leave days) may increase the chances of parent-child relationships that are harsh, unsupportive, or neglectful which in turn increase the risk of undesirable child outcomes (Repetti, 2005). Links between maternal employment and child well-being across the globe have been examined extensively. In meta-analyses, few if any associations are found (Goldberg, Prause, Lucas-Thompson, and Himsel, 2008; Lucas-Thompson, Goldberg, and Prause, 2010). Below we provide a brief review of empirical findings by child's age.

Maternal employment, particularly full-time employment, during a child's first year of life has been linked to modestly lower cognitive outcomes and modestly higher behavior problems (Baum, 2003; Baydar and Brooks-Gunn, 1991; Berger et al., 2008; Brooks-Gunn, Han, and Waldfogel, 2002; Cooksey, Joshi, and Verropoulou, 2009; Han, Waldfogel, and Brooks-Gunn, 2001; Hill, Waldfogel, Brooks-Gunn, and Han, 2005; Waldfogel, Han, and Brooks-Gunn, 2002). Studies that have focused on the first 9 to 12 months of a child's life have reported associations between full-time maternal employment and child cognitive development and executive function (Brooks-Gunn, Han, and Waldfogel, 2010; Conway, Han, Brooks-Gunn, and Waldfogel, 2017).

Different from the first year after birth, maternal employment during the second and third years of the children's life is associated with higher future achievement (Lucas-Thompson et al., 2010; Waldfogel et al., 2002). Some negative effects of employment could still be present at older ages, but Ruhm (2004) argued that the positive effects of maternal employment during the child's second and third years can offset negative effects. Indeed, this finding may be especially salient for low-income families who have more to gain from additional income. Results from one longitudinal study with low-income families found that preschool-age children whose mothers transitioned off welfare and into work did not suffer any negative outcomes (Chase-Lansdale et al., 2003). Furthermore, maternal earnings in low-income families reduce financial strain and thereby maternal depression, leading to an improvement in the quality of parenting behaviors (Jackson, Brooks-Gunn, Huang, and Glassman, 2000). In addition, recent studies using cohorts of children born after 2000 have found little or no effects of early maternal employment on child development associated with part-time or full-time employment, although these studies do not focus on the first 9 to 12 months of a child's life specifically (Coley and Lombardi, 2017; Coley and Lombardi, 2014). One possible explanation for differences in findings might be the timing of the cohorts. For earlier cohorts, differences between working and non-working mothers were greater than for more recent cohorts. That is, selection into maternal employment is different today than it was in prior decades (Hill et al., 2005).

Very little empirical information exists about middle childhood and the effects that maternal employment might have on children during this period of time. Researchers focus on early childhood and adolescence because these are important developmental periods during which environmental influences may be particularly salient in shaping or altering children's developmental trajectories. There are few theoretical reasons to hypothesize that parental employment would have a unique impact on children during middle childhood.

Similar to preschool-age children, adolescent children of working mothers experience some negative effects which are, on average, balanced with positive ones. The negative effects tend to result from less parental supervision, whereas the positive effects result from the availability of more resources and decreases in parental stress. In low-income families, improvements in adolescents' mental health associated with maternal employment have been observed, likely as a result of increased household income. Time diaries from low-income working mothers show significantly more time apart from adolescent children after entering the workforce. However, during the hours when mothers were not at work, time apart from children decreased. When mothers entered the labor force, they compensated for time away during work hours by spending more time together during non-work hours (Chase-Lansdale et al., 2003).

In the following sections we consider factors which are related to parenting behaviors with a particular focus on the first year. These include gender and ethnicity. Then, a series of mechanisms which may link early employment and parenting are considered. We primarily focus on associations between employment and parenting. In doing so, we highlight how parental employment influences parenting in both positive and negative ways while considering various contextual factors.

Employment and Parenting: Contextual Factors and Pathways

Contextual Factors

Child gender might influence how parent employment is linked with parenting and child development. Negative effects of first-year employment on child outcomes tend to be stronger for boys than girls because boys are more affected by early experiences (Rutter, 1979; Zaslow and Hayes, 1986), and specifically by non-maternal childcare (Bornstein, Gist, Hahn, Haynes, and Voigt, 2001; Bornstein, Hahn, Gist, and Haynes, 2006; Bornstein and Hahn, 2007; Crockenberg, 2003; Weinberg, Tonick, Cohn, and Olson, 1999). Boys are less likely to develop secure attachments to non-parental caregivers (Ahnert and Lamb, 2003) and may be less able than girls to self-regulate and cope with negative arousal (Crockenberg, 2003; Weinberg et al., 1999). Girls may also be better-equipped than boys to adapt to the large group sizes that often symbolize non-parental childcare (Bornstein and Hahn, 2007: Bornstein et al., 2006).

Parent *gender* might influence parental employment, parenting, and child development. Parent gender is one given consistently high employment rates among fathers historically compared to maternal employment. Less variation among fathers makes it more difficult to study the effects of paternal employment on child well-being. For example, many existing data sources do not provide sufficient numbers on fathers who are present in the home and not working to examine the variations in paternal employment. In addition, fathers who do not work tend to be a highly selected group with unique characteristics. Previous studies have often taken the presence of the father and characteristics of the father, such as earnings, into account, but have not focused on the effects of paternal employment on child outcomes, specifically. With data from the National Longitudinal Survey of Youth (NLSY), Han et al. (2001) constructed six categories to represent the joint pattern of the mother's working status with father's presence and working status in the first year of a child's life: working mother and no father, working mother and non-working father, working mother and working father, non-working mother and no father, non-working mother and non-working father, and non-working mother and working father. Children from two-parent families whose mothers worked in the first year had lower cognitive scores than those in two-parent families whose mothers did not work in the first year and whose fathers did. Furthermore, the negative associations of first-year maternal employment were largest for children whose fathers were present but not working. This finding suggests that there is a connection between mothers' and fathers' work in the first year and child outcomes. An earlier study using the NLSY suggests that father care when mothers are working is linked to negative child outcomes (Baydar and Brooks-Gunn, 1991). A second analysis, also with the NLSY data, found positive effects of paternal employment on child cognitive outcomes (Ruhm, 2004). Paternal employment was measured as the average weekly work hours of the father during years 1 through 3 after the child's birth. The number of hours worked by the father were positively associated with child cognitive outcomes. Currently it remains unclear why effects may differ between maternal and paternal employment. Given that a full-time working father and a non-working mother represent traditional family roles, it may be that fathers who stray from traditional roles are doing so not by choice, but because of some other factor that may impact employment status and child outcomes, biasing estimates between the two. For example, fathers who do not work may be sick, less qualified, recently fired or laid off, or experiencing other hardships. Such parental stress may translate into poorer parenting, strained family relationships, and lower quality home environments, in turn impacting child development. Given the recent trends of fathers spending more time on shared responsibilities with mothers for household chores and childrearing, results from existing research using cohorts before the 2000s may not necessarily be applicable to contemporary cohorts of children. Therefore, a new refined analysis is warranted on the association between paternal employment, parenting, and child well-being using contemporary cohorts of children.

Parental education is another context factor. Comparing mothers with college degrees to those without, estimates suggest that the former work 7 more weeks per year than the latter. Cumulating over several years of childhood, these differences may translate into more family resources for children of mothers with a college degree, but less time spent together (Carneiro, Meghir, and Parey, 2012). Family resources and time spent together can offset one another, but the association depends on the quality of the non-parental childcare. Parents with low levels of education often also have lower incomes and fewer skills (Marshall, 2004). As a result of these constraints, children from low-income families are more likely to be placed in low-quality, center-based, or informal care settings (Henly and Lyons, 2000). By contrast, for families living in poverty, the benefit of additional income, especially during the first year of a child's life, may be more than for families living above the poverty threshold (Baydar and Brooks-Gunn, 1991; Desai, Chase-Lansdale, and Michael, 1989; Han et al., 2001).

Some research suggests that negative effects of first-year employment on child outcomes differ by *ethnicity* and *culture*. Specifically, effects tend to be stronger for Latin American families and European American families than for African American families (Berger et al., 2008). There is some indication that European American mothers are more likely to engage in activities such as book reading and verbal communication with their infants (Raikes et al., 2006). If European American mothers spend more time talking to their children compared to mothers of other groups, their children may have more to lose in terms of language exposure when placed in non-parental care. Some evidence also suggests that first-year maternal employment results in behavior problems for Latin American children but not European American or African American children (Berger et al., 2008), at least as reported by mothers. Because Latin American mothers tend to be more physically involved with infants, providing more hands-on support with tasks such as feeding (Carlson and Harwood, 2003; Ispa et al., 2004), first-year employment may then be a greater disruption for Latin American infants than for infants of other groups. Another possibility is that the greater involvement of relatives in the rearing of African American children from birth may mean that maternal employment would not bring as much disruption for African American infants (see Stack, 1974).

Single female-headed households can alter how employment affects parenting and children compared to two-parent households. Major demographic shifts have contributed to a dramatic increase in the number of single female-headed households, largely explained by increased rates of divorce and of children being born to single mothers. Although findings on the effects of single-parenthood on child development are mixed, on average, children growing up with one parent fare worse than their peers in two-parent homes (Waldfogel, Craigie, and Brooks-Gunn, 2010; Weinraub and Bowler, 2019). The link between single-parenthood and child development is possibly due to limited financial and time-related resources. Single-parent families tend to have lower incomes and only one parent's time to make available to children. With no external support, a single-parent must take on the role of the breadwinner as well as the caregiver, often requiring single mothers of young children to be employed full time (Pilkauskas, Waldfogel, and Brooks-Gunn, 2016).

The link between parental employment and parenting can also vary based on parents' *work characteristics*. If parents work in jobs with overwhelming demands, menial tasks, instability, and little flexibility or support, the benefit of the work might be less compared to a higher quality job. Working conditions and job complexity can influence parent-child relationships and parenting styles. It is likely that parents with more mundane and less flexible occupations provide less appropriate and less stimulating home environments than those whose work is more complex (Menaghan and Parcel, 1995). In contrast, parents whose work is more autonomous and self-directing are more likely to practice a more adaptive, flexible, and authoritative parenting style, encouraging more autonomy and self-control in their children (Menaghan, 2005).

Parents' work schedules may also influence children's development by shaping familial resources, such as parental time available for children, income, and parental physical and psychological well-being. Whereas working nonstandard hours, particularly night and evening shifts, may allow more parent-child time during the day, such schedules may lead to fatigue and stress and hence diminish parents' physical and psychological capacity for providing quality parenting (Heymann, 2000). A growing body of research has explored how nonstandard work schedules influence individuals' physical, psychological, and social well-being, which may, in turn, compromise family and children's well-being (Li et al., 2014; Presser, 2003).

For example, nonstandard schedules take a physical, psychological, and social toll on workers that may compromise a parent's ability to provide a supportive and warm home environment (e.g., parental warmth and sensitivity, enriching and stimulating activities) that can positively shape children's well-being (Han, 2005, 2008; Han, Miller, and Waldfogel, 2010; Kalil, Ziol-Guest, and Epstein, 2010; Presser, 2003). Parental nonstandard work schedules have also been found to compromise, to a certain degree, children's cognitive and socioemotional well-being and to increase risky behavior amongst adolescents (for a review, see Li et al., 2014). The effects of nonstandard work schedules vary, depending on the specific schedule. Evening, night, or rotating work hours tend to have more adverse associations with children's cognitive and socioemotional well-being than when parents work standard daytime hours (e.g., 8 a.m. to 4 p.m.). Gassman-Pines (2011) and Han et al. (2010) both showed that working nonstandard hours, particularly night hours, can cause parents to feel stressed and too emotionally and physically drained to have consistently warm and supportive interactions with their children. In turn, the parent-child relationship and the quality of the home environment, as well as parental knowledge of children's whereabouts, can be compromised, all of which can negatively affect child well-being (Crouter, Bumpus, Davis, and McHale, 2005; Han et al., 2010). These associations have been observed throughout children's developmental stages from infancy to adolescence but may be more acute during the preschool and adolescent years (Li et al., 2014).

In contrast, parental nonstandard work schedules might be positively associated with child well-being, although we have relatively little data on this topic. On time-use data, parents who work non-standard schedules tend to compensate for lost time in other ways, such as reducing sleep and leisure to protect time with children (Wight, Raley, and Bianchi, 2008). This line of research highlights the importance of joint arrangements between parents to provide the best care for their children.

Some adverse effects associated with parental nonstandard work schedules on child well-being may have to do with whether or not parent(s) (in)voluntarily choose to work at such hours and/or at such high intensity in addition to parents' occupational status (Han, 2008). For example, no adverse effects on child well-being were found when parents worked at professional jobs versus service-sector jobs, and such findings may have to do with the fact that parents with professional jobs may either voluntarily work at nonstandard hours to accommodate the demand from a 24/7 economy or have resources (e.g., purchasing quality care and educational-related activities) to cushion the potential adverse effects of long and nonstandard hours on their children's well-being (Han, 2008).

These job characteristics affect the quantity and quality of time available for children, and the amount of resources parents could have to invest in their children's well-being. An important association between a number of aspects of parental work and child and family well-being include access to paid sick leave, paid parental leave, schedule flexibility, employment stability, and sufficient income (Devine et al., 2006; Han, Ruhm, and Waldfogel, 2009; Heymann, 2000). These benefits may bring a great deal of resources and support to cushion the hardship parents may encounter to provide quality parenting.

We now turn to various pathways through which employment might influence parenting in both direct and indirect ways.

Direct Pathway

Parental employment can be both rewarding and taxing; rewarding if parental employment increases family income, enhances parental self-confidence and satisfaction that in turn affect parenting positively, and consequently, optimal child development; and taxing if parental employment induces parental stress, income instability, and family conflict that may affect parenting negatively.

The *parental relationship* may be one pathway through which employment influences parenting. As a result of consistent, sensitive, and responsive parenting, infants develop a sense of security and subsequently form an attachment to their parents. Therefore, on one hand, some have argued that separations for employment between parents and children particularly during the first year of life may adversely affect the processes of the interactions (Jaeger and Weinraub, 1990; Owen and Cox, 1988) and consequently parenting. On the other hand, others have argued that under the right circumstances, infants can form secure attachments to parents regardless of separations due to employment. If parents provide sensitive caregiving during time spent together and non-parental caregivers also provide sensitive care during periods of separation from parents, children can develop and benefit from multiple secure attachments (Goossens and van IJzendoorn, 1990).

In analyses with National Institute of Child Health and Human Development (NICHD) Study of Early Child Care (SECC) data, mothers were rated as providing less sensitive care by age 3 if they worked full time by the first 9 months of their child's life than those who had not worked at all in the first 9 months (Brooks-Gunn et al., 2002). Mothers who worked part time had higher maternal sensitivity scores than mothers who did not work or worked full time (Brooks-Gunn et al., 2010).

Similar to the mother-child relationship, children can develop an attachment relationship with a father through sensitive interactions. Indeed, children with employed mothers might rely more heavily on father-child relationships (Staines and Pleck, 1986). While some studies have found families with working mothers have more involved fathers, others have found that fathers exhibit more negative affect and parenting behaviors (Grych and Clark, 1999). Yet the converging trend regarding labor force participation and time devoted to household tasks and childcare responsibilities (Galinsky, Aumann, and Bond, 2011; Haas and Hwang, 2008; Huerta et al., 2013) reflects mothers working more and fathers increasingly taking on childcare and home responsibilities. These shifts appear to be positively associated with child development (Huerta et al., 2013).

Indirect Pathways

In the following sections we discuss the mechanisms through which parental employment might influence parenting. These mechanisms offer explanations for how employment and parenting might be linked. We describe these associations and how the nature of the link might depend on contextual factors. We draw upon Ecological System Theory (Bronfenbrenner, 1979) and Family Systems perspective (Kerig, 2019; McLoyd, 1998) in addition to the economic investment model (Mayer, 1997; Ruhm, 2004) and Family Stress Model (Conger, Conger, and Martin, 2010; McLoyd, Jayaratne, Ceballo, and Borquez, 1994) to inform our understanding of the mechanisms linking parental employment with parenting. Whereas Ecological System theory and Family Systems perspective inform us about how parent-child interactions may help develop children's cognitive and socioemotional well-being, theories of parental investment underscore the time and material resources parents spend engaging their children in activities that promote children's optimal development (Foster, 2002). The family stress model highlights how parental stress from work (e.g., demanding schedules, unsociable hours) may compromise the quality of parenting to place children at risk for socioemotional and behavioral difficulties (Yeung, Linver, and Brooks-Gunn, 2002). These theoretical perspectives support opposing mechanisms, suggesting that parental employment will increase economic resources and possibly increase parental stress and reduce parental time devoted to parenting.

Emotional distress. Parental emotional distress may be an important mechanism between employment and parenting. Emotional distress oftentimes is measured by depressive and anxious symptoms as well as by parenting stress, which overlap with the Family Stress Model. A history of empirical findings describes the link between depression and parenting emphasizing greater hostile, negative, and withdrawn behaviors in depressed parents (Dix and Moed, 2019; Lovejoy, Graczyk, O'Hare, and Neuman, 2000; Lyons-Ruth, Wolfe, and Lyubchik, 2000), which are linked to negative developmental outcomes through the course development (Dodge, 1990; Downey and Coyne, 1990; Goodman and Gotlib, 2002; Phares and Compas, 1992). Whereas the link between depression and parenting is clear, two competing perspectives can be applied to the link between employment and depression. The first suggests that, if work is rewarding, parents may be less depressed and also more sensitive and responsive in their parenting style. This perspective is referred to as the enhancement or expansion hypothesis. Multiple roles are hypothesized to enhance individual well-being and expand a feeling of self-worth and sense of identity (Marks, 1977). Energy is not seen as fixed; rather, each role offers additional sources of self-esteem, stimulation, and identity (Hock and Demeis, 1990). The contrasting perspective contains two separate, but overlapping, theories: role strain theory (Barnett and Hyde, 2001) and the scarcity hypothesis (Rosenfield, 1989). Role strain theory purports that multiple roles such as that of employee and that of mother held by the same individual could come into conflict, and can result in stress and depression. The scarcity hypothesis proposes that individuals have a limited supply of energy. The more roles an individual holds, the greater the likelihood of role overload, which in turn, leads to psychological distress.

Stress resulting from work may function in a similar way, increasing conflict and tension in the parent-child relationship. A negative mood spillover process may bring stress from the workplace into the home and into parent-child interactions (Repetti, Wang, and Saxbe, 2009). For example, long work hours and nonstandard work hours may have important implications for the energy, time, and resources that parents can draw on to rear their children (Heymann, 2000). Literature on work-family spillover effects (Repetti, 2005) and on work-family balance (Menaghan, 2005; Perry-Jenkins, Repetti, and Crouter, 2000) suggests that parents' experiences at the workplace may spill over to the home by affecting their personal well-being, which in turn influences relationships with their children (Bumpus, Crouter, and McHale, 1999, 2006; Crouter, Bumpus, Maguire, and McHale, 1999). In particular, the stressful job conditions associated with working long hours (e.g., 50+ hours per week) or a nonstandard schedule may in turn lead to less warm and supportive family dynamics, including not being able to help children with homework, participate in children's school events, lower parental knowledge of children's whereabouts, and lower quality home environments (Menaghan and Parcel, 1991, 1995). Moreover, even if they are able to find the time to spend with their children, parents working long hours or evening or night hours may not have the energy to foster a positive parent-child relationship (Han, 2008; Han et al., 2010; Presser, 2003).

The nature of the association between employment and depression can depend on the quality of the work. Low-income parents are more likely to have lower-quality employment than their higher income counterparts. Low-quality jobs are characterized by overwhelming work demands, menial tasks, instability, and little flexibility or support (Karasek and Theorell, 1990; Rosenfield, 1989). Job characteristics such as these may lead to depression as challenges such as inadequate childcare, the demands of low-wage work, and competing demands on time accumulate (Edin and Lein, 1997; Wilson, Ellwood, and Brooks-Gunn, 1995; Zaslow, Oldham, Moore, and Magenheim, 1998).

Women who return to work earlier in the first year after the birth of a child have higher levels of subsequent depressive symptoms (Chatterji and Markowitz, 2005). Also, depressive symptoms partially mediate, or explain, the association between first year maternal nonstandard work hours and child socioemotional outcomes (Daniel, Grzywacz, Leerkes, Tucker, and Han, 2009). Taken together, theory and empirical evidence suggest that the association between employment and depression and stress, and subsequently parenting, depend not only on the characteristics of the child (e.g., a child's developmental age) and the parent, but also have a lot to do with the nature of the work.

The mediating role of childcare in the association between employment and parenting depends on the type and quality of the available care and the emphasis the care places on developing relationships with families. The circumstances surrounding employment and how they might impact parenting are closely linked to the *type of childcare* available. For example, low-income employed parents, on average, have fewer childcare options and also jobs with less flexibility, fewer benefits, and more nonstandard work hours (Marshall, 2004). As a result of these constraints, children from low-income families are more likely to be placed in informal care settings (Henly and Lyons, 2000). On average, children of employed parents are more likely to receive center-based care than their counterparts, but this link may vary by ethnicity, family income, and the nature of parental work. For example, children of Latin American origin are less likely, in general, to be placed in center-based care than in in-home-based care (Berger et al., 2008; Waldfogel et al., 2002). Children of low-income families, particularly single-mother families, tend to be cared for by grandparents (Berger et al., 2008). Children whose parents with nonstandard work schedules tend to be cared for by either fathers or grandparents (Han, 2004). Prior studies with the NICHD SECCYD data (NICHD ECCRN, 2002, 2004, 2006) have found that children who attended center-based care had higher cognitive scores but worse behavioral outcomes than their comparable counterparts. Similar results have also been found in analyses with the Early Childhood Longitudinal Study–Kindergarten Cohort (Loeb, Bridges, Fuller, Rumberger, and Bassok, 2007; Magnuson, Meyers, Ruhm, and Waldfogel, 2004). High-quality care has also been associated with children's cognitive development (Burchinal et al., 2000; NICHD ECCRN, 2002, 2005, 2006; Vandell and Wolfe, 2000). Findings regarding links between socioemotional outcomes and childcare have been mixed (Belsky et al., 2007; Bornstein et al., 2006; Langlois and Liben, 2003: Loeb et al., 2007; Love et al., 2003; Magnuson, Ruhm, and Waldfogel, 2007; NICHD ECCRN, 2003, 2004, 2005, 2006).

Additional attention has been paid to the influence of *quality center-based care* might have on families, the parent–child relationship, and parenting skills directly. For example, Head Start, a preschool program primarily serving low-income families, has always placed an emphasis on the participation of parents in program activities. The program has taken actions to develop and use strategies to make parent and family engagement activities systematic and integrated within Head Start programs. In fact, family engagement is now defined as more than just parent involvement in program activities. Instead, the emphasis is on the ongoing relationship between parents and staff, staff and children, and parents and children. These changes in Head Start practices are supported by a body of literature that has provided evidence for links between the alignment between practices in the home and the care setting and strong parent-staff relationships with parenting and children's development (McWayne, Hampton, Fantuzzo, Cohen, and Sekino, 2004; Blue-Banning, Summers, Frankland, Nelson, and Beegle, 2004; Spielberg, 2011). For children who are enrolled in Head Start or other similar comprehensive care settings, employed parents might receive direct support to improve parenting.

Parental income. A large body of literature exists suggesting that household income, generally, during early childhood, is positively associated with children's cognitive outcomes (Dearing, McCartney, and Taylor, 2001; Duncan and Brooks-Gunn, 1997; Duncan, Yeung, Brooks-Gunn, and Smith, 1998; Repetti and Wang, 2009). For example, studies that draw from the Family Stress Model (Conger, Ge, Elder, Lorenz, and Simons, 1994) have shown that economic hardship is associated with increased emotional pressure and emotional distress among parents (Conger et al., 1992; Elder, Liker, and Cross, 1984; Whitbeck et al., 1991). Parental emotional distress, in turn, may affect the parent-child relationship and result in disrupted parenting which may increase behavioral problems in children (McLoyd, 1998; NICHD ECCRN, 2005). In addition, studies using samples from British Household Panel Survey have found that children's long-term educational attainment is negatively associated with mothers' full-time employment (Ermisch and Francesconi, 2000), and such findings might have to do with increased parental stress from moving into low-paid employment (and reductions in parental time with children) without significantly increasing income. In contrast, the additional income due to parental employment would allow parents to purchase resources to engage their children in activities that promote children's optimal development, which might be particularly true for children in relatively socioeconomic disadvantaged families (Ruhm, 2008).

Few studies have specifically examined links between mothers' and fathers' individual income contributions and parenting or, consequently, child outcomes (Cabrera, Mincy, and Um, 2018). Some evidence suggests that fathers who earn very little or experience unemployment have poorer connections with their children (Bianchi and Milkie, 2010); poorer connections with children may have to do with the fact that these fathers are a highly selected group. In contrast, the association between maternal income and parenting may depend on marital status and poverty levels. Specifically, maternal employment in the first year is most beneficial for single mothers living in poverty who cannot rely on another source of income (Coley and Lombardi, 2013). For low-income mothers, paid employment can increase income, foster stable routines in the family, and increase the quality of the home environment (Vandell and Ramanan, 1992). Parental employment may affect the home environment in two ways. First, employment may increase resources necessary to meet children's needs through housing, food, safety, clothing, and the purchase of learning materials and opportunities (Ross and Mirowsky, 1992). Second, providing for children may affect a parent's personal sense of well-being, control, and self-esteem leading to improved parenting and parent-child interactions (Ross and Mirowsky, 1992). Whereas income is generally positively associated with child outcomes, empirical evidence suggests that the degree to which parental income is associated with positive parenting may depend on the gender of the parent, marital status, family income, and poverty level.

Implications for Policy: Employment and Parenting

Increases in maternal employment have been dramatic since the 1950s. In most developed countries, increases in maternal employment are probably due to changes in the economic, social, and political environments. First, families often rely on two incomes to cover rising housing and living costs. Second, many view women's participation in the labor market as a primary component of gender equity. Third, demographic shifts have contributed to a dramatic increase in the number of single female–headed households. Changes such as these prompt parents to enter or return to the workforce soon after the birth of a child. Fourth, and only relevant for low-income families living in the United States, the 1996 welfare reform legislation required that low-income mothers be employed or engaged in an approved job-related activity to receive welfare benefits (even mothers of young children). For example, the Temporary Assistance for Needy Families (TANF) program in the United States that resulted from the 1996 Personal Responsibility and Work Opportunity Reconciliation Act (PRWORA) aimed at increasing parents' self-sufficiency by promoting employment. These policy changes also limited the length of time that families can receive welfare assistance, and in many states required mothers to participate in the labor force as soon as 6 months after the birth of a child. These policy changes have resulted in large increases in rates of maternal employment, specifically among low-income, single mothers (Moffitt, 2002). States differ in when mothers are required to work after the child's birth, as the 1996 welfare reform law stipulated that mothers who receive welfare benefits are to go back to work within the first year of a child's birth, and some states were allowed to relax this rule. Using this variation, Herbst (2017) examined links between work in the first year of a child's life for welfare-eligible mothers and child's cognitive scores at 9 and 24 months of age. Negative associations were found for earlier return to work in the first year of a child's life. Possible mechanisms were explored. Specifically, earlier return to work was associated with more maternal depressive symptoms, lower incidence of breastfeeding, and more use of non-relative care (but not center-based care), and these associations in turn lead to negative child outcomes.

The three primary policy approaches in place in the United States are assistance with childcare, financial support, and leave. The first policy area provides help with childcare expenses either indirectly or directly. Indirect childcare assistance exists in the form of tax relief or childcare subsidies (often vouchers), both of which target low-income working parents. Direct childcare refers to government funding of non-parental childcare such as Head Start. The second policy area, financial support, is government funding to help families offset the general cost of childrearing. For example, all working families with children are eligible for a child tax credit. Additionally, low-income working parents are able to claim the Earned Income Tax Credit (EITC), currently the government's largest cash transfer program. In addition, means-tested financial assistance is available to the lowest-income working parents with children through TANF, or welfare. Many other in-kind benefit programs are also available to low-income working families. For example, the Supplemental Nutrition Assistance Program (SNAP, which replaced the "Food Stamp" program) and the Women, Infants, and Children (WIC) program are designed to help with the costs of food for low-income families. Medicaid and the State Children Health Insurance Program (SCHIP) are available to offset health care costs for both working and unemployed low-income parents. The third policy area is family leave, which provides parents with job security during the birth of a child. The Family and Medical Leave Act (FMLA) allows parents job-protected, unpaid time off from work. The FMLA applies to all public employers and to private employers with 50 or more employees, resulting in about 10% of all private employers and about 60% of all private sector employees (U.S. Department of Labor, 2000). Within qualifying places of employment, workers who have been employed for at least 12 months and who have worked a minimum of 1,250 hours in the past year are eligible for leave pursuant to the FMLA. Following the birth or adoption of a child, eligible workers can take up to 12 weeks of job-protected leave during the first year. The 12 weeks can be claimed by both an eligible mother and father in the same family, unless both parents have the same employer. In addition to leave for the care of new children, the FMLA also grants leave for other family needs. The FMLA does not provide wage replacement, but does require that employers continue worker's health insurance during covered periods of leave.

The United States is among the over 30 most economically developed countries in the world, which together form the OECD. Most OECD countries provide a safety net of social welfare policies focused on childcare, financial assistance, flexible work schedules, and job-protected time away from work to support working parents. The United States does not have any statutory paid leave policies, in addition to a welfare system offers minimum assistance and heavily depends on means-tested measures instead of universal policy. On a national level, FMLA is offered with 12 weeks of unpaid leave after childbirth (Han and Waldfogel, 2003; Heymann and McNeill, 2013). Some workers may have access to employer-based leave programs, but these benefits usually apply only to professional high-ranking employees. In contrast, most OCED countries provide paid parental leave, with 96% of countries providing paid maternity leave and 44% of countries providing paid paternity leave (Heymann and McNeill, 2013). Additionally, because the leave in most other countries is paid, eligible parents are more likely to take the leave that is offered. Countries with longer, paid, and job-protected leaves tend to have children and mothers who exhibit better outcomes during pregnancy, labor, birth, and the neonatal and post-neonatal periods (Tanaka, 2005). The piecemeal U.S. system prevents many workers from having access to leave, as 40%–50% of employees are not eligible for leave under FMLA and only 17% of companies offer paid paternity leave to some employees (Melamed, 2014).

Some OECD countries have explored other options to support working parents. For example, the United Kingdom has implemented policies allowing parents the "right" to request part-time or flexible work schedules (Waldfogel, 2010). Under this policy a parent may request a change in work hours and the employer must give the request significant consideration. Because of the large percentage of parents who have taken advantage of this policy, the United Kingdom has extended it to all parents, not just those of young children.

Conclusion

In the United States and other developed countries, trends in maternal employment are occurring simultaneously with other social trends. The past decades have witnessed the substantial rise of women obtaining equal or more education than men. Contemporary fathers also hold more equalitarian gender role attitudes than those of prior generations and this gender-equality attitude and the rise of dual-earner families have pushed many fathers to be more involved in family and childrearing tasks (Galinsky et al., 2011; Lamb and Lewis, 2010). Looking forward, we expect to see these patterns continuing, and policies and programs to support families with children become ever more important.

To address work-family conflicts and provide support to families with children when families need it the most (e.g., during infancy and toddlerhood), many countries in Europe (e.g., Demark, France, Norway, Sweden, United Kingdom) have instituted inclusive family-friendly policies, including an average of 10 months (across OECD countries) paid maternity and paternity leave, universal childcare after parents reenter the workforce, and child and/or family benefits (e.g., monthly income support to families with newborns). There is a growing consensus about the importance of the first several years of a child's life and how they can lead to optimal child development for years to come. To this end, policies in most OECD countries endorse the importance of providing children with high-quality care and education with the government fund. Preschool is increasingly seen as education and is moving toward being universal such that a free or low-cost preschool places are being offered to all children aged 3 and older.

A comprehensive family-friendly policy approach is needed to support families with young children. Research suggests that parental employment can both positively and negatively influence the parent and the child. Parental employment may be associated with less time spent with the child, but more income can also promote parental and family well-being; maternal employment may be more or less stressful depending on workplace policies, and childcare costs, quality, and options. The quality of time spent with a child is equally important than the overall quantity of time for promoting optimal child development. The availability of part-time employment, flexible work schedules, telework arrangements, and family-friendly work environments may serve as important measures to allow parents to participate in the workforce while also care for their children. Enhancing policies aimed to support working families may provide parents with more choice and flexibility during the most vulnerable and malleable phase of their children's development.

References

Aguiar, M., and Hurst, E. (2007). Measuring trends in leisure: The allocation of time over five decades. *Quarterly Journal of Economics, 122*(3), 969–1006.

Aguiar, M., Hurst, E., and Karabarbounis, L. (2013). Time use during the great recession. *American Economic Review, 103*(5), 1664–1696.

Ahnert, L., and Lamb, M.E. (2003). Shared care: Establishing a balance between home and child care settings. *Child Development, 74*(4), 1044–1049.

Barnett, R.C., and Hyde, J.S. (2001). Women, men, work, and family: An expansionist theory. *American Psychologist, 56*(10), 781–796.

Baum, C.L. II. (2003). Does early maternal employment harm child development? An analysis of the potential benefits of leave taking. *Journal of Labor Economics, 21*(2), 409–448.

Baydar, N., and Brooks-Gunn, J. (1991). Effects of maternal employment and child-care arrangements on pre-schoolers' cognitive and behavioral outcomes: Evidence from the children of the National Longitudinal Survey of Youth. *Developmental Psychology, 27*(6), 932–945.

Belsky, J., Burchinal, M., McCartney, K., Vandell, D.L., Clarke-Stewart, K.A., Owen, M.T., and the NICHD Early Child Care Research Network. (2007). Are there long-term effects of early child care? *Child Development, 78*(2), 681–701.

Berger, L., Brooks-Gunn, J., Paxson, C., and Waldfogel, J. (2008). First-year maternal employment and child outcomes: Differences across racial and ethnic groups. *Children and Youth Services Review, 30*(4), 365–387.

Bianchi, S.M. (2000). Maternal employment and time with children: Dramatic change or surprising continuity? *Demography, 37*(4), 401–414.

Bianchi, S.M. (2011). Changing families, changing workplaces. *The Future of Children, 21*(2), 15–36.

Bianchi, S.M., and Milkie, M.A. (2010). Work and family research in the first decade of the 21st century. *Journal of Marriage and Family, 72*(3), 705–725.

Bianchi, S.M., Robinson, J.P., and Milkie, M.A. (2006). *Changing rhythms of American family life.* New York, NY: Russell Sage Foundation.

Bivens, J. (2016). *Why is recovery taking so long—and who's to blame?* Washington, DC: Economic Policy Institute. Retrieved from www.epi.org/files/pdf/110211.pdf

Blau, D.M., and Currie, J. (2006). Pre-school, day care, and after school care: Who's minding the kids? In E. Hanushek and F. Welch (Eds.), *Handbook of the economics of education* (pp. 1163–1278). Amsterdam, The Netherlands: Elsevier.

Blue-Banning, M., Summers, J.A., Frankland, H.C., Nelson, L.L., and Beegle, G. (2004). Dimensions of family and professional partnerships: Constructive guidelines for collaboration. *Exceptional Children, 70*(2), 167–184.

Bornstein, M.H. (2002). *Handbook of parenting: Children and parenting* (2nd ed., Vol 1). Mahwah, NJ: Lawrence Erlbaum Associates.

Bornstein, M., and Hahn, C-S. (2007). Infant child care settings and the development of gender-specific adaptive behaviors. *Early Child Development and Care, 177*(1), 15–41.

Bornstein, M.H., Gist, N.F., Hahn, C.S., Haynes, O.M., and Voigt, M.D. (2001). *Long-term cumulative effects of daycare experience on children's mental and socioemotional development.* Washington, DC: National Institute of Child Health and Human Development.

Bornstein, M., Hahn, C-S., Gist, N., and Haynes, O. (2006). Long-term cumulative effects of child care on children's mental development and socioemotional adjustment in a non-risk sample: The moderating effects of gender. *Early Child Development and Care, 176*(2), 129–156.

Brand, J.E. (2015). The far-reaching impact of job loss and unemployment. *Annual Review of Sociology*, *41*(1), 359–375.

Brand, J.E., and Thomas, J.S. (2014). Job displacement among single mothers: Effects on children's outcomes in young adulthood. *American Journal of Sociology*, *119*(4), 955–1001.

Bronfenbrenner, U. (1979). *The ecology of human development: Experiments by nature and design.* Cambridge, MA: Harvard University Press.

Bronfenbrenner, U. (Ed.). (2005). *Making human beings human: Bioecological perspectives on human development.* Thousand Oaks, CA: Sage.

Brooks-Gunn, J., Han, W.-J., and Waldfogel, J. (2002). Maternal employment and child cognitive outcomes in the first three years of life: The NICHD study of early child care. *Child Development*, *73*(4), 1052–1072.

Brooks-Gunn, J., Han, W.-J., and Waldfogel, J. (2010). First-year maternal employment and child development in the first seven years. *Monographs of the Society for Research in Child Development (SRCD)*, *75*(2), 1–147.

Brooks-Gunn, J., Schneider, W., and Waldfogel, J. (2013). The Great Recession and the risk for child maltreatment. *Child Abuse and Neglect*, *37*, 721–729.

Brundage, V. (2014, November). *Trends in unemployment and other labor market difficulties.* Beyond the Numbers: Employment and Unemployment (Vol. 3, No. 25), U.S. Bureau of Labor Statistics. Retrieved from www.bls.gov/opub/btn/volume-3/trends-in-unemployment-and-other-labor-market-difficulties.htm

Bumpus, M.F., Crouter, A.C., and McHale, S.M. (1999). Work demands of dual-earner couples: Implications for parents' knowledge about children's daily lives in middle childhood. *Journal of Marriage and the Family*, *61*(2), 465–475.

Bumpus, M.F., Crouter, A.C., and McHale, S.M. (2006). Linkages between negative work-to-family spillover and mothers' and fathers' knowledge of their young adolescents' daily lives. *Journal of Early Adolescence*, *26*(1), 36–59.

Burchinal, M.R., Roberts, J.E., Riggins, R., Jr., Zeisel, S.A., Neebe, E., and Bryant, D. (2000). Relating quality of center-based child care to early cognitive and language development longitudinally. *Child Development*, *71*(2), 339–357.

Bureau of Labor Statistics. (2007). *Changes in men's and women's labor force participation rates.* The Economics Daily, U.S. Department of Labor. Retrieved from www.bls.gov/opub/ted/2007/jan/wk2/art03.htm

Bureau of Labor Statistics. (2016a). *Facts over time.* U.S. Department of Labor. Retrieved from www.dol.gov/wb/stats/facts_over_time.htm

Bureau of Labor Statistics. (2016b). *Employment characteristics of families-2015.* U.S. Department of Labor. Retrieved from www.bls.gov/news.release/pdf/famee.pdf

Cabrera, N. J., Mincy, R. B., and Um, H. (2018). The long-reach of fathers' earnings on children's skills in two-parent families: Parental investments, family processes, and children's language skills. Fragile Families Working Paper, WP18-06-FF. https://fragilefamilies.princeton.edu/sites/fragilefamilies/files/wp18-06-ff.pdf

Cabrera, N.J., Tamis-LeMonda, C.S., Bradley, R.H., Hofferth, S., and Lamb, M.E. (2000). Fatherhood in the twenty-first century. *Child Development*, *71*(1), 127–136.

Carlson, V., and Harwood, R. (2003). Attachment, culture, and the caregiving system: The cultural patterning of everyday experiences among Anglo and Puerto Rican mother-infant pairs. *Infant Mental Health Journal*, *24*(1), 53–73.

Carneiro, P., Meghir, C., and Parey, M. (2012). Maternal education, home environments, and the development of children and adolescents. *Journal of European Economic Association*, *11*(suppl_1), 123–160.

Chase-Lansdale, L., Moffit, R., Lohman, B., Cherlin, A., Coley, R., Pittman, L., Roff, J., and Votruba-Drzal, E. (2003). Mothers' transitions from welfare to work and the well-being of preschoolers and adolescents. *Science*, *299*(5612), 1548–1552.

Chatterji, P., and Markowitz, S. (2005). Does the length of maternity leave affect maternal health? *Southern Economic Journal*, *72*(1), 16–41.

Chatterji, P., Markowitz, S., and Brooks-Gunn, J. (2013). Effects of early maternal employment on maternal health and well-being. *Journal of Population Economics*, *26*(1), 285–301.

Coelli, M. (2011). Parental job loss and the education enrollment of youth. *Labor Economics*, *18*(1), 25–35.

Coley, R.L., and Lombardi, C.M. (2013). Does maternal employment following childbirth support or inhibit low-income children's long-term development? *Child Development*, *84*(1), 178–197.

Coley, R.L., and Lombardi, C.M. (2014). Early maternal employment and children's school readiness in contemporary families. *Developmental Psychology*, *50*, 2071–2084.

Coley, R.L., and Lombardi, C.M. (2017). Early maternal employment and children's academic and behavioral skills in Australia and the United Kingdom. *Child Development*, *88*, 263–281.

Conger, L., and Elder, G.H., Jr. (1994). *Families in troubled times adapting to change in rural America.* Hawthorne, NJ: Aldine de Gruyter.

Conger, R.D., Conger, K.J., and Martin, M.J. (2010). Socioeconomic status, family processes, and individual development. *Journal of Marriage and Family, 72*(3), 685–704.

Conger, R.D., Ge, X., Elder, G.H., Lorenz, F.O., and Simons, R.L. (1994). Economic stress, coercive family process, and developmental problems of adolescents. *Child Development, 65*(2), 541–561.

Conger, R.D., Ge, X., Elder, G.H., Lorenz, F.O., Simons, R.L., and Whitbeck, L.B. (1992). A family process model of economic hardship and adjustment of early adolescent boys. *Child Development, 63*(3), 526–541.

Conway, A., Han, W-J., Brooks-Gunn, J., and Waldfogel, J. (2017). First-year maternal employment and adolescent externalizing behavior. *Journal of Child and Family Studies, 26*(8), 2237–2251.

Cooksey, E., Joshi, H., and Verropoulou, G. (2009). Does mothers' employment affect children's development? Evidence from the children of the British 1970 Birth Cohort and the American NLSY79. *Longitudinal and Life Course Studies, 1*(1), 95–115.

Crockenberg, S.C. (2003). Rescuing the baby from the bathwater: How gender and temperament (may) influence how child care affects child development. *Child Development, 74*(4), 1034–1038.

Crouter, A.C., Bumpus, M.F., Maguire, M.C., and McHale, S.M. (1999). Linking parents' work pressure and adolescents' well-being: Insights into dynamics in dual-earner families. *Developmental Psychology, 35*(6), 1453–1461.

Crouter, A.C., Bumpus, M.F., Davis, K.D., and McHale, S.M. (2005). How do parents learn about adolescents' experiences? Implications for parental knowledge and adolescent risky behavior. *Child Development, 76*(4), 869–882.

Cummings, E. M., and Warmuth, K. A. (2019). Parenting and attachment. In M. H. Bornstein (Ed.), *Handbook of parenting Vol. 4: Social conditions and applied parenting* (3rd ed., pp. 374–400). New York, NY: Routledge.

Daniel, S.S., Grzywacz, J.G., Leerkes, E., Tucker, J., and Han, W-J. (2009). Nonstandard maternal work schedules during infancy: Implications for children's early behavior problems. *Infant Behavior and Development, 32*(2), 195–207.

Dearing, E., McCartney, K., and Taylor, B.A. (2001). Change in family income-to-needs matters more for children with less. *Child Development, 72*(6), 1779–1793.

Desai, S., Chase-Lansdale, P.L., and Michael, R.T. (1989). Mother or market? Effects of maternal employment on the intellectual ability of 4-year old children. *Demography, 26*(4), 545–561.

Devine, C.M., Jastran, M., Jabs, J.A., Wethington, El., Farrell, T.J., and Bisogni, C.A. (2006). A lot of sacrifices: Work-family spillover and the food choice coping strategies of low-wage employed parents. *Social Science and Medicine, 63*(10), 2591–2603.

Dix, T., and Moed, A. (2019). Parenting and depression. In M. H. Bornstein (Ed.), *Handbook of parenting Vol. 4: Social conditions and applied parenting* (3rd ed., pp. 449–482). New York, NY: Routledge.

Dodge, K.A. (1990). Developmental psychopathology in children of depressed mothers. *Developmental Psychology, 26*(1), 3–6.

Downey, G., and Coyne, J. (1990). Children of depressed parents: An integrative review. *Psychological Bulletin, 108*(1), 50–76.

Duncan, G., and Brooks-Gunn, J. (Eds.). (1997). *Consequences of growing up poor.* New York, NY: Russell Sage Foundation.

Duncan, G., Yeung, W.J., Brooks-Gunn, J., and Smith, J.R. (1998). How much does childhood poverty affect the life chances of children? *American Sociological Review, 63*(3), 406–423.

Edin, K., and Lein, L. (1997). *Making ends meet how single mothers survive welfare and low-wage work.* New York, NY: Russell Sage Foundation.

Elder, G.H. (1974). *Children of the great depression: Social change in life experience.* Chicago: University of Chicago Press. (Reissued as 25th Anniversary Edition, Boulder, CO: Westview Press, 1999).

Elder, G.H., Liker, J.K., and Cross, C.E. (1984). Parent-child behavior in the Great Depression: Life course and intergenerational influence. In P.B. Baltes and O.G., Jr. Brim (Eds.), *Life-span development and behavior* (Vol. 6, pp. 109–158). New York, NY: Academic Press.

Ermisch, J., and Francesconi, M. (2000). *The effect of parents' employment on children's educational attainment.* Working Papers of the Institute for Social and Economic Research, Paper 2002–2021. Colchester: University of Essex. Retrieved from www.iser.essex.ac.uk/files/iser_working_papers/2002-21.pdf

Foster, E.M. (2002). How economists think about family resources and child development. *Child Development, 73*(6), 1904–1914.

Fox, L., Han, W-J., Ruhm, C., and Waldfogel, J. (2013). Time for children: Trends in the employment of parents, 1967–2009. *Demography, 50*(1), 25–49.

Fullerton, H.N., Jr. (1999). Labor force participation: 75 years of change, 1950–1998 and 1998–2025. *Monthly Labor Review, 122*(12), 3–12.

Galinsky, E., Aumann, K., and Bond, J.T. (2011). *Times are changing: Gender and generation at work and at home.* 2008 National Study of the Changing Workforce, Families and Work Institute. Retrieved from http://familiesandwork.org/downloads/TimesAreChanging.pdf

Gassman-Pines, A. (2011). Low-income mothers' nighttime and weekend work: Daily associations with child behavior, mother-child interactions, and mood. *Family Relations, 60*(1), 15–29.

Goldberg, W.A., Prause, J., Lucas-Thompson, R., and Himsel, A. (2008). Maternal employment and children's achievement in context: A meta-analysis of four decades of research. *Psychological Bulletin, 134*(1), 77–108.

Goodman, S.H., and Gotlib, I.H. (2002). Transmission of risk to children of depressed parents: Integration and conclusions. In S.H. Goodman and I.H. Gotlib (Eds.), *Children of depressed parents: Mechanisms of risk and implications for treatment* (pp. 307–326). Washington, DC: American Psychological Association.

Goossens, F.A., and van IJzendoorn, M.H. (1990). Quality of infants' attachments to professional caregivers: Relation to infant-parent attachment and day-care characteristics. *Child Development, 61*(3), 832–837.

Grych, J.H., and Clark, R. (1999). Maternal employment and development of the father-infant relationship in the first year. *Developmental Psychology, 35*(4), 893–903.

Gyamfi, P., Brooks-Gunn, J., and Jackson, A. (2001). Associations between employment and financial and parental stress in low-income single black mothers. *Women and Health, 32*(1–2), 119–135.

Haas, L., and Hwang, C.P. (2008). The impact of taking parental leave on fathers' participation in childcare and relationships with children: Lessons from Sweden. *Community, Work, and Family, 11*(1), 85–104.

Han, W-J. (2004). Nonstandard work schedules and child care choices: Evidence from the NICHD Study of Early Child care. *Early Childhood Research Quarterly, 19*(2), 231–256.

Han, W-J. (2005). Maternal nonstandard work schedules and child cognitive outcomes. *Child Development, 76*(1), 137–154.

Han, W-J. (2008). Shift work and child behavioral outcomes. *Work, Employment, and Society, 22*(1), 67–87.

Han, W-J., Miller, D.P., and Waldfogel, J. (2010). Parental work schedules and adolescents' risky behaviors. *Developmental Psychology, 46*(5), 1245–1267.

Han, W-J., Ruhm, C., and Waldfogel, J. (2009). Parental leave policies and parents' employment and leave-taking. *Journal of Policy Analysis and Management, 28*(1), 29–54.

Han, W-J., Ruhm, C., Waldfogel, J., and Washbrook, E. (2008). The timing of mothers' employment after childbirth. *Monthly Labor Review, 131*(6), 15–27.

Han, W-J., and Waldfogel, J. (2003). Parental leave: The impact of recent legislation on parents' leave-taking. *Demography, 40*(1), 191–200.

Han, W-J., Waldfogel, J., and Brooks-Gunn, J. (2001). The effects of early maternal employment on later cognitive and behavioral outcomes. *Journal of Marriage and the Family, 63*(2), 336–354.

Henly, J.R., and Lyons, S. (2000). The negotiation of child care and employment demands among low-income parents. *Journal of Social Issues, 56*(4), 683–706.

Henwood, K., and Procter, J. (2003). The "good father": Reading men's accounts of paternal involvement during the transition to first time fatherhood. *British Journal of Social Psychology, 42*(3), 337–355.

Herbst, C.M. (2017). Are parental welfare work requirements good for disadvantaged children? Evidence from age-of-youngest-child exemptions. *Journal of Policy Analysis and Management, 36*(2), 327–357.

Heymann, J. (2000). *The widening gap: Why America's working families are in jeopardy and what can be done about it.* New York, NY: Basic Books.

Heymann, J., and McNeill, K. (2013). *Children's chances: How countries can move from surviving to thriving.* Cambridge, MA: Harvard University Press.

Hill, H.D., Morris, P.A., Castells, N., and Walker, J.T. (2011). Getting a job is only half the battle: Maternal job loss and child classroom behavior in low-income families. *Journal of Policy Analysis and Management, 30*(2), 310–333.

Hill, J., Waldfogel, J., Brooks-Gunn, J., and Han, W-J. (2005). Maternal employment and child development: A fresh look using newer methods. *Developmental Psychology, 41*(6), 833–850.

Hock, E., and Demeis, D.K. (1990). Depression in mothers of infants—the role of maternal employment. *Developmental Psychology, 26*(2), 285–291.

Huerta, M.C., Adema, W., Baxter, J., Han, W-J., Lausten, M., Lee, R., and Waldfogel, J. (2013). *Fathers' leave, fathers' involvement and child development: Are they related? Evidence from four OECD countries.* OECD Social, Employment, and Migration Working Papers (No. 140). Paris, France: OECD. Retrieved from www.oecd.org/officialdocuments/publicdisplaydocumentpdf/?cote=DELSA/ELSA/WD/SEM(2012)11&docLanguage=En

Isaacs, J. (2013). *Unemployment from a child's perspective.* Washington, DC: The Urban Institute. Retrieved from www.urban.org/sites/default/files/publication/23131/1001671-Unemployment-from-a-Child-s-Perspective.PDF

Ispa, J.M., Fine, M.A., Halgunseth, L.C., Harper, S., Robinson, J., Boyce, L., Brooks-Gunn, J., and Brady-Smith, C. (2004). Maternal Intrusiveness, maternal warmth, and mother-toddler relationship outcomes: Variations across low-income ethnic and acculturation groups. *Child Development, 75*(6), 1613–1631.

Jackson, A., Brooks-Gunn, J., Huang, C., and Glassman, M. (2000). Single mothers in low-wage jobs: Financial strain, parenting, and preschoolers' outcomes. *Child Development, 71*(5), 1409–1423.

Jaeger, E., and Weinraub, M. (1990). Early nonmaternal care and infant attachment: In search of process. *New Directions for Child Development, 1990*(49), 71–90.

Johnson, R.C., Kalil, A., and Dunifon, R.E. (2012). Employment patterns of less-skilled workers: Links to children's behavior and academic progress. *Demography, 49*(2), 747–772.

Kalil, A. (2013). Effects of the great recession on child development. *Annals of the American Academy of Political and Social Science, 650*(1), 232–249.

Kalil, A., and Ziol-Guest, K.M. (2005). Single mothers' employment dynamics and adolescent well-being. *Child Development, 76*(1), 196–211.

Kalil, A., and Ziol-Guest, K.M. (2008). Parental employment circumstances and children's academic progress. *Social Science Research, 37*(2), 500–515.

Kalil, A., Ziol-Guest, K.M., and Levin Epstein, J. (2010). Nonstandard work and marital instability: Evidence from the National Longitudinal Survey of Youth. *Journal of Marriage and Family, 72*(5), 1289–1300.

Karasek, R.A., and Theorell, T. (1990). *Healthy work: Stress, productivity and the reconstruction of working life.* New York, NY: Basic Books.

Kerig, P. (2019). Parenting and family systems. In M. H. Bornstein (Ed.), *Handbook of parenting Vol. 3: Being and becoming a parent* (3rd ed., pp. 3–35). New York, NY: Routledge.

Lamb, M.E., and Lewis, C. (2010). The development and significance of father-child relationships in two-parent families. In M.E. Lamb (Ed.), *The role of the father in child development* (5th ed., p. 94). New York, NY: John Wiley & Sons.

Langlois, J.H., and Liben, L.S. (2003). Child care research: An editorial perspective. *Child Development, 74*(4), 969–975.

Lareau, A., and Weninger, E.B. (2008). Time, work and family life: Reconceptualizing gendered time patterns through the case of children's organized activities. *Sociological Forum, 23*(3), 419–454.

Lee, D., Brooks-Gunn, J., McLanahan, S., Notterman, D., and Garfinkel, I. (2013). The Great Recession, genetic sensitivity, and maternal harsh parenting. *Proceedings of the National Academy of Sciences, 110*, 13780–13784.

Levin, P.B. (2011). How does parental unemployment affect children's educational performance. In G.J. Duncan and R.J. Murnane (Eds.), *Whither opportunity? Rising inequality, schools, and children's life chances* (pp. 315–338). New York, NY: Russell Sage Foundation.

Li, J., Johnson, S.E., Han, W.-J., Andrews, S., Kendall, G., Strazdins, L., and Dockery, A. (2014). Parent's nonstandard work schedules and child wellbeing: A critical review of the literature. *Journal of Primary Prevention, 35*(1), 53–75.

Loeb, S., Bridges, M., Bassok, D., Fuller, B., and Rumberger, R. (2007). How much is too much? The influence of preschool centers on children's social and cognitive development. *Economics of Education Review, 26*(1), 52–66.

Love, J.M., Harrison, L., Sagi-Schwartz, A., Van IJzendoorn, M.H., Ross, C., Ungerer, J.A., . . . Chazan-Cohen, R. (2003). Child care quality matters: How conclusions may vary with context. *Child Development, 74*(4), 1021–1033.

Lovejoy, M., Graczyk, P.A., O'Hare, E., and Neuman, G. (2000). Maternal depression and parenting behavior: A meta-analytic review. *Clinical Psychology Review, 20*(5), 561–592.

Lu, Y., Wang, J.S.H., and Han, W.J. (2017). Women's short-term employment trajectories following birth: Patterns, determinants, and variations by race/ethnicity and nativity. *Demography, 54*(1), 93–118.

Lucas-Thompson, R.G., Goldberg, W., and Prause, J. (2010). Maternal work early in the lives of children and its distal associations with achievement and behavior problems: A meta-analysis. *Psychological Bulletin, 136*(6), 915–942.

Lyons-Ruth, K., Wolfe, R., and Lyubchik. A. (2000). Depression and the parenting of young children: Making the case for early preventative mental health services. *Harvard Review of Psychiatry, 8*(3), 148–153.

Maccoby, E.E., and Martin, J.A. (1983). Socialization in the context of the family: Parent-child interaction. In P.H. Mussen (Series Ed.) and E.M. Hetherington (Vol. Ed.), *Handbook of child psychology: Socialization, personality and social development* (Vol. 4, pp. 1–101). New York, NY: Wiley-Blackwell.

Magnuson, K., Meyers, M., Ruhm, C., and Waldfogel, J. (2004). Inequality in preschool education and school readiness. *American Educational Research Journal, 41*(1), 115–157.

Magnuson, K., Ruhm, C., and Waldfogel, J. (2007). Does prekindergarten improve school preparation and performance? *Economics of Education Review, 26*(1), 33–51.

Marks, S.R. (1977). Multiple roles and role strain: Some notes on human energy, time and commitment. *American Sociological Review, 42*(6), 921–936.

Marshall, N.J. (2004). The quality of early child care and children's development. *Current Directions in Psychological Science, 13*(4), 165–168.

Mayer, S.E. (1997). *What money can't buy: Family income and children's life chances.* Cambridge, MA: Harvard University Press.

McLoyd, V.C. (1998). Socioeconomic disadvantage and child development. *American Psychologist, 53*(2), 185–204.

McLoyd, V.C., Jayaratne, T.E., Ceballo, R., and Borquez, J. (1994). Unemployment and work interruption among African American single mothers: Effects on parenting and adolescent socioemotional functioning. *Child Development, 65*(2), 562–589.

McWayne, C., Hampton, V., Fantuzzo, J., Cohen, H.L., and Sekino, Y. (2004). A multivariate examination of parent involvement and the social and academic competencies of urban kindergarten children. *Psychology in the Schools, 41*(3), 363–377.

Melamed, A. (2014). Daddy warriors the battle to equalize paternity leave in the United States by breaking gender stereotypes: A fourteenth amendment equal protections analysis. *UCLA Women's Law Journal, 21*(1), 53–87.

Menaghan, E.G. (2005). Work-family challenges for low-income parents and their children. *Journal of Marriage and Family, 67*(2), 537–538.

Menaghan, E.G., and Parcel, T.L. (1991). Determining children's home environments: The impact of maternal characteristics and current occupational and family conditions. *Journal of Marriage and the Family, 53*(2), 417–431.

Menaghan, E.G., and Parcel, T.L. (1995). Social sources of change in children's home environments: The effects of parental occupational experiences and family conditions. *Journal of Marriage and the Family, 57*(1), 69–84.

Morrill, M., and Pabilonia, S. (2012). *What effect do macroeconomic conditions have on families time together?* BLS Working Papers 454, U.S. Bureau of Labor Statistics, Washington, DC: U.S. Department of Labor. Retrieved from www.bls.gov/ore/pdf/ec120030.pdf

Moffitt, R.A. (2002, January). *From welfare to work: What the evidence shows.* Policy Brief (No. 13), Welfare Reform and Beyond. Washington, DC: Brookings Institution. Retrieved from www.brookings.edu/research/from-welfare-to-work-what-the-evidence-shows/

NICHD Early Child Care Research Network. (2002). Child-care structure-process-outcome: Direct and indirect effects of child-care quality on young children's development. *Psychological Science, 13*(3), 199–206.

NICHD Early Child Care Research Network. (2003). Does amount of time spent in childcare predict socioemotional adjustment during the transition to kindergarten? *Child Development, 74*(4), 976–1005.

NICHD Early Child Care Research Network. (2004). Type of child care and children's development at 54 months. *Early Childhood Research Quarterly, 19*(2), 203–230.

NICHD Early Child Care Research Network. (2005). Early child care and children's development in the primary grades: Follow-up results from the NICHD study of early childcare. *American Educational Research Journal, 42*(3), 537–570.

NICHD Early Child Care Research Network. (2006). Child care effect sizes for the NICHD study of early child care and youth development. *American Psychologist, 61*(2), 99–116.

OECD. (2007). *Babies and bosses: Reconciling work and family life, a synthesis of findings for OECD countries.* Paris: Organisation for Economic Co-operation and Development. Retrieved from www.oecd.org/els/family/39689983.pdf

OECD Social Policy Division. (2010, March). *Gender brief.* Retrieved from www.oecd.org/social/family/44720649.pdf

Oreopoulos, P., Page, M., and Stevens, A.H. (2008). The intergenerational effect of worker displacement. *Journal of Labor Economics, 26*(3), 455–483.

Owen, M.T., and Cox, M.J. (1988). Maternal employment and the transition to parenthood. In A.E. Gottfried and A.W. Gottfried (Eds.), *Maternal employment and children's development: Longitudinal research* (pp. 85–119). New York, NY: Plenum Press.

Parker, K., and Wong, W. (2013, March). *Modern parenthood: Roles of moms and dads converge as they balance work and family.* Washington, DC: Pew Research Center. Retrieved from www.pewsocialtrends.org/files/2013/03/FINAL_modern_parenthood_03-2013.pdf

Perry-Jenkins, M., Repetti, R.L., and Crouter, A.C. (2000). Work and family in the 1990s. *Journal of Marriage and the Family, 62*(4), 981–998.

Pew Research Center. (2015). *Parenting in America: Outlook, worries, aspirations are strongly linked to financial situations.* Retrieved from www.pewsocialtrends.org/2015/12/17/1-the-american-family-today/

Phares, V., and Compas, B.E. (1992). The role of fathers in child and adolescent psychopathology: Make room for daddy. *Psychological Bulletin, 111*(3), 387–412.

Pilkauskas, N., Waldfogel, J., and Brooks-Gunn, J. (2016). Maternal labor force participation and differences by education in an urban birth cohort study—1998–2010. *Demographic Research, 34*(14), 407–420.

Pilkauskas, N., Waldfogel, J., and Brooks-Gunn, J. (In press). Maternal employment stability in early childhood: Links with child behavior and cognitive skills. *Developmental Psychology.*

Presser, H.B. (1989). Can we make time for children? The economy, work schedules, and child care. *Demography, 26*(4), 523–543.

Presser, H.B. (2003). *Working in a 24/7 economy: Challenges for American families.* New York, NY: Russell Sage Foundation.

Presser, H.B., Gornick, J.C., and Parashar, S. (2008). Gender and nonstandard work hours in 12 European countries. *Monthly Labor Review, 131*(2), 83–103.

Raikes, H., Pan, B.A., Luze, G., Tamis-LeMonda, C.S., Brooks-Gunn, J., Constantine, J., Tarullo, L.B., Raikes, H.A., and Rodriquez, E.Y. (2006). Mother-child bookreading in low-income families: Correlates and outcomes during the first three years of life. *Child Development, 77*(4), 924–953.

Raver, C.C. (2003). Does work pay psychologically as well as economically? The role of employment in predicting depressive symptoms and parenting among low-income families. *Child Development, 74*(6), 1720–1736.

Rege, M., Telle, K., and Votruba, M. (2011). Parental job loss and children's school performance. *Review of Economic Studies, 78*(4), 1462–1489.

Repetti, R.L. (2005). A psychological perspective on the health and well-being consequences of employment experiences for children and families. In S. Bianchi, L. Capser, and R. King (Eds.), *Work, family, health, and well-being* (pp. 245–258). Mahwah, NJ: Lawrence Erlbaum Associates.

Repetti, R.L. and Wang, S. (2009). Parent employment and chaos in the family. In G.W. Evans and T.D. Wachs (Eds.), *Chaos and its influence on children's development: An ecological perspective* (pp. 191–208). Washington, DC: American Psychological Association.

Repetti, R.L., Wang, S., and Saxbe, D. (2009). Bringing it all back home: How outside stressors shape families' everyday lives. *Current Directions in Psychological Science, 18*(2), 106–111.

Rosenfield, S. (1989). The effects of wives' employment: Personal control and sex differences in mental health. *Journal of Health and Social Behavior, 30*(1), 77–91.

Ross, C., and Mirowsky, J. (1992). Households, employment, and the sense of control. *Social Psychology Quarterly, 55*(3), 217–235.

Ruhm, C.J. (2004). Parental employment and child cognitive development. *Journal of Human Resources, 39*(1), 155–192.

Ruhm, C.J. (2008). Maternal employment and adolescent development. *Labour Economics, 15*(5), 958–983.

Rutter, M. (1979). Protective factors in children's responses to stress and disadvantage. In W.W. Dent and J.E. Rolf (Eds.), *Primary prevention of psychopathology: Social competence in children* (Vol. 3, pp. 49–74). Hanover, NH: University Press of New England.

Sandberg, J.F., and Hofferth, S.L. (2001). Changes in children's time with parents: United States, 1981–1997. *Demography, 38*(3), 423–436.

Schildberg-Hörisch, H. (2016). *Parental employment and children's academic achievement.* IZA World of Labor. Retrieved from https://wol.iza.org/articles/parental-employment-and-childrens-academic-achievement/long

Schneider, W., Waldfogel, J., and Brooks-Gunn, J. (2015). The Great Recession and behavior problems in 9-year old children. *Developmental Psychology, 51*(11), 1615–1629.

Schneider, W., Waldfogel, J., and Brooks-Gunn, J. (2017). The Great Recession and risk for child abuse and neglect. *Children and Youth Services Review, 72*, 71–81.

Shonkoff, J.P., and Phillips, D.A. (Eds.). (2000). *From neurons to neighborhoods: The science of early childhood development.* Washington, DC: National Academy Press.

Sinno, S.M., and Killen, M. (2011). Social reasoning about 'second-shift' parenting. *British Journal of Developmental Psychology, 29*(2), 313–329.

Spielberg, L. (2011). *Successful family engagement in the classroom: What teachers need to know and be able to do to engage families in raising student achievement.* Flamboyan Foundation. Cambridge, MA: Harvard Family Research Project. Retrieved from http://flamboyanfoundation.org/wp/wp-content/uploads/2011/06/FINE-Flamboyan_Article-March-2011.pdf

Sroufe, L.A. (1979). The coherence of individual development: Early care, attachment, and subsequent developmental issues. *American Psychologist, 34*(10), 834–841.

Stack, C. (1974). *All our kin.* New York, NY: Basic Books.

Staines, G., and Pleck, J. (1986). Work schedule flexibility and family life. *Journal of Occupational Behaviour, 7*(2), 147–153.

Strazdins, L., Baxter, J.A., and Li, J. (2017). Long hours and longings: Australian children's views of fathers' work and family time. *Journal of Marriage and Family, 79*(4), 965–982.

Tanaka, S. (2005). Parental leave and child health across OECD countries. *The Economic Journal, 115*(501), F7–F28.

Thompson, R.A. (2006). The development of the person: Social understanding, relationships, conscience, self. In W. Damon (Series Ed.), R.M. Lerner (Series Ed.), and N. Eisenberg (Vol. Ed.), *Handbook of child psychology: Social, emotional, and personality development* (6th ed., Vol. 3, pp. 24–98). Hoboken, NJ: John Wiley & Sons.

U.S. Department of Labor. (2000). *Balancing the needs of families and employers: Family and medical leave surveys.* Retrieved from www.dol.gov/whd/fmla/cover-statement.pdf

Vandell, D.L., and Ramanan, J. (1992). Effects of early and recent maternal employment on children from low-income families. *Child Development, 63*(4), 938–949.

Vandell, D. L., Simpkins, S., and Wegemer, C. (2019). Parenting and children's organized activities. In M. H. Bornstein (Ed.), *Handbook of parenting Vol. 5: The practice of parenting* (3rd ed., pp. 347–379). New York, NY: Routledge.

Vandell, D.L., and Wolfe, B. (2000). *Child care quality: Does it matter and does it need to be improved?* Report prepared for the Office of the Assistant Secretary for Planning and Evaluation, Washington, DC: U.S. Department of Health and Human Services. Retrieved from https://aspe.hhs.gov/report/child-care-quality-does-it-matter-and-does-it-need-be-improved-full-report

Waldfogel, J. (2010). *Britain's war on poverty.* New York, NY: Russell Sage Foundation.

Waldfogel, J., Craigie, T-A., and Brooks-Gunn, J. (2010). Fragile families and child well-being. *Future of Children, 20*, 87–112.

Waldfogel, J., Han, W-J., and Brooks-Gunn, J. (2002). The effects of early maternal employment on child cognitive development. *Demography, 39*(2), 369–392.

Weinberg, M.K., Tronick, E.Z., Cohn, J.F., and Olson, K.L. (1999). Gender differences in emotional expressivity and self-regulation during early infancy. *Developmental Psychology, 35*(1), 175–188.

Weinraub, M., and Kaufman, R. (2019). Single parenthood. In M. H. Bornstein (Ed.), *Handbook of parenting Vol. 3: Being and becoming a parent* (3rd ed., pp. 271–310). New York, NY: Routledge.

Whitbeck, L.B., Simons, R.L., Conger, R.D., Lorenz, F.O., Huck, S., and Elder, G.H., Jr. (1991). Family economic hardship, parental support, and adolescent self-esteem. *Social Psychology Quarterly, 54*(4), 53–363.

Wight, V.R., Raley, S.B., and Bianchi, S.M. (2008). Time for children, one's spouse and oneself among parents who work nonstandard hours. *Social Forces, 87*(1), 243–271.

Williams, J.C., Blair-Loy, M., and Berdahl, J.L. (2013). Cultural schemas, social class and the flexibility stigma. *Journal of Social Issues, 69*(2), 209–234.

Wilson, J.B., Ellwood, D.T., and Brooks-Gunn, J. (1995). Welfare to work through the eyes of children: The impact on parenting of movement from AFDC to employment. In P.L. Chase-Lansdale and J. Brooks-Gunn (Eds.), *Escape from poverty: What makes a difference?* (pp. 63–86). New York: Cambridge University Press.

Yeung, W.J., Linver, M.R., and Brooks-Gunn, J. (2002). How money matters for young children's development: Parental investment and family processes. *Child Development, 73*(6), 1861–1879.

Zaslow, M.S., and Hayes, C.D. (1986). Sex differences in children's responses to psychosocial stress: Toward a cross-context analysis. In M. Lamb and B. Rogoff (Eds.), *Advances in developmental psychology* (Vol. 4, pp. 289–337). Hillsdale, NJ: Erlbaum.

Zaslow, M.J., Oldham, E., Moore, K.A., and Magenheim, E. (1998). Welfare families' use of early childhood care and education programs, and implications for their children's development. *Early Childhood Research Quarterly, 13*(4), 535–563.

5

THE TRIPLE P – POSITIVE PARENTING PROGRAM

A Community-Wide Approach to Parenting and Family Support

Matthew R. Sanders, Karen M. T. Turner, and Jenna McWilliam

Author Note

The Triple P – Positive Parenting Program is owned by The University of Queensland. The university, through its main technology transfer company, UniQuest Pty Ltd, has licensed Triple P International Pty Ltd to publish and disseminate the program worldwide. Royalties stemming from published Triple P resources are distributed in accordance with the University's intellectual property policy and flow to the Parenting and Family Support Centre, School of Psychology, Faculty of Health and Behavioural Sciences, and contributory authors. No author has any share or ownership in Triple P International Pty Ltd. Drs Sanders and Turner are authors of various Triple P programs and are members of the Triple P Research Network. Jenna McWilliam is an employee of Triple P International Pty Ltd.

Brief Overview of the Program

The Triple P – Positive Parenting Program is a preventively oriented multi-level system of family intervention which aims to promote positive, caring relationships between parents and their children, and to help parents develop effective management strategies for dealing with a variety of childhood behavioral and emotional problems, and common developmental issues (Sanders, 2012). The Triple P system draws on social learning theory (Bandura, 1977; Patterson, 1982), applied behavior analysis (Baer, Wolf, & Risley, 1968), research on child development and developmental psychopathology (Hart & Risley, 1995; Rutter, 1985a, 1985b), social information processing models (e.g., Dodge, 1986), and public health principles (e.g., Farquhar et al., 1985). It has many distinguishing features in its flexibility, varied delivery modalities, multi-disciplinary approach, and focus on self-regulation and generalization of parenting skills.

Triple P teaches parents strategies to encourage their child's social and language skills, emotional self-regulation, independence, and problem-solving ability. Attainment of these skills promotes family harmony, reduces parent–child conflict and risk of child maltreatment, fosters successful peer relationships, and prepares children for successful experiences at school and later in life. This reduces the risk for a developmental trajectory leading to poor outcomes such as school failure, substance abuse, juvenile offending, and risk taking, including sexually risky behavior (Guajardo, Snyder, & Petersen, 2009; Moffitt et al., 2011; Stack, Serbin, Enns, Ruttle, & Barrieau, 2010).

Target Populations

Triple P incorporates five levels of intervention of increasing strength for parents of children from birth to age 16. The interventions encompass universal, selective, and indicated prevention as well as treatment programs, and include variants for specific populations such as children with a developmental disability and families at risk for child maltreatment. While positive parenting methods are relevant to all parents, parents of children who are demanding, disobedient, defiant, aggressive, or generally disruptive are particularly likely to benefit from more intensive Triple P interventions (Sanders, Markie-Dadds, Tully, & Bor, 2000). Although the Triple P system has been designed as an early intervention strategy within a prevention framework, many of the principles and techniques have been successfully used in intervention programs for clinically diagnosed children with severe behavior problems (particularly children with oppositional defiant disorder, conduct disorder, or attention-deficit/hyperactivity disorder).

The Triple P Multi-level System

Table 7.1 summarizes the multi-level Triple P approach, which aims to provide the "minimally sufficient" effective intervention to meet a family's needs in order to maximize efficiency and ensure that support becomes widely available to all parents.

Level 1: Universal Triple P aims to use health promotion and social marketing strategies to deter the onset of child behavior problems by: promoting the use of positive parenting practices and decreasing dysfunctional parenting in the community; increasing parents' receptivity towards participating in a parenting program; increasing favorable community attitudes towards parenting programs and parenting in general; de-stigmatizing and normalizing the process of seeking help for parenting issues; increasing the visibility and reach of effective programs; and countering alarmist, sensational, or parent-blaming messages in the media.

Level 2: Selected Triple P/Brief Primary Care Triple P is delivered through primary care or community services as brief 10–20 minute individual sessions on a specific concern (e.g., disobedience, bedtime problems) or a 90-minute

TABLE 7.1 The Triple P Multi-level System

Level of intervention	Target population	Intervention methods	Facilitators
Level 1 Media and communications strategy (very low intensity) • *Universal Triple P* • *Stay Positive*	All parents interested in information about parenting and promoting their child's development.	Coordinated communications strategy raising awareness of parent issues and encouraging participation in parenting programs. May involve electronic and print media (e.g., brochures, posters, websites, television, talk-back radio, newspaper and magazine editorials).	Typically coordinated by communications, health or welfare staff.
Level 2 Health promotion strategy/brief selective intervention (low intensity) • *Selected Triple P* • *Selected Teen Triple P* • *Selected Stepping Stones Triple P*	Parents interested in parenting education or with specific concerns about their child's development or behavior.	Health promotion information or specific advice for a discrete developmental issue or minor child-behavior problem. May involve a 90-minute group seminar format or brief (up to 20 minutes) telephone or face-to-face clinician contact.	Practitioners who provide parent support during routine well-child health care (e.g., health, education, allied health, and childcare staff).
Level 3 Narrow focus parent training (low–moderate intensity) • *Primary Care Triple P* • *Triple P Discussion Groups* • *Primary Care Teen Triple P* • *Teen Triple P Discussion Groups*	Parents with specific concerns as above who require consultations or active-skills training.	Brief program (about 80 minutes over four sessions, or 2-hour discussion groups) combining advice, rehearsal and self-evaluation to teach parents to manage a discrete child problem behavior. May involve telephone contact.	Same as for Level 2.
• *Primary Care Stepping Stones Triple P*	Parents of children with disabilities, with concerns as above.	A parallel program with a focus on disabilities.	Same as above.

Level / Program	Target population	Description	Practitioner
Level 4 Broad focus parent training (moderate–high intensity) • *Standard Triple P* • *Group Triple P* • *Self-Directed Triple P* • *Triple P Online Standard* • *Standard Teen Triple P* • *Group Teen Triple P* • *Self-Directed Teen Triple P*	Parents wanting intensive training in positive parenting skills. Typically parents of children with behavior problems such as aggressive or oppositional behavior.	Broad focus program (about 10 hours over 8–10 sessions) focusing on parent–child interaction and the application of parenting skills to a broad range of target behaviors. Includes generalization-enhancement strategies. May be self-directed, online, involve telephone or face-to-face clinician contact, group sessions.	Intensive parenting intervention workers (e.g., mental health and welfare staff, and other allied health and education professionals who regularly consult with parents about child behavior).
• *Standard Stepping Stones Triple P* • *Group Stepping Stones Triple P* • *Self-Directed Stepping Stones Triple P*	Parents of children with disabilities who have or are at risk of developing behavioral or emotional disorders.	A parallel series of tailored programs with a focus on disabilities.	Same as above.
Level 5 Intensive family intervention (high intensity) • *Enhanced Triple P*	Parents of children with behavior problems and concurrent family dysfunction such as parental depression or stress, or conflict between partners.	Intensive individually tailored program with modules (60–90 minute sessions) including practice sessions to enhance parenting skills, mood management and stress coping skills, and partner support skills.	Intensive family intervention workers (e.g., mental health and welfare staff).
• *Pathways Triple P*	Parents at risk of child maltreatment. Targets anger-management problems and other factors associated with abuse.	Intensive individually tailored or group program with modules (60–120 minute sessions depending on delivery model) including attribution retraining and anger management.	Same as above.
• *Lifestyle Triple P*	Parents of overweight or obese children. Targets healthy eating and increasing activity levels as well as general child behavior.	Intensive 14-session group program (including telephone consultations) focusing on nutrition, healthy lifestyle and general parenting strategies. Includes generalization enhancement strategies.	As above plus dieticians/nutritionists with experience in delivering parenting interventions.
• *Family Transitions Triple P*	Parents going through separation or divorce.	Intensive 12-session group program (including telephone consultations) focusing on coping skills, conflict management, general parenting strategies and developing a healthy co-parenting relationship.	Intensive family intervention workers (e.g., counselors, mental health, and welfare staff).

group seminar series. The seminar program is particularly useful as a universal transition program for parents enrolling their children in child care, kindergarten, or preschool, although it can also be used as a booster program or refresher course for parents who have completed a higher level of intervention such as Group Triple P.

Level 3: Primary Care Triple P/Triple P Discussion Groups comprise a more intensive (e.g., 3–4 half-hour individual sessions or 2-hour discussion groups), selective prevention strategy targeting parents who have mild and relatively discrete concerns about their child's behavior or development. This intervention level incorporates active skills training and the selective use of parenting tip sheets or workbooks covering common developmental and behavioral problems. It also builds in generalization enhancement strategies for teaching parents how to apply knowledge and skills gained to non-targeted behaviors and other siblings.

Level 4: Standard Triple P/Group Triple P/Self-Directed Triple P/Triple P Online Standard are indicated prevention/early intervention programs (e.g., 10 individual 60-minute sessions or eight interactive online modules) targeting families of higher risk children identified as having detectable sub-clinical problems, or who meet diagnostic criteria, with the aim of preventing the progression of problem behavior. Group (e.g., five 2-hour groups plus three brief telephone consultations) and self-directed (a 10-session workbook) variants at this level of intervention can also be offered to an entire population to improve parenting capacity and identify individual children at risk. Parents are taught a variety of child management skills including: monitoring problem behavior; building relationships through spending quality time, talking, and affection; providing brief contingent praise and attention for desirable behavior; arranging engaging activities in high-risk situations; establishing limits and rules; using directed discussion and planned ignoring for minor problem behavior; giving clear, calm instructions; and backing up instructions with logical consequences, quiet time (non-exclusionary time-out), and time-out. Parents learn to apply these skills both at home and in the community, and to generalize and maintain parenting skills across settings and over time. While all principles and strategies are introduced, content is individually tailored as families develop their own goals and select strategies to form their own personalized parenting plans.

Level 5: Enhanced Triple P is an indicated level of intervention for families with additional risk factors that have not changed as a result of participation in a lower level of intervention. It extends the intervention to include up to five modules (three 60–90 minute sessions each) that focus on areas such as partner support and communication, mood management and stress coping skills, and anger management skills for parents. Usually, at this level of intervention, children have behavior problems that are complicated by additional family adversity factors. Families typically complete a Level 3 or 4 intervention prior to Level 5, but practitioners may run Level 5 sessions concurrently with, or even prior to, parenting sessions based on their case formulation and family need.

Tailoring to Individual Needs

Within each level of intervention, considerable tailoring of the program to parents' particular circumstances is possible to enable specific risk and protective factors to be addressed. Indeed, even though the interventions are manualized, considerable practitioner ingenuity is required to adapt a program to parents' unique goals and family circumstances. With the exception of Level 1 media and communications strategies and Level 2 seminars, families commencing a face-to-face Triple P program complete a comprehensive intake interview and assessment process to determine the nature and history of the presenting problem, develop goals for change, determine the best approach to meet their needs and their capacity to complete program sessions and practice tasks, and negotiate an intervention plan. Families may also choose a self-directed program such as a self-help workbook or online program which may or may not be couched within a therapeutic relationship.

Program resources are designed to minimize potential barriers, such as targeting an average 6th grade reading level in parent resources to avoid difficulties with literacy, using video and live practitioner modeling to demonstrate parenting strategies, and including families from diverse ethnic and cultural backgrounds in video demonstration resources. It is our view that positive parenting principles and strategies can cross cultures. What may vary according to culture are the goals and target behaviors, practical implementation of strategies, and ways of sharing information. Triple P resources have to date had 22 language translations and have been disseminated in 25 countries, with surprisingly little need for adaptation (Morawska et al., 2011). Programs have been deployed in many different cultural contexts, including ethnically diverse populations in Australasia (e.g., Australia, New Zealand), the UK (e.g., England, Scotland), North America (e.g., Canada, the USA), Western Europe (e.g., Ireland, Sweden, Germany, Belgium, the Netherlands, Switzerland), the Middle East (e.g., Iran, Turkey), South America (e.g., Chile), Asia (e.g., Japan, Hong Kong, Singapore), and with Indigenous parents in Australia, Canada, New Zealand, and the USA.

The one major cultural adaptation of Triple P has been for Australian Indigenous families when the mainstream program was sought by Indigenous workers, but potential barriers for families were identified. Community consultation with elders, professionals, and parents resulted in the development of culturally adapted resources and minor program delivery variation, such as adding a preliminary session to the group program to discuss current and historical issues in the community and share stories about parents' experiences and attitudes relating to parenting (Turner, Richards, & Sanders, 2007). This adaptation has been adopted by other First Nations communities in Canada, New Zealand, and the USA.

Evidence for Triple P

Triple P research has incorporated a range of qualitative and quantitative methodologies to evaluate interventions, from single case experiments using interrupted time series designs (e.g., Sanders & Glynn, 1981) to randomized controlled efficacy trials (e.g., Sanders et al., 2000) to large-scale population-level effectiveness evaluations of Triple P as a multi-level system in communities (e.g., Prinz, Sanders, Shapiro, Whitaker, & Lutzker, 2009). A recent meta-analysis (Sanders, Kirby, Tellegen, & Day, 2013) reviewed research from 1970 to 2013 and quantitatively analyzed 101 Triple P evaluation studies (comprising 16,099 families). Statistically and clinically significant (Cohen's d) effects were found for all delivery formats and program variants, even with small sample sizes. Overall, across all intervention levels, significant short-term effects were found for: children's social, emotional, and behavioral outcomes ($d = 0.473$); parenting practices ($d = 0.578$); parenting satisfaction and efficacy ($d = 0.519$); parental adjustment ($d = 0.340$); parental couple relationship ($d = 0.225$); and observed child behavior ($d = 0.501$). Significant effects were found for all outcomes at longer-term follow-up, including observed parent behavior ($d = 0.249$). The positive family outcomes demonstrated for each of the five Triple P levels of intervention provide support for a multi-level, multi-disciplinary system of parenting programs, including prevention and treatment options, to increase timely access to cost-effective services promoting child, parent, and family wellbeing.

These findings are consistent with previous Triple P meta-analyses. Nowak and Heinrichs (2008) investigated 55 studies and found effect sizes for child problem behavior and parenting to range between 0.35 and 0.48 for between-groups and 0.45 and 0.57 for within-groups post-intervention comparisons. Thomas and Zimmer-Gembeck (2007) found effect sizes for 11 studies ranged from 0.31 to 0.73 for child behavior and 0.38 to 0.70 for parenting. In another series of meta-analyses, 15 studies resulted in an overall effect size of 0.42 for child behavior problems (de Graaf et al., 2008a), and 19 studies found an overall effect size of 0.54 for dysfunctional parenting (de Graaf et al., 2008b). Wilson et al. (2012) found an effect size of 0.61 for maternal-reported child behavior problems based on 23 RCTs.

Dissemination and Implementation Approach

The dissemination of Triple P is managed through an exclusive license agreement between The University of Queensland (the copyright holders) and Triple P International (TPI: a proprietary company established to disseminate Triple P). In recent years, TPI has developed a Triple P Implementation Framework (the Framework), drawing on best practice from the field of implementation science (e.g., The Active Implementation Frameworks: Fixsen, Naoom, Blase, Friedman,

& Wallace, 2005; the RE-AIM Framework: Glasgow, Vogt, & Boles, 1999) and 15 years of experience supporting organizations to adopt and implement Triple P.

The five phases of the Framework (see Figure 7.1) focus on the core elements of implementation, including: choosing the right practices and program; articulating desired outcomes; preparing the organization or community for effective implementation; ensuring practitioners and supervisors are prepared for training and service delivery; providing the training; and supporting the development of an evaluation and monitoring process to support maintenance and sustainability. Each phase contains a set of critical activities to be addressed by an organization or community. For each set of activities, guiding questions, discussion areas, tools, and resources are available. TPI Implementation Consultants (ICs) provide support to ensure that the implementation process is smooth, timely, and responds to the needs and constraints of the implementing organization and community.

Most community-wide roll outs of Triple P involve a number of organizations and sectors within a community. TPI uses the Framework to support communities to establish a collaborative approach and implementation systems that develop the capacity for effective, sustainable program implementation. Taking a systematic approach, the Framework addresses implementation considerations at each layer of a community system roll out, with a focus on self-regulation and minimal sufficiency, to scale up at a pace that allows for maximum

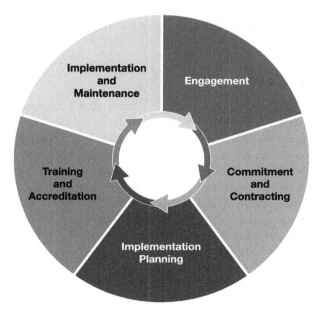

FIGURE 7.1 Triple P Implementation Framework. Source: www.triplep.net

community benefit. Promoting self-regulation at the systems level aims to build capacity for the system to self-sustain once full implementation has been achieved. Taking a minimally sufficient approach at the systems level involves ensuring that processes and implementation activities are context-specific and recognizing the existing capacity within the system. The five phases of the Framework and their application for a community-wide approach are described below in more detail.

Engagement

It is critical that the right programs and practices are chosen (the "fit") by implementing organizations. This requires a sound knowledge of the community and the organization as well as a good understanding of the Triple P system. Through dialogue and guided questions, organizations are assisted by an IC to assess which programs are the best fit for the outcomes they hope to achieve. During the engagement phase, the organization and TPI begin to develop an understanding of how the Triple P system may best suit the needs of their community and what may need to be considered for effective implementation and sustainability. Considerations include whether there are gaps within the existing services of the community, which Triple P services are the best fit for these gaps, how organizations could work collaboratively, and how referrals between services could happen. During this initial phase, organizations also consider the cultural acceptability of the program. When introduced into new countries, cultural acceptability research is encouraged to ensure programs are delivered in a culturally sensitive way.

Commitment and Contracting

Organizations that plan to deliver Triple P must clearly articulate who they would like to see served and what they would like to see achieved by providing Triple P. Given the breadth of interventions available in the Triple P system and the program's multi-disciplinary approach, there is no one right way to configure a community-wide roll out of the program. Organizations and ICs work together to develop a shared understanding of the scope of the implementation and the local capacity to implement and sustain the program. Key activities include determining the target population, how the proposed programs will fit within the community, and calculating the capacity needed to meet the initiative's intended reach and goals. TPI has developed a tool to assist this process for community-wide roll outs – the Capacity Calculator. This is an epidemiological planning tool designed to assist policy makers, funders, and organizations to plan the implementation of Triple P as a population approach, based on desired outcomes.

Organizations looking to adopt Triple P as a community-wide roll out are encouraged to establish partnerships with other organizations committed to the approach, goals, and methods used in the intervention. Establishing these partnerships helps to support the implementation of Triple P throughout a community by increasing the reach of the program to the populations served by different organizations. Through these partnerships and shared planning, the mix of programs is aligned with each organization's mandate, workforce, and service delivery methods, providing for broad and balanced availability of services throughout the community.

Implementation Planning

There are many examples of the successful implementation of Triple P in regular services following foundational efficacy trials; however, agencies have varying degrees of preparedness to adopt and maintain a new program or intervention system, and a thorough planning process is critical. Frequently, organizations move directly from training practitioners to expecting them to deliver the service within the unchanged context of the organization. This approach does not support long-term sustainability. For practitioners to successfully achieve the proven outcomes from Triple P, an organization must have the appropriate supports and infrastructure to sustain the program (e.g., providing time for practitioners to adequately prepare, engage in peer support, and establish effective data collection systems).

An organization or group of partner organizations (collaborative) must examine the match between their practices and the requirements of the levels of Triple P to be implemented. ICs support an organization or collaborative to assess their existing capacity and resources through five key activities: considering organization readiness; preparing to plan; organizational assessment; developing an implementation plan; and developing an evaluation plan. These activities are designed to ensure that an organization or collaborative develops awareness for their capacity to implement Triple P and puts in place the planning and implementation structures and processes required. They are encouraged to identify how existing functions operate within their organization and the changes needed to support effective implementation by considering the Active Implementation Drivers (see Fixsen et al., 2005). An organization or collaborative is then supported through the implementation planning process to identify the sequence of activities needed to support effective implementation and to develop an evaluation plan.

As part of this planning process, the practitioners who will deliver Triple P are carefully selected (e.g., considering their capacity to engage with families in different ways, such as groups versus individual programs) and prepared by their organization prior to undertaking any training. The organization's implementation planning process should also attend to logistical issues, such as planning to ensure that sufficient time is allocated in practitioners' work duties to deliver programs and anticipating potential barriers to the accessibility of programs (e.g., child care, transportation, location, hours). Other factors to consider include resource costs, future training support to allow for staff attrition, and administrative implications, which need to be considered at the outset to promote sustainability.

Romney and colleagues (Romney, Israel, & Zlatevski, 2014) found significantly better client completion rates and cost-effectiveness for those agencies that completed a site readiness process intended to prepare them for the implementation demands of successfully delivering Group Triple P (e.g., desire for and belief in the "fit" of the program, commitment to train at least three practitioners and commence delivering within 30 days of training completion, administrative support, and regular supervision). For agencies where administrators and staff completed the readiness process, the odds of parents completing the first Triple P group were 12.2 times greater than for those in groups run by sites that had not completed the readiness process. This meant the average cost-per-client was over seven times higher for the agencies that had not completed the readiness process.

Training and Accreditation

Practitioner training may be contracted by a commissioning agency seeking to have its staff trained, or may involve attendance of individual practitioners in open enrollment training courses conducted by TPI in different countries.

Training process

A standardized professional training program is available for all levels of the Triple P system (with the exception of Level 1). Triple P Provider Training Courses use an active skills training approach that involves a combination of didactic input by an accredited trainer, video and live demonstration of core consultation skills, small group exercises to practice skills, problem-solving exercises, course readings, and competency-based assessment. This assessment includes a written quiz and live or videotaped demonstration by participants to show mastery of core competencies specific to the level of training undertaken. Triple P training is designed to be relatively brief to minimize disruption to staff schedules and to reduce the need for relief workers while staff undertake training. The training experience comprises attendance at a 1–5 day training course (based on the level of intervention), a pre-accreditation day, and an accreditation.

A range of professionals deliver Triple P interventions to parents. To be eligible to undertake the training, participants are recommended to have professional training in psychology, medicine, nursing, social work, counseling, or other related fields so that they have some prior exposure to principles of child development, and experience working with families. However, there are some instances where Level 2 and 3 programs are delivered by paraprofessionals working in a family support role. Only practitioners who complete accreditation requirements can be considered properly trained to deliver the intervention. Follow-up studies of participants in Triple P training show that about 85% of practitioners who start training become accredited and, of those, about 90% implement Triple P (Seng, Prinz, & Sanders, 2006). While different professional groups have varying qualifications, from certificate to postgraduate training (Sethi, Kerns, Sanders, & Ralph, 2014) and number of years of previous experience (Turner, Nicholson, & Sanders, 2011), these have not been found to be significant predictors of program use.

Central training team

All Triple P Provider Training Courses are facilitated by Triple P trainers, who are Masters or PhD level professionals (mainly clinical or educational psychologists). Professionals invited to become trainers undergo an intensive 6-day Triple P Trainer Course that prepares them to conduct provider training and accreditation. The course involves simulated training sessions and ongoing peer review and feedback to develop trainer skills. After initial induction, trainers are awarded provisional status and can begin conducting Triple P Provider Training Courses under supervision from TPI (i.e., co-facilitating with another trainer). In order to receive full accreditation status they are required to receive satisfactory evaluations for at least two Triple P Provider Training Courses and complete the required Triple P Trainer Accreditation Quiz.

Although many agencies favor a train-the-trainer model, such an approach can lead to substantial program drift and poorer client outcomes. Program disseminators can quickly lose control of the training process and, as a result, find it harder to efficiently incorporate revisions that are required when ongoing research indicates changes need to be included in the program. Maintaining control over the initial training of providers, although not without its challenges, is achievable and helps to promote quality standards. Triple P trainers do not work independently; they are contracted by TPI and use standardized training materials which serve to ensure that program integrity is protected. While the majority of Triple P Provider Training occurs in English, training resources have been translated into eight additional languages to date.

Tailoring training methods to target groups

Triple P training is delivered to a broad range of service providers. The delivery of courses has to be customized to a certain extent to cater for the special characteristics of the service providers undergoing training. This can be accomplished by ensuring trainers are familiar with the local context, including where providers work, their role in providing parenting support, their professional backgrounds, and levels of experience. Quality training is flexible enough that the experience and learning styles of the group can be addressed while ensuring that essential content is properly covered. This tailoring can involve selection of relevant (to the audience) case examples and illustrations, drawing upon the knowledge, experience, and expertise of the group, being sensitive to the cultural background and values of the group, and by drawing the attention of the group to the variant and invariant (i.e. core content and process) features of the program.

Maintaining training quality

Maintaining the quality of the training process itself needs to be carefully managed by TPI to minimize program drift at source. To prevent drift, all trainers use standardized materials (including participant notes, training exercises, and training DVDs demonstrating core consultation skills), become part of a trainer network, and adhere to a quality assurance process as part of the maintenance of their ongoing accreditation. In order to maintain their fully accredited status, for each successive 2-year quality assurance period, Triple P trainers are required to: 1) complete at least one training or accreditation course per year; 2) maintain satisfactory course ratings; 3) participate in at least 10 hours of approved peer support groups using the Peer-Assisted Supervision and Support Model (PASS; Sanders & Murphy-Brennan, 2010); and 4) complete a minimum of 10 hours of relevant professional development (e.g., attendance at an annual Trainer's Day, other training update sessions, training observation and feedback, delivery of Triple P to parents, review of research papers, conference presentations).

TPI also directly manages all aspects of the professional training programs, including the initial practitioner training courses, pre- and post-training support for practitioners, an online provider network, and follow-up technical assistance.

Technical support

Positive child and parent outcomes are expected when practitioners deliver programs with fidelity (Little et al., 2012). This fidelity is often associated with practitioners receiving adequate supervision and implementation support, particularly during initial implementation. TPI encourages capacity building within organizations and has a range of support options available (e.g., a Triple P Workshop Series, with topics such as engaging hard to reach families, assessment, managing group processes).

An online provider network has also been established for accredited practitioners to make ongoing technical support available to Triple P practitioners (www.triplep-parenting.net/provider). This network provides practitioners with practice tips and suggestions as well as downloadable clinical tools and resources (e.g., monitoring forms, public domain questionnaires, session checklists), and keeps practitioners up to date with the latest research findings and new programs being released.

Implementation and Maintenance

Following training, practitioners begin to offer Triple P in their community. Sustaining the changes put in place during implementation planning requires support through all implementing organizations in a community. These changes occur at multiple levels within the organization, including with practitioners (e.g., delivering Triple P with fidelity, attending peer support sessions, accessing support as required), managers (e.g., encouraging service delivery, clarifying performance expectations and outcomes), organizations (e.g., reflecting on challenges and variances, implementing processes for peer support, coaching and supervision, funding), and at the systems level (e.g., using data to review support processes, service delivery, administrative support, and leadership structures).

It is essential that organizations and communities actively evaluate the impact of the implementation (e.g., Plan, Do, Study, Act Cycle; Deming, 1986). As a practice takes hold, an organization enters into an implementation evaluation stage for approximately 6–12 months to accumulate enough service delivery data for analyses. Ideally, the resulting performance evaluations demonstrate which systems can effectively sustain the successful delivery of Triple P. The data also show areas that need refinement, revision, or expansion for effective service delivery to continue over time.

Supporting implementation fidelity

Evidence-based programs achieve the best results when delivered with fidelity and competence (Beidas & Kendall, 2010), while incompetently delivered evidence-based programs may even be harmful (Henggeler, 2011). Fidelity of implementation of Triple P is promoted through the Framework and through standardized parent and practitioner resources. During the implementation planning phase, organizations consider how program fidelity checks will be embedded in core service delivery. In addition to the standardized professional training process described above, providers receive detailed written and video resources. Practitioner resources specific to each level of the intervention (levels 2–5) and program variants (e.g., Stepping Stones Triple P, Teen Triple P) include comprehensive manuals that detail each session's activities, PowerPoint presentations, DVDs demonstrating the parenting skills being introduced to parents, and self-report session fidelity checklists (e.g., Sanders, Markie-Dadds, & Turner, 2013). In addition, there are parent resources that include tip sheets and workbooks for specific program variants. Implementation fidelity can also be enhanced through the use of supervision and peer coaching (see supervision of providers section below).

Promoting flexible tailoring and responsive program delivery

Many manualized evidence-based programs have been criticized as being rigid and inflexible. Mazzucchelli and Sanders (2010) argued that delivering a program with fidelity does not mean inflexible delivery, and that there are high- and low-risk variations in content and process that can influence clinical outcomes. The training process encourages practitioners to work collaboratively with parents and to be responsive to client need and situational context while preserving the key or essential elements of the program. Core content, such as the positive parenting principles and strategies, must be presented to parents. However, adapting examples used to illustrate key teaching points, using customized homework tasks, and varying session length and number can be used to respond to the needs and goals of specific clients. Through this type of tailoring, core concepts and procedures are preserved but the idiosyncratic needs of particular parent groups are also addressed (e.g., parents of twins or triplets, parents of children with special needs).

Assessing program outcomes

Program outcome assessment for the Triple P system occurs at two different levels: program effects for individual families and changes at a whole population level. Each program level and program variant has a set of recommended outcome measures to assess child-, parent-, and family-level outcomes. As an example, recommended measures for Level 4 Standard Triple P are outlined in Table 7.2.

Organizations are encouraged to establish an evaluation plan and develop processes for how pre- and post-intervention data will be collected by practitioners in the context of their broader evaluation framework. A data scoring application is available to help practitioners score and track the most commonly used questionnaires. While a comprehensive assessment battery may not be possible for population-level evaluations, some population evaluations have the capacity to use a single standardized measure such as the Eyberg Child Behavior Inventory delivered universally to a target population (e.g., Sarkadi, Sampaio, Kelly, & Feldman, 2014), or a number of standardized measures (e.g., Salari et al., 2013). To assess population outcomes, various evaluation projects have conducted random population surveys, via telephone or face-to-face, using brief demographic and program awareness items as well as standardized measures such as The Strengths and Difficulties Questionnaire (e.g., Sanders et al., 2008; Fives et al., 2014). Other measures include independent community prevalence data such as substantiated child maltreatment cases recorded by child protective services, child out-of-home placements recorded through the foster care system, and child hospitalizations and emergency-room visits due to child maltreatment injuries (e.g., Prinz et al., 2009).

TABLE 7.2 Assessment Measures Commonly Used in Standard Triple P (Level 4)

Domain	Measure
Child adjustment	• Eyberg Child Behavior Inventory (Eyberg & Pincus, 1999). • Sutter-Eyberg Student Behavior Inventory – Revised (Eyberg & Pincus, 1999). • The Strengths and Difficulties Questionnaire (Goodman, 1997, 1999). • Child Adjustment and Parent Efficacy Scale (Morawska, Sanders, Haslam, Filus, & Fletcher, 2014).
Parenting and family adjustment	• Parenting Scale (Arnold, O'Leary, Wolff, & Acker, 1993). • Parenting Tasks Checklist (Sanders & Woolley, 2005). • Parent Problem Checklist (Dadds & Powell, 1991). • Parenting and Family Adjustment Scales (Sanders, Morawska, Haslam, Filus, & Fletcher, 2014).
Parent adjustment	• Depression-Anxiety-Stress Scales (Lovibond & Lovibond, 1995). • Relationship Quality Index, also known as the Quality Marriage Index (Norton, 1983).
Behavior monitoring (selected based on the nature of the target behavior)	• Behavior diary (episodic record) of the problem behavior, when and where it occurred, what happened before (triggers) and what happened afterwards (maintaining factors). • Frequency tally (event record) noting each occurrence of the target behavior. • Permanent product tally of the specific outcome of a behavior or series of behaviors. • Duration record tracking how long a behavior lasts in hours, minutes or seconds. • Partial interval time sample recording the presence or absence of a behavior in a specified time interval (e.g., 10-minute blocks). • Momentary time sample recording the behavior occurring at the moment a given time interval ends.
Direct observation	• Family Observation Schedule (Sanders, 2000). • Functional analysis: Competing behaviors (behaviors to increase and decrease).
Consumer satisfaction	• Consumer Satisfaction Questionnaire (Sanders, Markie-Dadds, & Turner, 2013).

Supervision of providers

Practitioners who have access to supervision and workplace support post-training are more likely to implement Triple P (Turner, Sanders, & Hodge, 2014). The PASS model (Sanders & Murphy-Brennan, 2010) was developed to provide practitioners with implementation support following training. The model is introduced during training so that practitioners can establish a supervision network in their workplace, with initial consultation support or facilitation by a TPI trainer if required. PASS involves practitioners meeting in small groups to review their sessions with parents. As different organizations have varying capacity for clinical supervision, this process is largely self-directed and applies a self-regulatory framework to promote reflective practice and to encourage practitioners to deliver sessions according to the standardized protocols in the manuals. Sessions are recommended to occur every two weeks for the first six sessions and then monthly thereafter. A manual and video demonstrating core skills for practitioners, peer mentors, and supervisors were created to aid training in the PASS model.

The self-regulation approach to supervision is an alternative to more traditional, hierarchically based clinical supervision with an experienced expert supervisor who provides feedback and advice to a supervisee. The self-regulation model utilizes the power and influence of the peer group to promote reciprocal learning outcomes for all participants in supervision groups, which means that peers become attuned to not only assessing their own clinical skills and those of fellow practitioners, but also to providing a motivational context to enable peer colleagues to change their own behaviors, cognitions, and emotions so they become proficient in delivering interventions.

Maintenance supports

Maintaining the implementation of Triple P requires intentional feedback loops to ensure that the practice, organizational, and systems changes put in place are achieving the desired outcomes. Organizations should use available data to revise support processes or service delivery, and to confirm that leadership structures and administrative support are operating effectively. Ongoing procedures should be established to maintain workforce staffing levels, support program fidelity, and promote a shared understanding of the overall initiative aims. An organization or collaborative implementing Triple P in a community-wide approach can work with an IC to estimate their impact to date in the community using the Triple P Capacity Calculator. This process can then help to inform goals to maintain, adjust, or expand service delivery.

Effectiveness of Dissemination and Implementation Efforts

Practitioners have been trained in 25 countries with large-scale roll outs (if not country-wide roll outs), including Australia, Canada, the UK, Ireland, the Netherlands, Belgium, Hong Kong, and the USA. At time of writing, 90,000 training attendances have involved over 60,000 unique practitioners (i.e., many practitioners attend training in more than one program variant).

Population Outcomes

Research evaluating the impact of Triple P on population-level indicators is in its infancy. To date, five population-level studies have been published documenting the effects of the multi-level system. These studies have occurred in Australia, the USA, Germany, Sweden, and Ireland. For example, the US Triple P Systems Trial conducted in 18 counties in South Carolina showed that the implementation of the Triple P system reduced several population-level indicators of child maltreatment including 16% fewer children in out-of-home placements, 17% fewer hospitalizations due to child maltreatment related injuries, and the growth of confirmed cases of child abuse slowed (22% lower; Prinz et al., 2009).

Another example of a large-scale implementation of the Triple P system was in two central Ireland counties and assessed the population level impact via 6000 random household surveys (3000 before and 3000 after the implementation) in the intervention and matched comparison counties. A significant population impact was demonstrated, with a 30% reduction in the population prevalence of "caseness" (i.e., clinical-level severity) for behavioral and emotional problems in children, and also reductions in parental psychological distress and stress. A number of other significant, small-to-medium population effects were found, including improvements in reporting a good relationship with one's child, appropriate parenting strategies, satisfaction with parenting information and services available, and likelihood of participation in future parenting programs (Fives et al., 2014).

Cost-effectiveness

Independent economic analyses of the Triple P system have shown the intervention to be very cost-effective. For example, for the US Triple P Systems Trial, the Washington State Institute for Public Policy has found that implementation of the Triple P system resulted in a $6 return per $1 invested based on child maltreatment costs alone (2011 data; Lee et al., 2012), and an $8.80 return based on child maltreatment, education, crime, property, and health care (major depression) costs (2012 data; Washington State Institute for Public Policy, 2014).

Policy Implications

Lessons for Policy Makers

The traditional approach, to concentrate parenting support only for those families in dire need or when there are well-established problems, is highly unlikely to reduce the prevalence rates of these problems at a population level. In contrast, the adoption of a population approach, in which services are more widely available, does not require all families to receive in-person services in order for a prevalence rate reduction to occur in child abuse and social and emotional problems in a community (Prinz et al., 2009).

In general, policy changes are needed so that agencies delivering family and mental health services to children can be reimbursed for delivering universal, selective, and targeted prevention programs to a wider range of parents. Typically, funding is dependent on clinical diagnosis and tertiary (treatment) service provision rather than prevention and early intervention programs. To ensure adequate reach of evidence-based programs and access for all families, funding models need to be altered to include prevention and early intervention services. Policy and funding models should also prioritize effective implementation practices to ensure that evidence-based programs can be funded and implemented effectively and in a sustained way.

While there are increasing policy imperatives for accountability, which can be assessed at an individual family level and aggregated for agencies, the movement towards universal population-level program roll outs requires better evaluation mechanisms, such as population surveys linking funding to outcome deliverables. Such evaluations can assure policy makers and funders of the practical benefit and dollar value of such approaches.

Influencing Policy

We have taken a multi-pronged approach to influence policy makers, including: conducting briefings for senior bureaucrats, policy makers, and politicians; making formal in-person and written submissions to various National and State Royal Commissions of Inquiry (e.g., Commission into Child Abuse; Carmody, 2013); joining advocacy groups seeking to change the law relating to use of corporal punishment by parents; making television programs and radio broadcasts to promote positive parenting messages in the community (e.g., Driving Mum and Dad Mad, UK); establishing a research blog documenting the latest research findings (triplepblog.net); and hosting an annual international conference for researchers, policy makers, and practitioners (www.helpingfamilieschange.org).

Influencing policy is a challenging and ongoing process. In many ways, having others not connected with a program advocate for the program is the most powerful form of policy influence. In our experience, support from service-based champions and independent expert committees who review available evidence (e.g., NICE, 2013; Blueprints for Healthy Youth Development, 2014) brings the approach to the attention of key decision makers. Ultimately, these decision makers need to be convinced that adoption of a program or system can be sold to their own parliamentary colleagues in treasury or cabinet and ultimately to the public, and that the adoption can be defended in the media.

Challenges and Barriers to Sustained Implementation

Capacity to Go to Scale

The capacity of an evidence-based program to be scaled up is crucial in a public health context. "Going to scale" means that program developers and disseminators (purveyors) have the relevant knowledge, experience and resources to roll out programs on a large scale, and the ability to respond to workforce training demands. When efforts to disseminate Triple P began in earnest in 1996, we could find no well-established exemplars of how to undertake the task. As noted earlier, to enable The program to go to scale, a purveyor organization, TPI, was licensed by The University of Queensland to disseminate the program worldwide. This has also required significant university investment and involvement in the development of intellectual property protocols, licenses, and contracts.

The breadth of Triple P dissemination would not have been achieved without a dedicated dissemination organization with the resources and expertise to manage the process internationally. Large-scale roll outs require the capacity to go to scale rapidly. This has involved responding quickly by having a training team ready to travel internationally to conduct training according to demand, as well as building a local workforce of trainers in countries where training demand warrants this. The development of the Implementation Framework and creation of a team of implementation consultants further enables TPI to respond quickly to support organizations and communities to take their implementation of Triple P to scale, no matter the size of the initiative. The team of ICs regularly communicates via peer networks, allowing for knowledge and experience from a wide range of implementations to be shared. This knowledge exchange allows organizations to benefit from learnings from other roll outs around the world.

Achieving Adequate Population Reach

Despite good intentions and formal written agreements between funders and delivery agencies, not all practitioners or agencies reach the number of families they intend to serve. Failure to achieve implementation targets adds to the cost of the intervention and reduces the return on investment in training. Several strategies have been developed to assist agencies to reach their intended number of families. These include providing templates for promotional material such as posters and brochures, and using a strong communications strategy known as "Stay Positive" that aims to normalize and de-stigmatize participation in parenting support services. Encouragement of "peer-to-peer" advocacy creates "pull demand" for Triple P. For example, Fives and colleagues (2014) showed that parents who had participated in Triple P commonly speak to people they know (friends, neighbors, and relatives) about their experiences. This peer-to-peer advocacy helps mobilize a social contagion which, in turn, attracts other parents to the program. This social network effect may be an important by-product of community-level implementation.

Future Directions

Triple P has evolved considerably over the past three decades, from a program for parents of disruptive preschoolers delivered individually through clinic-based and home coaching, to a multi-level system of intervention with varied delivery modalities and formats that is used around the world. This is due to an ongoing commitment to research and innovation, and a successful and evolving dissemination and implementation support mechanism.

Triple P continues to evolve in four directions concurrently: 1) ongoing research and development work to improve the existing intervention system, so that population-level change can be achieved; 2) the development, testing, and dissemination of additional targeted interventions for vulnerable populations (e.g., parents of children with fetal alcohol problems, parents of pre-term babies); 3) the development, testing, and dissemination of programs through new technology platforms such as responsive online programs (e.g., creating parallel online versions of varying levels of Triple P, evaluating an online triaging system into online programs of varying intensity); and 4) strategic initiatives to further strengthen the scientific basis of all aspects of the program (e.g., developing and testing a public health model of Triple P for deployment in low- and middle-income countries [LMICs]).

There is a complementary role of both developer-led and independent evaluations of Triple P (Sanders & Kirby, 2014). We have taken several quality assurance steps to promote high-quality research training in our doctoral program so that empirical findings on Triple P continue to be nourished by ongoing research and development. This feeds into other processes such as a robust scientific forum for researchers through an annual scientific retreat and international conference, a searchable evidence base of published studies on Triple P, a research blog for rapid dissemination on new findings, and an ongoing commitment to consumer and end-user input into the development of Triple P.

A commitment to provide parenting support for all families requires a major effort to ensure that programs are suitable and effective with a very diverse range of parent and family situations. With that goal in mind, to date, we have developed and tested programs for children from infancy to adolescents, for parents of children with a range of mental health and developmental problems (e.g., conduct problems, ADHD, anxiety disorders, feeding disorders, pain syndromes, autism spectrum disorders, traumatic brain injury, cerebral palsy), parents with a variety of adjustment difficulties (e.g., parents with a depressive disorder, intellectual impairment, anger management problems, marital distress), and families in a number of living circumstances (e.g., parents who are separated and divorced, single parents, grandparents, working parents suffering from occupational stress and burnout).

Although the growing reach of the program and associated research being conducted in multiple countries is encouraging, there is still much to do. Evidence-based parenting programs are under-developed and not accessible to the vast majority of the world population, particularly in low-resource environments. Recently the World Health Organization (2009) and United Nations Office on Drugs and Crime (2009) have called for evidence-based parenting programs to be implemented in LMICs. We are developing and testing Triple P in several of these countries, including sub-Saharan countries of Kenya and South Africa, and Latin American countries (e.g., Panama). This work involves a coalition of non-governmental and philanthropic organizations, and work has been done in some of the most challenging communities, such as urban ghettos. Current work also focuses on parenting programs with Indigenous populations including Aboriginal and Torres Strait Island populations in Australia, Maori and Pacific Island people in New Zealand, and First Nations populations in North America. Current large-scale implementation trials are also under way, testing the multi-level Stepping Stones Triple P intervention for parents of children with a disability. Other RCTs are under way with parents with bipolar disorder, parents of young children who are offenders, vulnerable first-time pregnant parents, and parents of children with chronic illnesses including diabetes, asthma, and eczema.

The goal is to develop the minimally sufficient number of additional program variants to ensure all parents can access a culturally and contextually relevant program suited to their needs. It is also important that Triple P programs continue to evolve for new generations of parents with very different circumstances and histories as compared to the generation who participated in the original trials. For example, many time-poor modern families and practitioners raised in a digital world may wish to access parenting programs advice and training through the Internet. This has the potential to increase reach, reduce costs, and enhance public health impact. However, this represents a major challenge and potential threat for developers and purveyor organizations and, indeed, practitioners who have relied on face-to-face intervention delivery and in-person training programs. The next generation of parenting programs will need to develop creative ways of preserving features of interventions that are highly valued, or seen as crucial mechanisms for change, while integrating technology-assisted ways of mobilizing the same mechanisms (e.g., peer support via closed social communities linked to online programs).

Finally, we are embarking on some new synergies between different disciplines to create new opportunities for prevention using population-based approaches. We have recently teamed with the field of Engineering and Global Change Scientists interested in energy poverty and promoting the sustainable use of natural resources to test whether the combination of engineering solutions (e.g., using cooking devices that burn gas instead of traditional methods using animal manure as a fuel source) and parenting and family-based population health interventions can concurrently produce healthier and more sustainable environments to raise children.

References

Arnold, D. S., O'Leary, S. G., Wolff, L. S., & Acker, M. M. (1993). The Parenting Scale: A measure of dysfunctional parenting in discipline situations. *Psychological Assessment, 5*, 137–144.

Baer, D. M., Wolf, M. M., & Risley, T. R. (1968). Some current dimensions of applied behavior analysis. *Journal of Applied Behavior Analysis, 1*(1), 91–97.

Bandura, A. (1977). *Social learning theory.* Englewood Cliffs, NJ: Prentice-Hall.

Beidas R. S., & Kendall, P. C. (2010). Training therapists in evidence-based practice: A critical review of studies from a systems-contextual perspective. *Clinical Psychology: Science and Practice, 17,* 1–30.

Blueprints for Healthy Youth Development (2014). *Triple P System fact sheet.* Boulder, CO: Institute of Behavioral Science, University of Colorado Boulder.

Carmody, T. (2013). *Taking responsibility: A roadmap for Queensland child protection.* Brisbane, Australia: State of Queensland (Queensland Child Protection Commission of Inquiry).

Dadds, M. R., & Powell, M. B. (1991). The relationship of interparental conflict and global marital adjustment to aggression, anxiety, and immaturity in aggressive nonclinic children. *Journal of Abnormal Child Psychology, 19,* 553–567.

de Graaf, I., Speetins, P., Smit, F., de Wolff, M., & Tavecchio, L. (2008a). Effectiveness of the Triple P Positive Parenting Program on parenting: A meta-analysis. *Journal of Family Relations, 57,* 553–566.

de Graaf, I., Speetjens, P., Smit, F., de Wolff, M., & Tavecchio, L. (2008b). Effectiveness of the Triple P-Positive Parenting Program on behavioral problems in children: A meta-analysis. *Behavior Modification, 32,* 714–735.

Deming, W. E. (1986). *Out of the crisis.* Cambridge, MA: Massachusetts Institute of Technology, Center for Advanced Engineering Study.

Dodge, K. (1986). A social information processing model of social competence in children. In M. Perlmutter (Ed.), *Minnesota Symposia on Child Psychology: Vol. 18. Cognitive perspectives on children's social and behavioral development* (pp. 77–125). Hillsdale, NJ: Lawrence Erlbaum.

Eyberg, S. M., & Pincus, D. (1999). *Eyberg Child Behavior Inventory and Sutter-Eyberg Student Behavior Inventory—Revised: Professional manual.* Odessa, FL: Psychological Assessment Resources.

Farquhar, J. W., Fortmann, S. P., Maccoby, N., Haskell, W. L., Williams, P. T., Flora, J. A., et al. (1985). The Stanford Five-City Project: Design and methods. *American Journal of Epidemiology, 122*(2), 323–334.

Fives, A., Pursell, L., Heary, C., Nic Gabhainn, S., & Canavan, J. (2014). *Parenting support for every parent: A population-level evaluation of Triple P in Longford Westmeath. Final report.* Athlone: Longford Westmeath Parenting Partnership (LWPP).

Fixsen, D. L., Naoom, S. F., Blase, K. A., Friedman, R. M., & Wallace, F. (2005). *Implementation research: A synthesis of the literature.* Tampa, FL: University of South Florida, Louis de la Parte Florida Mental Health Institute, The National Implementation Research Network.

Glasgow, R. E., Vogt, T. M., & Boles, S. M. (1999). Evaluating the public health impact of health promotion interventions: The RE-AIM framework. *American Journal of Public Health, 89*(9), 1322–1327.

Goodman, R. (1997). The Strengths and Difficulties Questionnaire: A research note. *Journal of Child Psychology and Psychiatry, 38,* 581–586.

Goodman, R. (1999). The extended version of the Strengths and Difficulties Questionnaire as a guide to child psychiatric caseness and consequent burden. *Journal of Child Psychology and Psychiatry, 40*(5), 791–799.

Guajardo, N. R., Snyder, G., & Petersen, R. (2009). Relationships among parenting practices, parental stress, child behaviour, and children's social-cognitive development. *Infant and Child Development, 18,* 37–60.

Hart, B. M., & Risley, T. R. (1995). *Meaningful differences in the everyday experience of young American children*. Baltimore, MD: Paul. H. Brooks.

Henggeler, S. W. (2011). Efficacy studies to large-scale transport: The development and validation of multisystemic therapy programs. *Annual Review of Clinical Psychology, 7*, 351–81.

Lee, S., Aos, S., Drake, E., Pennucci, A., Miller, M., & Anderson, L. (2012) *Return on investment: Evidence-based options to improve statewide outcome, April 2012*. (Document No. 12—4-4-12-1). Olympica: Washington State Institute for Public Policy.

Little, M., Berry, V., Morpeth, L., Blower, S., Axford, N., Taylor, R., Bywater, T., Lehtonen, M., & Tobin, K. (2012). The impact of three evidence-based programmes delivered in public systems in Birmingham, UK. *International Journal of Conflict and Violence, 6*, 260–272.

Lovibond, S. H., & Lovibond, P. F. (1995). *Manual for the Depression Anxiety Stress Scales (2nd Ed.)*. Sydney, NSW: Psychology Foundation of Australia.

Mazzucchelli, T. G., & Sanders, M. R. (2010). Facilitating practitioner flexibility within an empirically supported intervention: Lessons from a system of parenting support. *Clinical Psychology: Science and Practice, 17*(3), 238–252.

Moffitt, T. E., Arseneault, L., Belsky, D., Dickson, N., Hancox, R. J., Harrington, H., et al. (2011). A gradient of childhood self-control predicts health, wealth, and public safety. *Proceedings of the National Academy of Sciences of the USA, 108*, 2693–2698.

Morawska, A., Sanders, M., Goadby, E., Headley, C., Hodge, L., McAuliffe, C., et al. (2011). Is the Triple P-Positive Parenting Program acceptable to parents from culturally diverse backgrounds? *Journal of Child and Family Studies, 20*(5), 614–622.

Morawska, A., Sanders, M. R., Haslam, D., Filus, A., & Fletcher, R. (2014). Child Adjustment and Parent Efficacy Scale: Development and initial validation of a parent report measure. *Australian Psychologist, 49*(4), 241–252.

National Institute for Health and Care Excellence [NICE]. (2013). *Antisocial behaviour and conduct disorders in children and young people: The NICE guideline on recognition, intervention and management* (National Clinical Guideline Number 158). London: The British Psychological Society and The Royal College of Psychiatrists.

Norton, R. (1983). Measuring marital quality: A critical look at the dependent variable. *Journal of Marriage and the Family, 45*, 141–151.

Nowak, C., & Heinrichs, N. (2008). A comprehensive meta-analysis of Triple P-Positive Parenting Program using hierarchical linear modeling: Effectiveness and moderating variables. *Clinical Child Family Psychology Review, 11*, 114–144.

Patterson, G. R. (1982). *A social learning approach to family intervention: III. Coercive family process*. Eugene, OR: Castalia.

Prinz, R. J., Sanders, M. R., Shapiro, C. J., Whitaker, D. J., & Lutzker, J. R. (2009). Population-based prevention of child maltreatment: The U.S. Triple P system population trial. *Prevention Science, 10*, 1–12.

Romney, S., Israel, N., & Zlatevski, D. (2014). Exploration-stage implementation variation: Its effect on the cost-effectiveness of an evidence-based parenting program. *Zeitschrift für Psychologie, 222*(1), 37–48.

Rutter, M. (1985a). Family and school influences on cognitive development. *Journal of Child Psychology and Psychiatry and Allied Disciplines, 26*(5), 683–704.

Rutter, M. (1985b). Resilience in the face of adversity: Protective factors and resistance to psychiatric disorder. *British Journal of Psychiatry, 147*, 598–611.

Salari, R., Fabian, H., Prinz, R., Lucas, S., Feldman, I., Fairchild, A., & Sarkadi, A. (2013). The Children and Parents in Focus project: A population-based cluster-randomised controlled trial to prevent behavioural and emotional problems in children. *BMC Public Health, 13*, 961.

Sanders, M. R. (2000). *Family observation schedule.* Brisbane, Australia: Parenting and Family Support Centre, The University of Queensland.

Sanders, M. R. (2012). Development, evaluation, and multinational dissemination of the Triple P – Positive Parenting Program. *Annual Review of Clinical Psychology, 8,* 1–35.

Sanders, M. R., & Glynn, T. (1981). Training parents in behavioral self-management: An analysis of generalization and maintenance. *Journal of Applied Behavior Analysis, 14,* 223–237.

Sanders, M. R., & Kirby, J. N. (2014). Surviving or thriving: Quality assurance mechanisms to promote innovation in the development of evidence-based parenting interventions. *Prevention Science,* published online March 2014.

Sanders, M. R., Kirby, J. N., Tellegen, C. L., & Day, J. J. (2013). Towards a public health approach to parenting support: A systematic review and meta-analysis of the Triple P-Positive Parenting Program. *Clinical Psychology Review, 34*(4), 337–357.

Sanders, M. R., Markie-Dadds, C., Tully, L. A., & Bor, W. (2000). The Triple P-Positive Parenting Program: A comparison of enhanced, standard, and self-directed behavioral family intervention for parents of children with early onset conduct problems. *Journal of Consulting and Clinical Psychology, 68,* 624–640.

Sanders, M. R., Markie-Dadds, C., & Turner, K. M. T. (2013). *Practitioner's manual for Standard Triple P* (2nd ed.). Brisbane, Australia: Triple P International Pty Ltd.

Sanders, M. R., Morawska, A., Haslam, D. M., Filus, A., & Fletcher, R. (2014). Parenting and Family Adjustment Scales (PAFAS): Validation of a brief parent-report measure for use in assessment of parenting skills and family relationships. *Child Psychiatry and Human Development, 45*(3), 255–272.

Sanders, M. R., & Murphy-Brennan, M. (2010). Creating conditions for success beyond the professional training environment. *Clinical Psychology: Science and Practice, 17,* 31–35.

Sanders, M. R., Ralph, A., Sofronoff, K., Gardiner, P., Thompson, R., Dwyer, S., & Bidwell, K. (2008). Every Family: A population approach to reducing behavioral and emotional problems in children making the transition to school. *Journal of Primary Prevention, 29,* 197–222.

Sanders, M. R., & Woolley, M. L. (2005). The relationship between maternal self-efficacy and parenting practices: Implications for parent training. *Child: Care, Health and Development, 31*(1), 65–73.

Sarkadi, A., Sampaio, F., Kelly, M. P., & Feldman, I. (2014). A novel approach used outcome distribution curves to estimate the population-level impact of a public health intervention. *Journal of Clinical Epidemiology, 67*(7), 785–792.

Seng, A. C., Prinz, R. J., & Sanders, M. R. (2006). The role of training variables in effective dissemination of evidence-based parenting interventions. *International Journal of Mental Health Promotion, 8*(4), 20–28.

Sethi, S., Kerns, S. E. U., Sanders, M. R., & Ralph, A. (2014). The international dissemination of evidence-based parenting interventions: Impact on practitioner content and process self-efficacy. *International Journal of Mental Health Promotion, 16*(2), 126–137.

Stack, D. M., Serbin, L. A., Enns, L., Ruttle, P., & Barrieau, L. (2010). Parental effects on children's emotional development over time and across generations. *Infants and Young Children, 23,* 52–69.

Thomas, R., & Zimmer-Gembeck, M. J. (2007). Behavioral outcomes of parent–child interaction therapy and Triple P-Positive Parenting Program: A review and meta-analysis. *Journal of Abnormal Child Psychology, 35,* 475–495.

Turner, K. M. T., Nicholson, J. M., & Sanders, M. R. (2011). The role of practitioner self-efficacy, training, program and workplace factors on the implementation of an evidence-based parenting intervention in primary care. *Journal of Primary Prevention, 32*(2), 95–112.

Turner, K. M. T., Richards, M., & Sanders, M. R. (2007). Randomised clinical trial of a group parent education programme for Australian Indigenous families. *Journal of Paediatrics and Child Health, 43*(6), 429–437.

Turner, K. M. T., Sanders, M. R., & Hodge, L. (2014). Issues in professional training to implement evidence-based parenting programs: The needs of Indigenous practitioners. *Australian Psychologist.* Accepted 28 August, 2014.

United Nations Office on Drugs and Crime [UNODC] (2009). *Guide to implementing family skills training programmes for drug abuse prevention.* New York: United Nations.

Washington State Institute for Public Policy. (2014). *Child welfare benefit-cost results* (Document No. 11-07-1201). Olympia: Washington State Institute for Public Policy.

Wilson, P., Rush, R., Hussey, S., Puckering, C., Sim, F., Allely, C. S., et al. (2012). How evidence-based is an 'evidence-based parenting program'? A PRISMA systematic review and meta-analysis of Triple P. *BMC Medicine, 10*, 130.

World Health Organization [WHO] (2009). *Preventing violence through the development of safe, stable and nurturing relationships between children and their parents and caregivers. Series of briefings on violence prevention: The evidence.* Geneva, Switzerland: WHO.

6

THINKING SYSTEMATICALLY FOR ENDURING FAMILY CHANGE

Gregory M. Fosco, Brian Bumbarger, and Katharine T. Bamberger

Introduction

The family-centered prevention programs described in the previous chapters underscore (1) the importance of family systems and other theories for guiding the development of family-centered preventive programs; (2) the efficacy of such well-designed and theoretically informed programs for significantly improving outcomes for both children and parents; and (3) the robust, population-level public health benefits that can accrue from disseminating family-based programs that can simultaneously effect a wide range of risk outcomes by improving core aspects of family functioning. In addition to carefully considering change at the individual and family systems levels, the previous chapters demonstrate that there are important macro- and systems-level challenges to overcome before these types of programs can achieve their optimal reach and impact—to improve outcomes for whole populations over generations. The programs described in this volume have been uniquely successful at addressing many of these barriers, especially regarding dissemination, and in a few cases have achieved impressive scale. In many respects, the programs described in previous chapters can be viewed as the first generation of evidence-based family-centered prevention programs; they can serve as a guidepost for the development of the next generation of programs that will achieve even greater impact and scale, and do so more quickly and efficiently, and with larger effect sizes.

In this chapter, we discuss a number of the important challenges and potential barriers that remain, at both societal and family levels. At the societal level, this includes broad issues related to delivery and support capacity and infrastructure, which impact the reach and population-level impact that prevention programs can have (see Figure 14.1). At the family level, we discuss the importance of pushing the field toward testing the guiding theories of prevention programs

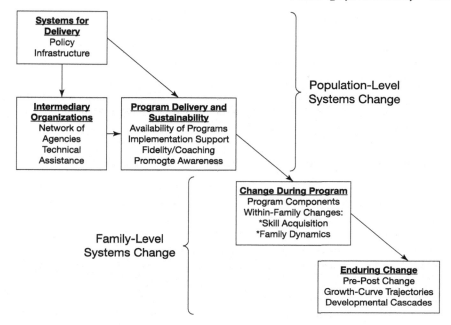

FIGURE 14.1 A Social-Ecosystems Model of Systems Change

by assessing both the prevention process *and* mechanisms that account for enduring changes for family and individual outcomes, which we think of as family-level systems change.

Population-Level Systems Change: Dissemination and Implementation of Evidence-Based Family Programs

Family systems theory and the evidence base for effective family-centered prevention can be considered recent innovations. As with any new technology or advancement, there has to be recognition of the incongruence with the larger culture or context when the innovation is first introduced. Consider the introduction of any important societal innovation: indoor plumbing, the automobile, television, the desktop computer, or e-mail. Each of these innovations was an exciting discovery, but without a supporting infrastructure, each would have been of limited use. All required a concomitant and complex infrastructure surrounding and supporting the innovation in order to take full advantage of the new technology (e.g., public water systems, highways and traffic signals, cable networks, LAN, and the internet). Thinking about the introduction of a generation of new family-focused prevention programs in the same way helps us to consider exactly what infrastructure is necessary and what systems change is required to take full advantage of this new "technology".

We can ask questions such as:

- What kind of prevention support and delivery systems are required?
- What policy and funding structures would be optimal?
- Who is responsible for developing this infrastructure?
- How can we measure and assess incremental change and improvement in this support and delivery infrastructure as part of the research agenda to assess the impact of these programs?

Systems for Delivery to Promote Dissemination and Adoption

A primary challenge relates to developing the necessary infrastructure to promote the adoption of effective family-based prevention programs by communities, including increasing demand and improving goodness of fit between programs and community-identified needs. As the evidence-based programs agenda has matured, there is increasing awareness of the need for improving communities' capacity to identify their unique service and programming needs and to support data-informed program selection. With increasing recognition and adoption of the public health risk-focused prevention paradigm (Hawkins, Catalano, & Arthur, 2002), more states and communities are implementing community-level risk-factor surveillance systems to empower the monitoring of risk and protective factors associated with or predictive of a wide range of health and behavior outcomes. These surveillance systems provide communities with the capacity to continually monitor underlying conditions across ecological domains (i.e. community, family, school, peer/individual) and at key developmental stages, and to promote informed decisions about the programs and strategies most likely to achieve population-level impact (Mrazek, Biglan, & Hawkins, 2007). Research has demonstrated that when communities have this surveillance and diagnostic capacity in place, they are more likely to adopt evidence-based programs, more likely to monitor implementation quality and implement with fidelity (i.e., less likely to make adaptations), more likely to achieve results across multiple health, education, and behavioral outcomes, and more likely to sustain programs beyond initial seed-funding (Feinberg, Jones, Greenberg, Osgood, & Bontempo, 2010; Tibbits, Bumbarger, Kyler, & Perkins, 2010; Rhoades, Bumbarger, & Moore, 2012). Having such diagnostic capacity can also help communities match program-targeted mechanisms to specific community needs or risk mechanisms, which can not only increase the likelihood of effectiveness but also create a better community fit and thus contribute to sustainability of program delivery (Cooper, Bumbarger, & Moore, 2013).

Quality in Program Delivery

Scale and quality of program delivery sometimes work in opposition. As dissemination and scale increase, so does the concern and challenge to maintain sufficient implementation quality and fidelity. Research has clearly established the correlation between high-quality implementation and better outcomes (Fixsen, Naoom, Blase, & Friedman, 2005; Durlak & DuPre, 2008), but there is continued call from practitioners and communities for greater sensitivity and adaptation to meet communities' cultural needs (Castro, Barrera, & Holleran Steiker, 2010). Although this demand for flexibility and tailored implementation must be recognized as valid and valuable, it should not be used to justify a laissez-faire approach in which practitioners are given carte-blanche to adapt theoretically well-defined programs at will. In fact, research has shown that as evidence-based programs (EBPs) go to scale, the majority of adaptation can be characterized not as thoughtful and proactive cultural tailoring, but more accurately as program "drift", which is reactive rather than proactive and likely to reduce program effectiveness (Moore, Bumbarger, & Cooper, 2013). Thus, the challenge is to maintain high-quality implementation as programs go to scale while still utilizing practitioners' indigenous knowledge and respecting local culture.

To address this challenge, the infrastructure for quality implementation must support capacity building within and across provider organizations to promote a *culture of excellence*. Among provider organizations, there is a need for a greater emphasis on and capacity to support workforce and leadership development and regular implementation monitoring and continuous quality improvement. Providers should be encouraged and supported to regularly reflect on the fundamental questions of "how well are we delivering prevention services?" and "what impact are we having on children and families?" Promoting this culture of excellence includes setting high standards for the workforce to whom we entrust the delivery of family-focused prevention programs. Perhaps as an artifact of historically naïve ideas about the simplicity of offering "parenting guidance", many family strengthening programs are still considered rather elementary, not requiring a particularly skilled or experienced workforce. It is not uncommon for entry-level human service workers with no specific training or experience, and without any minimum education requirements, to deliver these programs. Additionally, with very few exceptions, family-centered prevention programs are rarely delivered within an organizational context and culture of "clinical supervision". It is easiest to recognize this particular shortcoming of prevention delivery in comparison to some popular evidence-based therapeutic interventions, such as Multisystemic Therapy or Functional Family Therapy (Carr, 2000). In the case of both of these therapeutic interventions, implementers are required to be Master's level therapists, to have regular coaching and feedback from an experienced clinical supervisor, and to be certified through a structured training process. Both programs also have sophisticated national data infrastructure to support implementation quality and fidelity monitoring and the use of data feedback for continuous quality improvement. These models demonstrate the type of workforce and organizational capacity that is required to scale programs while maintaining sufficient quality and fidelity, and stand in stark contrast to the way family-focused prevention programs are typically disseminated.

Quality in program dissemination and implementation also requires a fundamental shift in the conventional training paradigm for scaling programs. The traditional model for training practitioners typically does not reflect best practices in teaching adult learners or incorporate decades of effective diffusion of innovation theory. The conventional approach to training for dissemination is proving ineffective and insufficient at achieving the level of mastery necessary for practitioners to achieve high-quality implementation. In our experience supporting the replication of nearly 300 EBPs over the last decade, very often the certification training offered by program developers is the wrong training at the wrong time. Specifically, in the conventional training model, there is too much emphasis on the *mechanics and logistics* of program delivery and too little emphasis on practitioners' depth of knowledge and understanding of the *underlying theory of prevention and behavior change*—both generally and as it relates to the particular program. Practitioners often leave training with a detailed script to read but without the necessary skills to effectively process and respond when realities force them to go off-script during program delivery. This may be at least partially due to the ongoing "black box" nature of many programs, as research to date on prevention mechanisms and participant learning processes is scarce (for a more in-depth discussion of this issue, see the section below on Family-Level Systems Change). Careful work evaluating these processes would help practitioners understand how exactly a given program's core elements lead to fundamental changes in risk or protective factors, skills, knowledge, attitudes, or intentions that have been hypothesized to ultimately lead to both proximal and distal behavior change outcomes.

Finally, in the conventional training model, training takes place well before implementation—often without any follow-up coaching, supervision or peer support during implementation; this leads predictably to skill and knowledge loss between training and implementation. Shifting to a model that instead emphasizes ongoing coaching and support during implementation, as exemplified by many of the model programs in this volume, is likely to not only increase practitioners' engagement, understanding, and mastery, but will quite likely reduce program implementation costs, since the typical face-to-face, large group pre-implementation training is the costliest aspect of many family-centered prevention programs.

Program Sustainability

In addition to dissemination and implementation, *sustainability* is another significant challenge for achieving (and maintaining) the scale necessary to affect population-level public health improvement. Even the most effective family-focused prevention programs must work across multiple generations to achieve their full potential (Haskins, Garfinkel, & McLanahan, 2014; Weisz, 2014). The sustainability challenge is especially great for programs that are *both* family-focused and preventive, since this combination presents specific challenges to scale and sustainability. The robust effects of family-based prevention programs in impacting a wide range of developmental outcomes is a double-edged sword. On one hand, it allows multiple developmental and behavioral outcomes to be targeted simultaneously, encouraging buy-in from a broad cross-section of service delivery organizations. On the other hand, current funding models tend to encourage a singular focus, which allows a diffusion of responsibility for family-strengthening across multiple service systems, where systems and policymakers "pass the buck" on promoting (and funding) these programs to other systems that may also be impacted by such a program. Because government systems are not naturally inclined to collaboration, a service that is everyone's responsibility can easily become no one's responsibility. Likewise, while the theoretical and empirical evidence clearly supports primary prevention approaches (Offord, Kraemer, Kazdin, Jensen, & Harrington, 1998), the practical and fiscal realities of short-term budget cycles are in opposition to the delayed "payoff" of programs that sometimes operate decades or generations in advance, and for which the cause–effect relationship between program outcomes and systems savings is more difficult to demonstrate.

Recently, however, there has been some reason for optimism that we may overcome these policy and funding conundrums. First, a new generation of more sophisticated economic analyses is helping to better articulate the return-on-investment equation, especially for family-focused prevention, and the cost-savings are often astounding even when using intentionally conservative calculations (Aos, Lieb, Mayfield, Miller, & Pennucci, 2004; Crowley, Coffman, Feinberg, Greenberg, & Spoth, 2014). Second, the passage of the Affordable Care Act has established a mechanism (and important legislative precedent) for supporting primary prevention—including family strengthening—through the same managed-care system that has been used to successfully scale family-focused treatment/therapy (Koh & Sebelius, 2010). Third, pioneering new Social Impact Bond initiatives are facilitating private sector venture capital investment in evidence-based programs as a way to 'kick-start' these programs in public systems without the need for public seed funding (Liebman, 2013; Pew-MacArthur, 2014).

The exemplar programs described in this volume have served as "proof-of-concept" that well-designed and theoretically informed family-focused prevention can achieve significant results beyond the controlled environments of research trials. This has led to increasing interest from state and federal agencies to take such programs to scale. Appreciating the complexity of the multiple macro-system challenges described in this chapter, there is growing recognition of the potential role of *intermediary organizations* as part of the necessary infrastructure for achieving scale. Representing an evolution of the traditional technical assistance provider, intermediaries facilitate productive interaction between researchers (including program developers and evaluators), policymakers (including funders and system leaders), and the practitioners and provider organizations responsible for program delivery. Wandersman and colleagues (2008) have described this interactive systems framework for promoting the dissemination and implementation of evidence-based practices (family-based and otherwise) and articulated the need for such intermediaries to function as a prevention support system. Intermediaries serve not only as technical assistance providers and knowledge brokers, but importantly connect these diverse stakeholder groups and facilitate the identification of barriers to dissemination and implementation, supporting cross-system problem-solving that might not otherwise be prioritized (Dymnicki, Wandersman, Osher, Grigorescu, Huang, & Meyer, 2014; Franks, 2010; Greenwood & Welsh, 2012). Some notable examples include Pennsylvania's Evidence-based Prevention and Intervention Support Center (EPISCenter) at Penn State University's Prevention Research Center (www.episcenter.psu.edu), the Connecticut Center for Effective Practice at the Child Health and Development Institute (www.kidsmentalhealthinfo.com), and the Centre for Effective Services in Ireland (www.effectiveservices.org). These intermediaries help to network practitioners, policymakers, and researchers; problem-solve barriers to the dissemination and high-quality implementation of evidence-based programs (family-focused and otherwise); and advance the research agenda to improve the efficiency and effectiveness of scaling evidence-based programs.

Family-Level Systems Change

Delivery and evaluation of family-based prevention programs, and the randomized controlled trial in particular, have historical roots in the medical model in which treatments are administered clinically to a patient. Accordingly, much of the research stemming from randomized controlled trials regards programs in a manner akin to giving a patient a medicine and comparing change in those who receive the medicine to those who did not. This approach overlooks the nuances of prevention programs and the reality that there are typically several distinct components to a given program, its delivery, and the processes by which families "absorb" the program components.

Indeed, change processes in family-based prevention programs reflect the intersection of family and developmental theory and prevention science. Building on strong theoretical foundations, family-based programs target specific dynamics and skills for change in an effort to promote protective factors and reduce risk factors in the service of improving the lives of the youth and families. Interestingly, this rich theory has largely been unevaluated within the context of prevention program evaluations that adhere closely to the gold-standard randomized controlled trial design in which random assignment to the prevention program is associated with improvements in targeted outcomes. With a premium placed on distal outcomes, there is a relative dearth of research that directly evaluates the theoretical models that guide these programs. The absence of such research has created a "black box" in our understanding of the effects of prevention programs (Chen & Rossi, 1983); that is, when change occurs due to a prevention program, there is little knowledge of the process of change. This "black box" problem creates limitations to our scientific understanding of program effectiveness and causes real-world problems in terms of practitioners' ability to gain a deep conceptual understanding and achieve high-quality delivery of a prevention program.

In the following sections, we discuss change processes in prevention programs in two timescales. We focus first on the traditional approach to testing change processes following prevention programs, which we refer to as *enduring change processes*. This approach typically examines the degree of change that occurs from pre-test to post-test and how such change predicts long-term outcomes for families and youth. In this section, we review methods that have been used and future directions for research that can show how prevention programs elicit change in proximal program targets (e.g., family relationships) and the subsequent enduring effects on distal outcomes (e.g., child misbehavior).

Second, we discuss research, methods, and future directions for the study of how families change during the course of the prevention program itself. This approach, which we consider to be *change during prevention programs*, makes use of new evaluation frameworks such as "components analysis", where programs are decomposed into their constituent parts, as well as related within-family research methods.

Mechanisms of Enduring Changes

It is a humbling exercise to stop and think for a moment about the enduring effects of the prevention programs summarized in this volume. In a way, it is quite impressive that a program that provides only a few hours of support each week and lasts only a couple of months would have such lasting effects that are detectable *years* later. This improbable result underscores the absolutely incredible impact that these programs have and the value of targeting family functioning as a means of creating a lasting impact on the lives of youth. At the same time, such impressive effects also raise important scientific questions about *how* these programs evoke such changes and *why* they are sustained for years after a program concludes. Such scientific questions call for a synthesis of developmental, family, and prevention science.

Traditional pre-post mediation analysis

Historically, tests of program mediators have typically involved examining whether randomization to the prevention program is associated with proximal outcomes, such as parenting practices or relationship quality at post-test, and that this proximal outcome accounts for the program effects on distal outcomes (e.g., adolescent substance use, children's school readiness); essentially, this approach applies principles of statistical tests of mediation to the randomized controlled trial design. Discussions elsewhere have expanded on best practices in testing mediation in prevention and intervention trials (e.g., Kazdin, 2007; Sandler, Schoenfelder, Wolchik, & MacKinnon, 2011). At a basic level, such studies offer valuable insight into why prevention programs cause improvements in outcomes. Unfortunately, very few programs have been subjected to tests of the causal mechanisms of change (Liddle, 2004; Sandler et al., 2011). Although it is unusual to find tests of even one mediator, Kazdin (2007) points out that testing multiple mediators is an important direction for future research. Studies with multiple mediators would allow for tests of specificity in the mechanisms of change (i.e., is it one process or another, or both?) and would create opportunities for tests of alternative hypotheses. Such tests can provide evidence for specificity in program effects, which in turn can lend support to the theoretical model. For example, a family program might have a parent and youth session that targets parenting skills and youth cognitions, respectively, but it may be unclear whether both of these proximal outcomes account for long-term youth outcomes (e.g., conduct problems). Only by testing both potential mediators (parenting skills and youth cognitions) is it possible to know if each have unique effects, or if one process is accounting for these outcomes.

Alternative hypothesis testing is also an important direction for evaluating prevention programs. When prevention programs are evaluated within the theoretical framework from which they were developed, it is common to ignore other potential mechanisms that may also account for change. Suppose for a moment that a program was developed using a behavioral parent training approach for reducing child noncompliance, and that this program focused on parenting practices such as establishing clear expectations, positive reinforcement of appropriate behavior, and using effective consequences for misbehavior. One would expect that a study testing mediators of this parenting program would test an index of these key parenting practices learned during the program as the mechanism accounting for changes in children's noncompliant behavior. However, an alternative hypothesis, drawing on a different theoretical model, might be that in the context of more consistent and effective parenting, parent–child bonding also improves. It is then plausible that parent–child bonding may be an alternative pathway by which the parenting program effects changes on noncompliance. However, neglecting to test such alternative hypotheses makes it more likely that findings will support the theory that guides the program, but only because other theories are not considered as alternatives.

Building on pre–post mediation approaches, studies that use intensive longitudinal methods, such as daily diary or ecological momentary assessment approaches, have several advantages in comparison to retrospective self-report methods. First, intensive longitudinal methods minimize recall bias because of the frequency of assessment (Stone, Shiffman, Atienza, & Nebeling, 2007), which is especially important for mundane day-to-day behaviors (e.g., using praise to reinforce good behavior), and for accuracy in reporting on the intensity of experiences (e.g., conflict), both of which are poorly recalled retrospectively (Schwarz, 2007). Second, intensive longitudinal methods offer greater ecological validity of the assessment—especially in comparison with laboratory assessments—because they are conducted frequently and in the context in which events have occurred (Stone et al., 2007). Third, intensive longitudinal methods can be used to evaluate dynamic within-person processes, which provide greater specificity of temporal events than do global, retrospective accounts (Collins, 2006; Stone et al., 2007). Because of these advantages, intensive longitudinal data are better-suited to address certain specific kinds of research questions and test theories involving processes and change (Collins, 2006), and can have enhanced predictive validity (Kumar et al., 2013) when compared to traditional methods. Although data collection is "intensive", instruments are often brief, relevant to the participant's current experience, and require little summarization across prior experiences. As a result, this approach is highly feasible and typically perceived as unobtrusive by participants (Smyth & Heron, 2014).

A powerful application of intensive longitudinal methods is the measurement-burst design, which can be flexibly applied to a variety of evaluation designs, depending on the expected timescale or constructs of interest (Shiffman, 2007; Sliwinski, 2008). In a measurement-burst design, there are periods of intense measurement "bursts", such as 14 consecutive daily assessments, with periods in between these bursts (e.g., one burst per year). In a prevention program evaluation, this might be applied such that the first measurement burst occurs at pre-test and a subsequent burst occurs at post-test. Such approaches are better able to accurately track daily behavior (e.g., use of parenting strategies) and fluctuations in behavior or emotions from day to day (Shiffman, 2007; Sliwinski, 2008; Smyth & Stone, 2003). There are many other possibilities in terms of dynamics within families that unfold in mutually influential interactions over time (e.g., Schermerhorn, Chow, & Cummings, 2010), or even the degree to which family members influence others' feelings or stress (Almeida, 2005). Overall, intensive longitudinal methods have the potential to capture families as systems (Larson & Almeida, 1999), and consequently, capture change in the family system as the result of a family-based prevention program.

Developmentally informed approaches to mediation

Many family-based prevention programs also draw upon a developmental psychopathology framework in their design. Such programs might target developmentally sensitive periods that have long-lasting repercussions developmentally, such as early childhood programs. Other approaches target periods of developmental transition (e.g., transition to school, transition into middle school, transitions following divorce). This same developmental framework can be applied to tests of program mechanisms. We highlight two major ways this can be done: developmental trajectory approaches, and developmental cascade model approaches.

Developmental trajectory approaches can be applied to the study of family or individual functioning that changes over a particular period of development, rather than limiting attention to a single post-test assessment. In these cases, latent growth curve modeling approaches (e.g., Duncan, Duncan, & Stryker, 2013) have been applied as a powerful strategy for evaluating the impact of family-based prevention programs on family or individual trajectories over time. For example, family-based programs implemented in early adolescence may be optimally timed for preventing adolescents from embarking on an escalating trajectory of substance use or problem behavior. Latent growth curve models, or growth mixture models, offer an assessment strategy that can identify the ways in which family-based programs can alter the developmental progression of problem behavior.

Similarly, family functioning may also correspond to a developmental trajectory perspective. For example, individual differences in family trajectories of parental monitoring and effective parenting practices have been identified in early adolescence (e.g., Dishion, Nelson, & Bullock, 2004). In this example, youth in families who experience rapid decreases in parental monitoring and involvement are at risk for substance use outcomes (e.g., Laird, Pettit, Bates, & Dodge, 2003). Thus, a prevention program would be effective if it helped families maintain their levels of parental monitoring and involvement over the years following the delivery of the program. Such nuanced theoretical models require appropriate design and analytic approaches. Using a latent growth curve modeling approach, it is possible to evaluate whether random assignment to a prevention or control group is associated with differences in rates of change in the proposed mediator over time. Following the parental monitoring and adolescent substance use example above, one would expect that participation in the prevention program would be associated with slower rates of decline in parental monitoring over time; in turn, slower rates of decline in monitoring over time would be associated with slower rates of escalation in substance use. In short, a program that prevented declines in monitoring would then place youth at reduced risk for later substance use. Some studies have used this approach with other family processes, such as family conflict (Van Ryzin & Dishion, 2012; Fosco, Van Ryzin, Stormshak, & Dishion, 2014) and family cohesion (Caruthers, Van Ryzin, & Dishion, 2014). More sophisticated bivariate growth modeling approaches could be used to test multiple mediators simultaneously, and within this multivariate framework, cross-lagged latent difference score modeling (McArdle, 2009) offers a powerful approach to explore the direction and timing of effects among potential mediators and between purported mediators and outcomes, acknowledging that processes of change may be reciprocal rather than exclusively unidirectional.

A second developmentally informed approach to mediation focuses on questions of how a prevention program might disrupt a developmental sequence toward long-term problematic adjustment. This perspective draws on a *developmental cascade* framework, which suggests that effects of individual functioning in one developmental period can set into motion a series of subsequent problems in other developmental periods (e.g., social problems in early childhood that continue into adulthood), expand into different developmental domains (e.g., behavioral problems leading to academic problems), and spill over into other developmental contexts (e.g., family dynamics predicting academic problems) (Dodge et al., 2009; Fosco & Feinberg, 2014; Masten & Cicchetti, 2010; Masten et al., 2005; Moilanen, Shaw, & Maxwell, 2010). Cascade processes may function in a unidirectional manner, or exhibit patterns of reciprocal influence over time (Masten & Cicchetti, 2010). Evaluating programs within a developmental cascade modeling framework can provide important insights into the degree to which program effects endure across developmental periods and the diffusion of program gains across domains and contexts.

Applications of developmental cascades to prevention programs can open up scientific inquiry to consider other influences on the long-term outcomes of youth in family-based prevention programs. Beyond program effects on targeted parenting skills or relationship enhancement, it is important to also think about broader systemic processes that might operate to support positive functioning, or that might, over time, work to erode the benefits from a prevention program. For example, the degree to which improvements in parenting practices are maintained over the long term may be explained by coparenting support processes (e.g., Feinberg, 2003). In families with strong coparenting support processes, positive parenting practices, such as praise for good behavior, may be easier to sustain within the family system. Moreover, from a family systems perspective, changes to any part of the family are thought to reverberate to other relationships in the family (Minuchin, 1985). This "ripple effect" may offer broader insight into change processes for programs that initially target a specific subset of the family system, such as parenting practices (Patterson, 2005), or it may broaden the range of program targets to maximize long-term maintenance. Of note, evidence is accruing to support the view that a parenting program designed to improve child behavior can have collateral benefits for parents' well-being and quality of life (Beach et al., 2008; DeGarmo, Patterson, & Forgatch, 2004; McEachern et al., 2013).

Cascade model approaches also offer unique insights into the long-term implications of a prevention program. For example, some programs may have long-term *indirect* effects on outcomes as a function of intermediary processes that warrant attention. Other programs may have "time-limited" effects because they do not alter the developmental sequence. This may be particularly relevant to high-risk families in which ecological factors may erode program effects over time. Such findings would provide important information that could, for example, promote a systematic use of booster sessions to support long-term program gains.

Change During Prevention Programs

The other domain of family change processes is change *during* prevention programs. Surprisingly little is known about how change occurs over the course of program delivery. There are some exceptions to this found in early work on parenting interventions that highlighted therapist techniques (e.g., Patterson & Forgatch, 1985), but much of what we "know" about how change in families is elicited in a matter of weeks or months is derived from extensive hands-on experience and trial-and-error approaches as programs were developed over time. Unfortunately, much of this work has been relegated to the applied expertise that accumulates within research groups and has not been disseminated broadly to inform the field. Although much of this work has been conducted through a systematic and iterative development process, it is often the case that empirical evaluations of how change occurs during prevention programs remain unpublished. The current state of the field is one where established and emerging programs alike would benefit from careful application of recent methodological innovations that can capture change processes in exciting new ways.

Component analysis

Essentially, component analysis focuses on whether all components of a prevention program are contributing to program benefits experienced by individuals or families. Early examples include dismantling designs of therapeutic intervention packages in which different combinations of components are administered to subgroups for comparison (Kazdin, 2007). Even in the context of theory-driven programs, surprising results can emerge. A notable example is found in a now-classic study in which cognitive-behavioral therapy was subjected to a component analysis that compared the full therapy package to two components: behavioral activation, and treatment of automatic cognitions (Jacobson et al., 1996). This study yielded surprising results, which indicated that those who received the full therapy did not exhibit better outcomes than those that received only one of the components of the therapy. This study, and subsequent work, has stimulated growth in our understanding of the presumed processes underlying therapeutic changes in depression.

Recently, meta-analytic techniques have been applied to consider a component analysis approach to family-based prevention programs (e.g., Kaminski, Valle, Filene, & Boyle, 2008). Using this approach, prevention programs are decomposed into logical units, which can include units of content or curricula (e.g., family management, conflict resolution, self-regulation, managing peer influences), program modalities (e.g., whether the program was delivered in-person or remotely, whether it was delivered individually or in a group setting), and/or the presence or absence of specific instructional techniques (e.g., role playing). Subsequently, all prevention programs included in a meta-analysis are coded for the presence or absence (or, in some cases, the amount) of each component, and these codes are used to predict program outcomes across studies. In Kaminski et al. (2008), for example, the authors found that curricula focusing on positive parent–child interactions and the use of role-playing activities were two components that predicted increased efficacy among family-based prevention programs targeting behavioral problems in young children. This approach can also include analysis of moderation of effects, in which specific components are evaluated with regards to specific subgroups (e.g., boys vs. girls, low-risk vs. high-risk families), or when the potential for synergistic (i.e., interactive) relationships between components is tested. This type of research can not only help to address questions of *how* programs achieve their effects, but *for whom* they are most effective. The knowledge generated can, in turn, contribute to the goals outlined at the beginning of this chapter, i.e., to develop a new generation of prevention programs that can achieve effects more quickly and efficiently, and with larger effect sizes.

These meta-analytic and early component analysis approaches under-score the importance of evaluating the "active ingredients" of prevention programs. This goal requires a diversification of evaluation designs that can complement the gold-standard randomized controlled trial. If we consider the possibility that program components may vary in their effects, then it is possible that, although some components may function as expected, others may have no effect at all, while some components may even have a deleterious effect, reducing the overall potency of a prevention program (Collins, Murphy, Nair, & Stretcher, 2005). Perhaps more concerning is the reality that these nuances are obscured by the traditional randomized trial design in which the prevention program is evaluated as a whole, rather than by random assignment to various components of the program (Collins, Murphy, & Stretcher, 2007).

Recently, innovative applications of factorial experimental designs have emerged as a response to the need for systematic evaluation of prevention programs (Collins, Dziak, Kugler, & Trail, 2014). Through random assignment to the different combinations of program components, it is possible to identify which components have a desired effect on outcomes and to test interactive (e.g., synergistic) effects of program components, which allows the investigator to determine the optimal subset of components for program effectiveness with a particular population (Collins, Dziak et al., 2014). Beyond evaluating com-ponents of prevention programs, these factorial experimental methods have been applied in new ways to aid in the development and optimization of programs. The multiphase optimization strategy (MOST; e.g., Collins et al.,

2011; Collins, Murphy, & Stretcher, 2007) is a methodological framework that guides researchers in drawing on a theoretical model to identify a set of program components, which is then evaluated and refined through factorial experiments, resulting in the assembly of a program package for evaluation and ultimately dissemination (Collins et al., 2011).

Another emerging perspective in prevention science is the problem of heterogeneity of family needs as they engage in prevention programs; this is a serious consideration at all levels, but is particularly salient for universal-level prevention programs. There is growing recognition that families differ in their needs and responsiveness to prevention programs (Weissberg & Greenberg, 1998). Some families may have broad support needs, while other families' needs may be more narrowly supported by specific components of a program. This issue presents a challenge for programs delivered as a standardized curriculum and has led some program designers to use adaptive strategies that modify the curriculum based on the unique needs of a given family. However, evidence-based application of adaptive programs requires that careful attention is given to the key characteristics of an individual or family that are related to program response (i.e., the "tailoring variables") and to the empirically guided decision rules for how and when to adapt programs (Collins, Murphy, & Bierman, 2004). Sequential multiple assignment randomized trial (SMART) designs have arisen as a way of developing and evaluating adaptive programs (Murphy, 2005). Briefly, this approach helps identify the tailoring variables, decision rules, and corresponding optimal program component sets and sequences that will allow for an empirically guided adaptive approach (for reviews, see Collins, Nahum-Shani, & Almirall, 2014; Collins et al., 2007; Murphy, 2005).

Within-family change processes

Few studies have examined family change processes as they occur over the course of a prevention program. Some intervention or therapy programs are beginning to think about daily timescales in which change begins during therapy sessions, which is related to changes between therapy sessions, and ultimately accumulates to explain the treatment outcome (Gelo & Manzo, 2015). With regard to family-based prevention programs, family members may participate in exercises to learn new skills, or participate in relationship enhancement training or exercises, and it is the use of new skills, or changes to relationship quality, that generally account for change in outcomes. However, the ways in which family members implement skills at home, or the ways relationships change, are generally unclear. Intensive longitudinal methods offer a powerful tool for understanding change processes that occur during the program. By following participants intensively through the process of change, it is possible to see what they are doing that contributes to change (e.g., engaging in sessions, practicing skills), in addition to seeing the change itself as it occurs. Specific research questions related to within-family change that could be addressed with intensive longitudinal methods during programs include: how family members' behaviors in daily life change as they participate in a family program (i.e., tracking change in outcomes to determine the timescale, rate, and "shape" of change between pre-test and post-test); identifying micro-timescale mechanisms of change in functioning/outcomes, such as increasing or heightened day-to-day feelings of coparenting support from a partner as a mechanism of change toward sensitive parenting; and pinpointing cascades of change among family members, such as which family members change first, who and what changes next, and whether that differs by participants' engagement in the program, family interactional patterns, or other characteristics (Smyth & Stone, 2003). In sum, using intensive longitudinal methods during a prevention program allows for a close look at ordering and mechanisms of change in family members with temporal specificity that is not possible with pre–post or even measurement burst designs that miss this time period marking the beginning of change.

Conclusions

Efforts at developing strong evidence for family-based prevention programs have paid off. There are now several programs that have demonstrated robust effects in the lives of youth and their families. The field has progressed tremendously in the science of development, evaluation, and dissemination of evidence-based prevention programs; the chapters in this volume serve as a testament to this fact. Of course, much remains to be done. This chapter offers a guiding framework for future research across two levels: (1) change in family prevention programs and (2) change in systems of support and delivery of family prevention programs.

An important direction for future research is to further our understanding of change processes in family-based prevention programs, which requires rigorous evaluation of the enduring effects of these programs as well as the ways in which change unfolds during program delivery. The importance of evaluating program mechanisms is by no means a new idea. However, with innovations in methodology and the growing availability of long-term data from established family-based prevention trials, there is a vast array of new information to be gained from these approaches. Not only do studies of these mechanisms allow us to understand *how* and *why* a program works, but it opens up new realms of evaluation, including the breadth of public health impact and ways that we can bolster these effects through systematic maintenance of program effects for those who need it most. Because of the important role it serves, evidence supporting theorized mediators of a prevention program should be a key criterion for establishing a prevention program as evidence-based (Kazdin, 2007; Sandler et al., 2011). In this chapter, we offer guidance for conceptualizing and implementing such studies.

Moreover, we discuss new directions in both domains. We give attention to the importance of branching out in new directions to measure and analyze change, including intensive measurement approaches, such as daily diary, ecological momentary assessment, or dynamic systems approaches. Through intensive longitudinal methods, it is possible to gather information about processes and interactions at multiple points over time (i.e., in measurement-burst designs) in order to evaluate change in those family processes affected by family-based programs. There are many relevant questions that intensive longitudinal data can address to advance the knowledge of family processes and program effectiveness and potentially inform future prevention programs in order to optimize program effects.

It is important to note, however, that these programs are only useful to the extent to which they are introduced to the lives of those who can benefit from such services. Reaching those families most in need of prevention services will require a paradigm shift in how we design, staff, train, and fund governmental service delivery organizations. The current delivery model, which suffers from inadequate training, high staff turnover, program churn, and competition for funds among organizations that should (ideally) be cooperating, has resulted in inappropriate or insufficient services that are not able to address our most important public health challenges. Recent innovations such as Social Impact Bonds hold a great deal of promise, as do recent advances in health care that have arisen out of the Affordable Care Act, which is pushing medical care providers to think more holistically about family health. In response, many providers that have traditionally focused only on physical health have broadened their focus to consider the emotional and psychological well-being of the patient *and his or her family*. Clearly, the next horizon for the field of family-based prevention is to be found in contexts such as these—the family medical practice, the juvenile justice court, the correctional facility. By bringing our knowledge and expertise into these contexts, supported by properly trained and qualified practitioners, we can envision a future in which the promise of family-based prevention is fulfilled.

References

Almeida, D. M. (2005). Resilience and vulnerability to daily stressors assessed via diary methods. *Current Directions in Psychological Science, 14*(2), 64–68.

Aos, S., Lieb, R., Mayfield, J., Miller, M., & Pennucci, A. (2004). *Benefits and costs of prevention and early intervention programs for youth* (No. 04–07, p. 3901). Olympia, WA: Washington State Institute for Public Policy.

Beach, S. R., Kogan, S. M., Brody, G. H., Chen, Y. F., Lei, M. K., & Murry, V. M. (2008). Change in caregiver depression as a function of the Strong African American Families Program. *Journal of Family Psychology, 22*(2), 241.

Carr, A. (2000). Evidence-based practice in family therapy and systemic consultation. *Journal of Family Therapy, 22*(1), 29–60.

Caruthers, A. S., Van Ryzin, M. J., & Dishion, T. J. (2014). Preventing high-risk sexual behavior in early adulthood with family interventions in adolescence: Outcomes and developmental processes. *Prevention Science, 15*, 59–69.

Castro, F. G., Barrera Jr., M., & Holleran Steiker, L. K. (2010). Issues and challenges in the design of culturally adapted evidence-based interventions. *Annual Review of Clinical Psychology, 6*, 213–239.

Chen, H.-T., & Rossi, P. H. (1983). Evaluating with sense: The theory-driven approach. *Evaluation Review, 7*(3), 283–302.

Collins, L. M. (2006). Analysis of longitudinal data: The integration of theoretical model, temporal design, and statistical model. *Annual Review of Psychology, 57*, 505–528.

Collins, L. M., Baker, T. B., Mermelstein, R. J., Piper, M. E., Jorenby, D. E., Smith, S. S. et al. (2011). The multiphase optimization strategy for engineering effective tobacco use interventions. *Annals of Behavioral Medicine, 41*(2), 208–226.

Collins, L. M., Dziak, J. J., Kugler, K. C., & Trail, J. B. (2014). Factorial experiments: Efficient tools for evaluation of intervention components. *American Journal of Preventive Medicine, 47*(4), 498–504.

Collins, L. M., Murphy, S. A., & Bierman, K. L. (2004). A conceptual framework for adaptive preventive interventions. *Prevention Science, 5*(3), 185–196.

Collins, L. M., Murphy, S. A., Nair, V. N., & Strecher, V. J. (2005). A strategy for optimizing and evaluating behavioral interventions. *Annals of Behavioral Medicine, 30*(1), 65–73.

Collins, L. M., Murphy, S. A., & Strecher, V. (2007). The multiphase optimization strategy (MOST) and the sequential multiple assignment randomized trial (SMART): New methods for more potent eHealth interventions. *American Journal of Preventive Medicine, 32*(5), S112–S118.

Collins, L. M., Nahum-Shani, I., & Almirall, D. (2014). Optimization of behavioral dynamic treatment regimens based on the sequential, multiple assignment, randomized trial (SMART). *Clinical Trials, 11*, 426–434.

Cooper, B. R., Bumbarger, B. K., & Moore, J. E. (2013). Sustaining evidence-based prevention programs: Correlates in a large-scale dissemination initiative. *Prevention Science*, 1–13.

Crowley, D. M., Coffman, D. L., Feinberg, M. E., Greenberg, M. T., & Spoth, R. L. (2014). Evaluating the impact of implementation factors on family-based prevention programming: Methods for strengthening causal inference. *Prevention Science, 15*(2), 246–255.

DeGarmo, D. S., Patterson, G. R., & Forgatch, M. S. (2004). How do outcomes in a specified parent training intervention maintain or wane over time? *Prevention Science, 5*(2), 73–89.

Dishion, T. J., Nelson, S. E., & Bullock, B. M. (2004). Premature adolescent autonomy: Parent disengagement and deviant peer process in the amplification of problem behaviour. *Journal of Adolescence, 27*(5), 515–530.

Dodge, K. A., Malone, P. S., Lansford, J. E., Miller, S., Pettit, G. S., Bates, J. E., Schulenberg, J. E., & Maslowsky, J. (2009). A dynamic cascade model of the development of substance use onset. *Monographs of the Society for Research in Child Development, 74*(3), 1–120.

Duncan, T. E., Duncan, S. C., & Strycker, L. A. (2013). *An introduction to latent variable growth curve modeling: Concepts, issues, and application.* New York: Routledge Academic.

Durlak, J. A., & DuPre, E. P. (2008). Implementation matters: A review of research on the influence of implementation on program outcomes and the factors affecting implementation. *American Journal of Community Psychology, 41*(3–4), 327–350.

Dymnicki, A., Wandersman, A., Osher, D., Grigorescu, V., Huang, L., & Meyer, A. (2014). *Willing, able → ready: Basics and policy implications of readiness as a key component for implementation of evidence-based practices.* ASPE Issue Brief, Office of the Assistant Secretary for Planning and Evaluation, Office of Human Services Policy, United States Department of Health and Human Services.

Feinberg, M. E. (2003). The internal structure and ecological context of coparenting: A framework for research and intervention. *Parenting: Science and Practice, 3*(2), 95–131.

Feinberg, M. E., Jones, D., Greenberg, M. T., Osgood, D. W., & Bontempo, D. (2010). Effects of the Communities That Care model in Pennsylvania on change in adolescent risk and problem behaviors. *Prevention Science, 11*(2), 163–171.

Fixsen, D. L., Naoom, S. F., Blase, K. A., & Friedman, R. M. (2005). *Implementation research: A synthesis of the literature.* Tampa, FL: University of South Florida.

Fosco, G. M., & Feinberg, M. E. (2014). Cascading effects of interparental conflict in adolescence: Linking threat appraisals, self-efficacy, and adjustment. *Development and Psychopathology, 27*(1), 239–252.

Fosco, G. M., Van Ryzin, M. J., Stormshak, E. A., & Dishion, T. J. (2014). Putting theory to the test: Examining family context, caregiver motivation, and conflict in the Family Check-Up model. *Development and Psychopathology, 26*, 305–318.

Franks, R. (2010). *Role of the intermediary organization in promoting and disseminating best practices for children and youth.* Farmington: Connecticut Center for Effective Practice, Child Health and Development Institute.

Gelo, O. C. G., & Manzo, S. (2015). Quantitative approaches to treatment process, change process, and process-outcome research. In O. Gelo, A. Pritz, & B. Rieken (Eds.), *Psychotherapy research* (pp. 247–277). Vienna: Springer.

Greenwood, P. W., & Welsh, B. C. (2012). Promoting evidence-based practice in delinquency prevention at the state level. *Criminology & Public Policy, 11*(3), 493–513.

Haskins, R., Garfinkel, I., & McLanahan, S. (2014). Introduction: Two-generation mechanisms of child development. *The Future of Children, 24*(1), 3–12.

Hawkins, J. D., Catalano, R. F., & Arthur, M. W. (2002). Promoting science-based prevention in communities. *Addictive Behaviors, 27*(6), 951–976.

Jacobson, N. S., Dobson, K. S., Truax, P. A., Addis, M. E., Koerner, K., Gollan, J. K. et al. (1996). A component analysis of cognitive-behavioral treatment for depression. *Journal of Consulting and Clinical Psychology, 64*(2), 295.

Kaminski, J. W., Valle, L. A., Filene, J. H., & Boyle, C. L. (2008). A meta-analytic review of components associated with parent training program effectiveness. *Journal of Abnormal Child Psychology, 36*(4), 567–589.

Kazdin, A. E. (2007). Mediators and mechanisms of change in psychotherapy research. *Annual Review of Clinical Psychology, 3*, 1–27.

Koh, H. K., & Sebelius, K. G. (2010). Promoting prevention through the Affordable Care Act. *New England Journal of Medicine, 363*(14), 1296–1299.

Kumar, S., Nilsen, W., Abernethy, A., Atienza, A., Patrick, K., Pavel, M. et al. (2013). Mobile health technology evaluation: The mHealth evidence workshop. *American Journal of Preventive Medicine, 45*(2), 228–236.

Laird, R. D., Pettit, G. S., Bates, J. E., & Dodge, K. A. (2003). Parents' monitoring-relevant knowledge and adolescents' delinquent behavior: Evidence of correlated developmental changes and reciprocal influences. *Child Development, 74*, 752–768.

Larson, R., & Almeida, D. M. (1999). Emotional transmission in the daily lives of families: A new paradigm for studying family process. *Journal of Marriage and Family, 61*(1), 5–20.

Liddle, H. A. (2004). Family-based therapies for adolescent alcohol and drug use: Research contributions and future research needs. *Addiction, 99*(s2), 76–92.

Liebman, J. (2013). *Building on recent advances in evidence-based policymaking.* Washington, DC: The Brookings Institution.

Masten, A. S., & Cicchetti, D. (2010). Developmental cascades. *Development and Psychopathology, 22*(3), 491–495.

Masten, A. S., Roisman, G. I., Long, J. D., Burt, K. B., Obradović, J., Riley, J. R. et al. (2005). Developmental cascades: Linking academic achievement and externalizing and internalizing symptoms over 20 years. *Developmental Psychology, 41*(5), 733.

McArdle, J. J. (2009). Latent variable modeling of differences and changes with longitudinal data. *Annual Review of Psychology, 60*, 577–605.

McEachern, A. D., Fosco, G. M., Dishion, T. J., Shaw, D. S., Wilson, M. N., & Gardner, F. (2013). Collateral benefits of the family check-up in early childhood: Primary caregivers' social support and relationship satisfaction. *Journal of Family Psychology, 27*(2), 271–281.

Minuchin, P. (1985). Families and individual development: Provocations from the field of family therapy. *Child Development, 56*, 289–302.

Moilanen, K. L., Shaw, D. S., & Maxwell, K. L. (2010). Developmental cascades: Externalizing, internalizing, and academic competence from middle childhood to early adolescence. *Development and Psychopathology, 22*(3), 635–653.

Moore, J. E., Bumbarger, B. K., & Cooper, B. R. (2013). Examining adaptations of evidence-based programs in natural contexts. *The Journal of Primary Prevention, 34*(3), 147–161.

Mrazek, P. B., Biglan, A., & Hawkins, J. D. (2007). *Community-monitoring systems: Tracking and improving the well-being of America's children and adolescents.* Falls Church, VA: Society for Prevention Research.

Murphy, S. A. (2005). An experimental design for the development of adaptive treatment strategies. *Statistics in Medicine, 24*(10), 1455–1481.

Offord, D. R., Kraemer, H. C., Kazdin, A. E., Jensen, P. S., & Harrington, R. (1998). Lowering the burden of suffering from child psychiatric disorder: Trade-offs among clinical, targeted, and universal interventions. *Journal of the American Academy of Child & Adolescent Psychiatry, 37*(7), 686–694.

Patterson, G. R. (2005). The next generation of PMTO models. *The Behavior Therapist, 28*(2), 25–32.

Patterson, G. R., & Forgatch, M. S. (1985). Therapist behavior as a determinant for client noncompliance: A paradox for the behavior modifier. *Journal of Consulting and Clinical Psychology, 53*(6), 846–851.

Pew-MacArthur Results First Initiative (2014). *Evidence-based policymaking: A guide for effective government.* Washington, DC: The Pew Charitable Trusts.

Rhoades, B. L., Bumbarger, B. K., & Moore, J. E. (2012). The role of a state-level prevention support system in promoting high-quality implementation and sustainability of evidence-based programs. *American Journal of Community Psychology, 50*(3–4), 386–401.

Sandler, I. N., Schoenfelder, E. N., Wolchik, S. A., & MacKinnon, D. P. (2011). Long-term impact of prevention programs to promote effective parenting: Lasting effects but uncertain processes. *Annual Review of Psychology, 62*, 299–329.

Schermerhorn, A. C., Chow, S. M., & Cummings, E. M. (2010). Developmental family processes and interparental conflict: Patterns of microlevel influences. *Developmental Psychology, 46*(4), 869–885.

Schwarz, N. (2007). Retrospective and concurrent self-reports: The rationale for real-time data capture. In A. A. Stone, S. Shiffman, A. A. Atienza, & L. Nebeling (Eds.), *The science of real time data capture: Self-reports in health research* (pp. 11–26). New York: Oxford University Press.

Shiffman, S. (2007). Designing protocols for ecological momentary assessment. In A. A. Stone, S. Shiffman, A. A. Atienza, & L. Nebeling (Eds.), *The science of real time data capture: Self-reports in health research* (pp. 27–53). New York: Oxford University Press.

Sliwinski, M. J. (2008). Measurement-burst designs for social health research. *Social and Personality Psychology Compass, 2*, 245–261.

Smyth, J. M., & Heron, K. E. (2014). Ecological momentary assessment (EMA) in family research. In S. McHale, P. Amato, & A. Booth (Eds.), *Emerging methods in family research* (pp. 145–161). New York: Springer.

Smyth, J. M., & Stone, A. A. (2003). Ecological momentary assessment research in behavioral medicine. *Journal of Happiness Studies, 4*, 35–52.

Stone, A. A., Shiffman, S., Atienza, A. A., & Nebeling, L. (2007). Historical roots and rationale of ecological momentary assessment (EMA). In A. A. Stone, S. Shiffman, A. A. Atienza, & L. Nebeling (Eds.), *The science of real time data capture: Self-reports in health research* (pp. 3–10). New York: Oxford University Press.

Tibbits, M. K., Bumbarger, B. K., Kyler, S. J., & Perkins, D. F. (2010). Sustaining evidence-based interventions under real-world conditions: Results from a large-scale diffusion project. *Prevention Science, 11*(3), 252–262.

Van Ryzin, M. J., & Dishion, T. J. (2012). The impact of a family-centered intervention on the ecology of adolescent antisocial behavior: Modeling developmental sequelae and trajectories during adolescence. *Development and Psychopathology, 24*, 1139–1155.

Wandersman, A., Duffy, J., Flaspohler, P., Noonan, R., Lubell, K., Stillman, L. et al. (2008). Bridging the gap between prevention research and practice: The interactive systems framework for dissemination and implementation. *American Journal of Community Psychology, 41*(3–4), 171–181.

Weissberg, R. P., & Greenberg, M. T. (1998). Prevention science and collaborative community action research: Combining the best from both perspectives. *Journal of Mental Health, 7*, 479–492.

Weisz, J. R. (2014). Short-term treatment as long-term prevention: Can early intervention produce legacy effects? *American Journal of Psychiatry, 171*(6), 600–602.

7

CULTURAL AND GENDER ADAPTATIONS OF EVIDENCE-BASED FAMILY INTERVENTIONS

Karol L. Kumpfer, Catia Magalhães, Jing Xie, and Sheetal Kanse

This chapter will review culturally and gender-adapted evidence-based family prevention and intervention programs. The growing ethnic populations in the USA and other Western countries have created the need for the development and evaluation of culturally adapted programs. The rapid spread worldwide of Western youth culture has also made effective parenting more critical to youth outcomes in non-Western cultures, requiring an extension of the evidence base for family programs to include populations in Asia, the Americas and Africa.

Research also points out that these problem behaviors are growing among teenage girls and women (Kumpfer, 2014), creating a demand for programs specifically tailored to their needs. The increase in delinquency and substance abuse in girls began in the United States in the mid-1990s with a desire among young girls to be liberated from sex role stereotypes and to be able to engage in the same "adult" behaviors exhibited by boys (Kumpfer, Alvarado, & Whiteside, 2003). The question of how best to prevent problem behaviors in girls and whether the existing evidence-based prevention programs were effective for girls was initially raised in the late 2000s (Kumpfer, Smith, & Summerhays, 2008). To find out if the current programs were as effective for girls as for boys, the authors conducted a survey for the United Nations Office on Drugs and Crime (UNODC) in Vienna. The survey concluded that most program developers had never conducted a gender analysis. Of the few that had done so and published their results, all of the family-based programs were effective for both girls and boys, but the youth-only programs primarily worked only for boys and not for girls (Kumpfer, 2014; Kumpfer & Magalhães, in press). Given the paucity of research on these topics, this chapter will end with recommendations for further research on the effectiveness of family-based programs for different ethnic populations and genders.

Cultural Adaptations of Family-Based Programs

The Need for Cultural Adaptation of Evidence-Based Family Programs

Effectiveness research involves the implementation and outcome evaluation of programs in different contexts and with new populations, including new cultures (i.e., type 2 translational research; Ferrer-Wreder, Adamson, Kumpfer, & Eichas, 2012). Effectiveness research can also involve controlled replication studies of family-based programs in new populations whose utility has already been established for a particular sample in an efficacy trial (Valentine et al., 2011).

Many practitioners doubt the value of using evidence-based programs (EBPs) developed for different cultures or in other countries, because they believe effective programs must be developed locally using principles of effective prevention. This chapter stresses that "principles of effective prevention", while useful in designing new programs, do not in themselves guarantee that a prevention program works. Proof is reserved for programs tested in multiple randomized controlled trials and field trials with different populations and replicated by independent research teams. The best programs are those with the largest effect sizes and not just those with statistically significant results. It is our belief that culturally adapting and testing existing EBPs is the best way to create effective prevention programs that will work for diverse ethnicities, cultures, or countries.

The resistance to adopting EBPs from other countries often arises because of the perceived difficulties of adapting them to new cultures or new situations. Many manualized evidence-based programs have been criticized as being too rigid and inflexible. This is partially by design, given that the first mandate for replication in prevention science is to maintain fidelity by implementing the program exactly as written. Resistance to such strict replications often resulted in poorer outcomes with different cultures. Program developers with experience in dissemination research have argued against this rigid interpretation of "fidelity" (Kumpfer et al., 2012a; Mazzucchelli & Sanders, 2010), stressing that delivering a program with fidelity does not mean inflexible delivery. Every EBP can be locally and culturally adapted within bounds, as long as core content (i.e., the themes and structure of program sessions) is left intact. Learning the boundaries between desirable cultural adaptation and undesirable structural modification should be part of training and supervision. Implementers should be encouraged to work collaboratively with program developers, supervisors, and families to adapt programs to the unique needs and situational context while preserving the program's core content.

The evidence-based family programs presented in this book were, for the most part, developed in the United States and tested in randomized controlled trials (RCTs) funded by federal government research agencies within the National Institutes of Health (NIMH). Only one program, Triple P, was developed in another English language country—Australia. Consequently, until recently, few of these family programs had been translated into other languages or culturally adapted, and even fewer were evaluated in RCTs for efficacy in non-English-speaking and non-Western cultures. Program developers were also mainly of Western cultural roots. Though some EBPs are in use in different countries, these culturally adapted versions have rarely been evaluated for effectiveness or efficacy. For example, many have only non-experimental pre- and post-test designs. Because of the lack of information on the extent and effectiveness of dissemination and evaluation of these evidence-based family programs in non-Western cultures, a review of program results will be presented in this chapter.

More Ethnic Minority Families Need Family Services

Worldwide, families are increasingly mobile and moving to new communities or countries in search of work and a better life for themselves (Kumpfer, Pinyuchon, Baharudin, Nolrajsuwat, & Xie, in press). This increase in refugee and immigrant families has created an increasing need for effective prevention and treatment services in far-flung locations around the world.

In the United States, ethnic minorities now comprise 37% of the US population; by 2060, due to the higher birthrates and immigration rates of minority families, particularly Latin and Asian families (CDC, 2013; US Census Bureau, 2012), minority families are expected to grow to 57% of the population and become the majority. Unfortunately, these minority families rarely seek prevention and treatment services, except when mandated by the courts because of suspected child abuse, drug abuse, or crime. In more traditional non-Western cultures, fear of bringing shame on the family by divulging family problems, as well as a belief that problems should be solved within the family, often deters at-risk families from seeking help. Insufficient family resources to pay for services are also an issue for many minority families. Lack of trained family services workers who are from minority cultures and speak their language compounds the problem. This is changing rapidly, however, as more ethnic students are graduating from Western universities in these fields with a desire to help families in their own countries or within their own cultures in this country.

Lack of culturally tailored family programs for minorities

Research suggests that it is difficult to engage minority families because most programs do not fit their culture and are not taught in their primary language (Biglan & Metzler, 1999; McLean & Campbell, 2003; Watson, 2005). Participation of ethnic families can be as low as 10% in family programs (Kumpfer, Alvarado, Smith, & Bellamy, 2002). Most universal prevention programs are developed for the general American population, focusing mostly on White, middle-class values that could be culturally inappropriate and not address the needs of ethnic families. For example, traditional ethnic families often favor family systems change approaches for prevention (see Van Ryzin and Fosco, this volume) as compared to individual change approaches, because their cultural values stress interconnection, reciprocity, and filial responsibility as contrasted with the Western value of individual achievement (Boyd-Franklin, 2001; Kumpfer et al., 2002). Thus, family-based interventions could be more appealing, and potentially more effective, for minority families if they were appropriately adapted for minority cultures.

Because of growing minority populations in this country and other Western countries, ethnic families will need increased attention from services providers, policy makers, and government funding agencies to identify and prevent behavioral health problems. Majority families in countries outside of the United States also need access to effective parenting and family programs. The simplest way to provide these effective family services is to culturally adapt proven evidence-based parenting and family programs rather than starting from scratch. Starting with a proven program increases the chances for success. Unfortunately, few governments are willing to invest the funds to conduct randomized controlled trials to determine the efficacy of newly adapted programs. Although early cultural adaptations have not been able to improve outcomes significantly, they have dramatically increased the attendance and retention of minority families (Kumpfer et al., 2002), which is a key first step in creating a significant public health impact.

To more fully realize a significant public health impact, however, the field must move beyond simple language translation of EBPs; unfortunately, it is often unclear what sorts of cultural adaptations are required. Given the high costs of program development and evaluation, the paucity of research on the cost/benefit of culturally adapted programs is unsurprising. To make family-based programs work better for minority families, the field requires more research on the primary family issues in minority cultures, as well as a better understanding by Western family program developers of cultural and family traditions, health disparities, and existing culturally appropriate and effective family services in minority communities.

Specific risk and protective factors in ethnic families

Making family interventions more effective for ethnic families requires understanding their most salient risk and protective factors. Testing of etiological or causal models for major adolescent problems (e.g., substance abuse, delinquency, school failure, teen pregnancy) has been conducted using structural equation models (SEM) on large data sets of general populations of youth (Ary, Duncan, Biglan, Metzler, Noell, & Smolkowski, 1999) and for each major ethnic population of youth in the USA (Center for Substance Abuse

Pathways to Substance Use for High Risk Youth

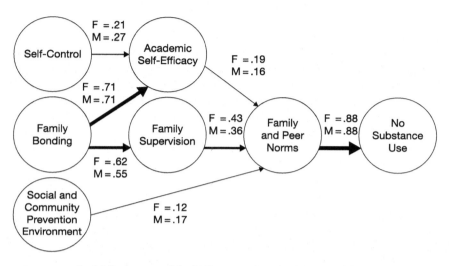

FIGURE 12.1 Social Ecology Model of Substance Abuse by Gender (Males/Females)

Prevention, 2000; Kumpfer et al., 2003; Sales, Sambrano, Springer, & Turner, 2003). As shown in Figure 12.1, the strongest pathway to poorer adolescent development is through the family (e.g., family bonding or parent/child attachment, supervision, and communication of positive family values and norms). The latter set of variables (i.e., values and norms) was merged into a latent construct representing parent/peer influence, which was the final pathway predicting a variety of problem behavior. It was equally powerful for different ethnic groups and for girls and boys (Sales et al., 2003). Family bonding and parental supervision, however, have a slightly greater impact on minority youth and also on girls' choice of substance-using or non-using friends. Behavioral and emotional self-control had a slightly larger role among boys, possibly because boys seem more prone to difficulties in this area. Girls were more influenced by their academic performance and self-efficacy than boys. The community and neighborhood environment has a greater influence on minority youth as well as on boys.

A similar model was tested for school failure, delinquency, and teen pregnancy as well as alcohol and drug use, with similar results (Ary et al., 1999). The authors found that low parental supervision had a greater influence on adolescent girls' alcohol and drug use than on boys'. Also, in a sample of African-American youth, Fothergill and Ensminger (2006) found that school bonding was a stronger protective factor for boys than for girls.

These tested theoretical models provide suggestive evidence that minority youth have similar risk and protective factors, but the strength of these factors varies somewhat by ethnic group and gender. For example, minority youth and girls are slightly more influenced by family protective factors than are non-minority boys, and girls seem to be more dependent on a positive relationship with their parents and friends to define their self-worth. In contrast, girls appear to be slightly less influenced by their community environment than are boys, but minority youth of both genders are more influenced by the community environment. These models supported the notion that many of the core family protective factors are similar for minority and Euro-Western families, including parent/child attachment, supervision or monitoring, and communication of family values and expectations.

Outside of these models, research has identified other key risk and protective factors. A key family risk factor found in ethnic minority families is increased differential generational acculturation, which can lead to increased family conflict and negatively impact family relationships (Rodnium, 2007). Other major ethnic minority family risk factors include discrimination, increased poverty, and parents working more than one job, implying a lack of time with children (Kumpfer, Magalhães, & Kanse, in press). Commonly identified protective factors include religiosity, family connectedness, and the presence of extended family members to provide emotional and fiscal support (Domenech Rodríguez & Bernal, 2012). Additional youth protective factors to be stressed in culturally adapted family prevention programs include maintaining cultural pride and family traditions and learning multicultural competencies, which support better psychological and academic adjustment (Beauvais & Trimble, 2006; Berkel et al., 2010; Guilamo-Ramos, 2009).

Acculturation among minority groups

Acculturation stress and differential generational acculturation are major family risk factors for minority families (Rodnium, 2007). Acculturation is "the extent to which individuals have maintained their culture of origin or adapted to the larger society" (Phinney, 1996, p. 921). This mainly pertains to families who immigrate to countries with different majority cultures and have to learn a new language and new rules for behavior. The level of acculturation among minority populations depends on many factors such as age, circumstances, socio-economic status, the reasons for immigration, length of stay, location of residence, and exposure to the new host culture in work or community activities (Farver, Bhadha, & Narang, 2002). Assimilation into the new culture is always much more difficult for families who are isolated or only associate with members of their own culture. Because education is generally mandatory, children in immigrant or refugee families typically assimilate much faster than their parents or grandparents. Immigrant parents are torn between retaining their original cultural identities or accepting and assimilating into the dominant host culture (Inman, Howard, Beaumont, & Walker, 2007). Previous research among Hispanic immigrants suggested that acculturation stress, deviation from the original cultural norms (e.g., daily contacts and social interaction with family and friends), language barriers, lower self-esteem, social isolation, boredom, and loneliness can result in increased alcohol consumption among immigrants (Gonzalez-Guarda, Ortega, Vasquez, & De Santis, 2010).

Because children generally assimilate more quickly than their parents to the majority culture (which is called "differential generational acculturation"), increased family conflict arising due to the clash of cultural values can alienate children from their parents and lead to children's developmental problems (e.g., delinquency, substance abuse, anxiety, depression, suicidal tendencies, violence, and prostitution; Dow, 2011; Farver et al., 2002; Feldman & Rosenthal, 1993). In our own research, Structural Equations Modeling (SEM) was used on youth self-report survey data to test the Social Ecology Model (Kumpfer et al., 2003) in four areas of Thailand with youth in retention and correctional facilities. Differential generational acculturation (i.e., adapting to Western culture as compared to maintaining traditional Thai culture) was found to be a major risk factor leading to increased family conflict, which then reduced family protective factors such as family bonding, supervision, and communication of positive family values and influence (Rodnium, 2007). Youth most in favor of adopting Western cultural values and behaviors were most prone to delinquency and drug use.

An additional risk factor in this context is role reversal, which occurs when children can speak the new language much more proficiently and must act as the mediator between the parents and the majority culture, taking on some aspects of the parental role. These youth then tend to reject parental authority and feel that their parents are "old fashioned". The risk posed by differential acculturation, as well as the other culture-specific issues documented above, call for clear models or frameworks that can be used to adopt existing family-based programs for minority populations.

Cultural Adaptation Models or Frameworks

Cultural adaptations of evidence-based family programs are needed to serve the growing minority population and to attract and engage more minority families (Biglan & Metzler, 1999; Kumpfer et al., in press). There is consequently a need for models or ideas on how to best culturally adapt family-based programs. Models for cultural adaptation have been proposed by a number of prevention researchers, namely Bernal, Ferrer-Wreder, Kumpfer, and others. In general, there are two types of cultural adaptation frameworks: those that inform *what* to modify in the intervention content and those that inform *how* to conduct the adaptation process (Ferrer-Wreder, Sundell, & Mansoory, 2012). The Ecological Validity Model (EVM) by Bernal, Bonilla, and Bellido (1995) is an example of *what* to adapt in eight domains: language, persons, metaphors, content, concepts, goals, methods, and context. A similar content model is the cultural sensitivity model, which distinguishes deep structure versus surface structure adaptations of program content (Resnicow, Soler, Braithwaite, Ahluwailia, & Butler, 2000).

The second set of frameworks focus on the *process* of adaptation, where decisions about when to adapt, how to adapt, and which stakeholders should be involved in the process are outlined. A number of frameworks fall into this category and vary in how prescriptive they are (i.e., whether they have a set of a priori steps that guide the process) and whether they are focused on the adaptation of one specific EBP. Several of these models have been described elsewhere (e.g., Bernal & Domenech Rodríguez, 2012); generally, they recommend adaptations to be informed by the expertise of program developers, past experience with similar populations, key stakeholders (e.g., funding project officers, members of local service delivery organizations), and members of the new population. They recommend the use of formative research methods such as focus groups and interviews, as well as formal outcome evaluations of the adapted intervention (Cabassa & Baumann, 2013; Domenech Rodríguez & Bernal, 2012). Unfortunately, many cultural adaptations are done informally "on the spot" by implementers to make the program concepts more understandable and acceptable to participants. Because of lack of time and failure to appreciate the need for replication, these informal adaptations are rarely documented sufficiently to enable outsiders to understand exactly what was delivered (unless the entire program was videotaped).

Kumpfer and UNODC steps to cultural adaptation

Kumpfer and associates (2012b) have developed over the past twenty years a recommended system for culturally adapting their Strengthening Families Program (SFP). These steps have been found to result in outcomes similar to or better than the original outcomes. The key is not to do any major adaptations before the program has been piloted with the new population. Also critical is that the implementers are from the participant population and understand cultural differences. Adaptations of content are recommended rather than modifications of program structure that would include shortening the number of sessions or lesson length, moving the topics or sessions around, or eliminating the basic format (i.e., parents and youth attend initial classes separately and then come together as a family). Participants from minority cultures sometimes object to experiential role plays as just "not done in our culture". However, they generally discover that, once given permission to do the role plays in a safe and non-judgmental setting, they actually enjoy these "fun and games" that are so critical to practicing new parenting and communication behaviors.

Cultural adaptation teams are encouraged to follow the steps to implementation and cultural adaptation found to produce the most effective outcomes, described in the recent UNODC publication (UNODC, 2009) and in journal publications (Kumpfer, Pinyuchon, de Melo, & Whiteside, 2008; Kumpfer, Magalhães, & Xie, 2012). These steps include: 1) conduct a local family needs assessment; 2) review EBP family programs and select the best program for age, ethnicity, and risk level of families (e.g., universal, selective, or indicated prevention); 3) create a cultural adaptation team, including family members, implementer (or group leader in the SFP), and the original program developer; 4) translate into the local language; 5) implement at first with minimal cultural adaptation; 6) make gradual cultural changes based on input from the adaptation team (e.g., culturally appropriate stories, songs); 7) test the adapted program with multiple replications; 8) conduct annual pre- and post-test evaluations to determine if the evolving cultural adaptations are making the program better or worse by comparing to the appropriate SFP age norms for the original program; 9) make adjustments as needed by adding or dropping new cultural adaptations; and 10) disseminate to similar cultural groups if the outcome evaluations show it to be as effective as the original SFP.

Family Programs with Cultural Adaptations

Many family-based programs have done at least one implementation in another country requiring language translations and evaluations of new programs outcomes. However, few of these programs document or disseminate a formal process of cultural adaptation. The family-based programs with the highest number of culturally adapted implementations include the SFP, which has been found effective for five major ethnic groups in the USA (Kumpfer et al., 2002) and 35 countries (Kumpfer, Pinyuchon, Baharudin, Nolrajsuwat, & Xie, in press), Triple P from Australia (to date in 25 countries), Incredible Years (three major US ethnic groups and in 22 countries), Parent Management Training— Oregon (in six countries), and Family Matters (in three countries). Several of these most widely disseminated family programs and their cultural adaptation processes are discussed in their own chapters in this book.

Indicated family prevention or treatment programs

Several indicated family-based prevention or treatment programs for higher risk youth with diagnosed behavioral health problems have been implemented internationally but not included in this book; hence, their cultural adaptations are discussed briefly below:

• *Multisystemic Therapy for Delinquents and Substance Abusing Youth* is an intensive family- and community-based treatment for juvenile offenders who have committed serious offences and their families. Most of the treatment is conducted in the home. It has been implemented internationally in 12 countries.

- *Multidimensional Family Therapy* is a manual-driven intervention with specific assessment and treatment modules for drug abusing youth. MDFT helps the youth develop more effective coping and problem-solving skills for better decision making and helps the family improve interpersonal functioning as a protective factor against substance abuse and related problems. MDFT has language and cultural adaptations for five countries.

There are other parent training programs with cultural adaptations, such as Bavolek's *Nurturing Program*, the first parent training program for child maltreatment adapted for Hispanics and the military; Miller-Hyle's *Dare To Be You*, implemented with Navajos, Hispanics, and Whites; Schinke's web-delivered *Mothers and Daughters Program* with separate versions for Hispanic, African American, and Asian families; McDonald's *Families and Schools Together* (FAST) being disseminated by the UNODC to developing countries from a compendium of evidence-based family programs (UNODC, 2010); and Brody's *Strong African American Families* (SAAF) adapted from SFP 10–14 (see Brody, this volume).

The Strengthening Families Program (SFP)

Multiple age and cultural adaptations of the SFP have been found robust in producing positive outcomes when implemented for new populations outside the United States (Kumpfer, Pinyuchon et al., 2008). The UN Office on Drugs and Crime (UNODC) is disseminating SFP to developing countries in four regions of the world (Balkans, Central America, Brazil, and Southeast Asia), along with the Pan American Health Organization (PAHO) in Latin America, the International Rescue Committee (IRC) for refugees, and many international governments. An RCT study funded by the Thai government found that if both mothers and fathers attend, compared with only mothers, the outcomes are improved significantly (Pinyuchon, 2010). The outcome effectiveness results in Serbia with about 350 families have been excellent (Malouf, 2014). A survey of implementers of SFP and other evidence-based substance abuse prevention programs in Europe (Burkhart, 2013) found unanimous belief that SFP can be culturally adapted with excellent outcomes if implemented with fidelity and the recommended steps to SFP cultural adaptations are followed (Kumpfer, Pinyuchon et al., 2008; Kumpfer, Magalhães et al., 2012; UNODC, 2009).

Within the United States, culturally specific SFP versions for five major ethnic populations (Hispanic/Latino, African American, Pacific Islander/ Hawaiian, Asian, and American Indian) were initially developed and evaluated in five separate 5-year phase-in studies using federal grants. The trials reported 40% better recruitment and retention for the culturally adapted versions, but overall the SFP outcomes were not a significant improvement compared to the non-culturally adapted SFP implemented with the same types of families (Kumpfer et al., 2002). Although we have no direct evidence, we can speculate about the reasons for this lack of improvement. Perhaps, given the robust program design and content of SFP, the additional cultural adaptations didn't add much except to increase attendance. We should not downplay the significant enhancements to recruitment and retention; we continue to recommend cultural adaptations for SFP and other family-based programs even if they do nothing more than increase family engagement. However, the time and cost of continuously updating culturally specific versions for each different age, risk level, or specific target populations has prompted the SFP developers as well as those for other EBPs to move to culturally sensitive, multi-ethnic versions rather than multiple culturally specific versions. A culturally sensitive SFP manual includes unique graphics for each ethnic group and changes names and examples as well, but the additional cultural tailoring and local language translation is done in the way the group leaders explain and present the SFP family skills.

Another issue is that a culturally specific version may not be specific enough for different ethnic subgroups and may still need considerable local adaptation even for White families, such as isolated Appalachian families (Marek, Brock, & Sullivan, 2006). None of the major categories of ethnicity in the US (e.g., Hispanic, Asian, American Indian, African American, Pacific Islanders) are homogeneous cultures, but differ in family traditions, values, historical and local issues in child raising, and language variations. For example, even among Hispanic families there is no uniform Spanish language to use for translations because each culture has different words for concepts. About five different language translations of SFP into Spanish (Mexican, Argentinian, Columbian, Puerto Rican, and El Salvadorian) were tried in an attempt to find a universally acceptable Spanish to most Hispanic and Latino families. However, each time the local Hispanic families would complain about inappropriate language in the manuals. For Asian and Pacific Islander families, it was clear that different language translations were needed in addition to local adaptations for each country and cultural group. For American Indians, several tribe-specific SFP versions were developed with funding by particular tribes, but these specific versions couldn't be used with other tribes; as a result, only the richest tribes could afford their own culturally specific version of SFP.

The SFP developers recently moved to a culturally sensitive SFP curriculum for each of the different age groups (SFP 3–5, 6–11, 12–16, 7–17, and new 0–3) by producing manuals that were free of any cultural-specific material. The new gold standard practice is for each SFP implementation team to use the culturally sensitive curricula as a starting point and to follow the recommended steps for cultural adaptation presented earlier and recommended by the UNODC Guidelines (UNODC, 2009) to make their own cultural adaptations over time using feedback from local families. In this scenario, cultural adaptations by culturally sensitive group leaders then became a mandated element of fidelity. At the very least, surface structure content should be altered to suit local cultural mores (i.e., incorporating songs, music, foods, games, and stories that reflect local culture). The involvement of consultants from the local population is essential for success, along with the approval of the program developer for any changes outside of these minor alterations. However, the SFP developers stress that, beyond these types of changes, implementation should closely adhere to the manual content, session order, and theoretical underpinnings in order to maintain fidelity and achieve similar outcomes to those obtained previously.

International SFP outcome results

Replications of SFP in randomized control trials (RCTs) and quasi-experimental studies in different countries (Canada, Ireland, the United Kingdom, Netherlands, Spain, Thailand, and Italy) with different cultural groups by independent evaluators have found SFP to be an effective program in reducing multiple risk factors for later alcohol and drug abuse, mental health problems, and delinquency by increasing family strengths, children's social competencies, and improving parenting skills (Kumpfer et al., 2002; Kumpfer & Johnson, 2007; Onrust & Bool, 2006; Orte, March, Ballester, &Touza, 2007). For summary of SFP outcomes from foreign studies see Kumpfer and associates (2012a).

Among the 13 countries in Europe that have culturally adapted and evaluated SFP are four that have one to five years of pre-to-post-test outcome results conducted independently by researchers: Orte et al. (2007) at the University of the Balearic Islands, Spain; Onrust and Bool (2006) at Trimbos Institute in Utrecht, Netherlands; Kimber (2005) at the Karolinska Institute in Stockholm, Sweden; and Foxcroft, Allen, and Coombes (2005; Coombes, Allen & Foxcroft, 2012) at Oxford Brookes University, United Kingdom. These studies were all non-experimental or quasi-experimental designs, but their positive results suggest that SFP can be culturally adapted and replicated in other countries with positive results. The Spanish and Irish results have been excellent, with even slightly higher effect sizes for the outcomes than the SFP US norms, possibly because they were implemented with higher risk families.

Excellent results have also been found in other countries (Portugal, Ireland, Northern Ireland, Italy, France, Slovenia, and Austria) with semi-independent replications where the implementing agencies have sent their data to the Strengthening Families Foundation, the SFP-recommended evaluation team that includes Dr. Kumpfer, the program developer and evaluator. These have all been quasi-experimental pre-to-post-test designs with a comparison to the norms for that country or the SFP international norms. In addition, the agencies used the recommended SFP testing instruments. Portugal and the Azores have implemented *SFP 6–11 Years* (see Kumpfer et al., earlier in this volume) and have excellent outcomes using the standardized SFP instruments. Norway has been implementing the *SFP 6–11 Years* and *SFP 10–14 Years* version, as has the United Kingdom.

A multi-county quasi-experimental evaluation of an Irish cultural adaptation of *SFP 12–16 Years* for *indicated* youth in Ireland (Kumpfer, Xie, & O'Driscoll, 2012) has produced some of the largest effect sizes (Cohen's d = .50 to 1.11). These effect sizes were about 20% larger than the comparison group (US) SFP norms, possibly because the families were so needy and alcohol use rates were higher at pre-test. All 21 measured teen, parent, and family outcomes were significantly improved in the 288 families. They used a unique collaborative recruitment and staffing model that included probation services, local drugs task forces, schools, garda (police), and substance abuse treatment agencies. Each agency sending a staffing member was allowed to reserve 2 to 3 slots for families on their waiting lists for family services.

Reduced SFP effectiveness when not culturally adapted or implemented with fidelity

When local implementers do not address issues of cultural differences, program effectiveness can be attenuated. For example, a NIDA-funded RCT of the standard SFP among 715 primarily high-risk African Americans in the Washington, DC region still found good results but reduced effect sizes, recruitment, and retention compared to other SFP RCTs (Gottfredson et al., 2006), likely due to the lack of appropriate cultural adaptations.

Program modifications that go beyond language to change format and length can reduce program fidelity and overall effectiveness. An unfortunate Swedish modification of the 7-session *SFP 10–14 Years* resulted in non-significant outcomes (Skärstrand, Larsson, & Andreasson, 2008). To save money after making expensive new videos, they eliminated all but two of the weekly family sessions and some of the parenting classes at night. Meals, incentives for homework completion, and babysitting were also not offered, reducing parent attendance to only 33% of the families. School teachers offered a longer SFP, with more drug education classes, to their full classroom of students, thus increasing the possibility of an "iatrogenic" effect described by Dishion and Mauricio (this volume) when implementers are not skillful in maintaining control over the youth. This natural experiment demonstrated that a critical core component of SFP's success is bringing the family together to improve communication and relationship quality by eating together, learning the same family skills, and playing games and role plays together to practice their new interaction skills.

Gender Adaptations of Family Programs

Need for Gender-Adapted Family EBP Intervention

Despite more effective prevention programs, behavioral health problems including delinquency, crime, teen pregnancy, eating disorders, depression, and substance use in girls have increased more than for boys worldwide beginning with a dramatic increase in the United States in 1992 (Kumpfer, 2014). Traditionally, girls in Western countries have used alcohol, tobacco, and drugs less than boys; however, the gender gap has almost disappeared in the US and other developed countries (Kumpfer & Magalhães, in press). This gender gap is related to a complex interaction of genetic and environmental causes. The consequences have been costly to governments, with increased numbers of women needing drug treatment, many of them mothers who are losing their children to foster care. Also the social, emotional, and health consequences for their children are tremendous, particularly in the light of recent epigenetic research stressing the need for nurturing parenting to prevent the phenotypic expression of inherited diseases (Jirtle, 2010; Brody et al., 2010, 2012).

Genetic risks

The increase in girls' substance abuse is occurring despite research suggesting that men appear to have twice as high a genetic risk of alcohol dependency compared to women, according to early twin adoption studies conducted in Sweden, Denmark, and the USA (Pickens et al., 1991). These genetic risks help to explain why addiction appears to be a "family disease" with children of parents with substance use disorders at much higher genetic risk (Kumpfer & Johnson, 2009). Recently, several gene variants have been identified related to increased risk for depression, anxiety, substance abuse, delinquency, and HIV risk, namely one or two short alleles of the 5-HTTLPR serotonin transporter gene or the 7-repeat dopamine gene (Brody et al., 2010, 2012). These are found in 40% of White and 60% of Asian groups. Nurturing parenting has been found to reduce occurrence of these behavioral health diagnoses in mice or children with these genes (Jirtle, 2010; Champagne, 2010). There is also recent epigenetic research suggesting that gene/environment interactions due to maternal stress can cause changes in genes *in utero* that may be passed into the next generation (Champagne, 2010). Since genetic risk has not changed drastically in girls, the recent increase in substance use prevalence in girls is more likely due to the significant changes in social environments, such as reductions in parental involvement and major changes in social roles for girls and women.

Environmental risks

The increases in girls' behavioral health problems worldwide are likely to be related to the export of Western values through movies, music, and clothing, and adolescent freedoms for girls that include more violent behavior, sexualization, and positive norms toward drinking and drug use (Kumpfer, Magalhães, & Kanse, in press). With increased access to jobs, affluence, and social freedoms, young girls have begun to behave more like boys, including their vices. Kumpfer,

Smith, and Summerhays (2008) called this the "Virginia Slims Effect" related to sexual and social role liberation.

In many societies, girls are being exposed to media and societal pressures to conform to an unrealistically thin body ideal (Reel & Beal, 2009; Sypeck, Gray, & Ahrens, 2004). Significantly more females than males begin using tobacco and drugs because they believe it helps them to stay thin (Califano, 2001). In the USA, the use of amphetamines among Caucasian girls is linked to the desire to lose weight (NCASA, 2003). In addition, substance use and disordered eating can co-occur. Research suggests that one in six students have admitted to restricting caloric intake in order to amplify the effects of alcohol (Cofsky, 2012). In one study (Burke, Cremeens, Vail-Smith, & Woolsey, 2010), the 30% of students that restricted calories also reported binge drinking. Girls who combine disordered eating with binge drinking are more at risk for violence, risky sexual behavior, alcohol poisoning, substance abuse, and chronic diseases later in life, such as cirrhosis of the liver (Baker, Mitchell, Neale, & Kendler, 2010).

Reduced poverty and parental controls, with more parents working more hours, are likely contributing to these increases in behavioral health problems in girls more than boys (Annenberg Institute of School Reform, 2009). Another important risk factor is the increasing divorce rates in modern society and the loss of fathers in girls' lives (Kumpfer & Magalhães, in press). According to the Social Ecology Model shown earlier (Kumpfer et al., 2003), girls are slightly more influenced by their parents than are boys in terms of parent/child relationship quality and monitoring. Also, peer pressure may be more strongly associated with drinking for girls than it is for boys (Donovan, 2002). When several of a girl's closest friends smoke or drink, they are more than seven times more likely to smoke and drink, whereas boys are only three times more likely (Barber, Bolitho, & Bertrand, 1999). Finally, early maturing girls who have older friends appear to be at an elevated risk for substance misuse, truancy, delinquency, and sexual activity (Caspi, Lynam, Moffitt, & Silva, 1993; Lanza & Collins, 2002).

High rates of comorbidity exist between substance use and depression in girls (Kloos, Weller, Chan, & Weller, 2009). Substance abusing girls are more likely to be depressed, and, likewise, depression leads to increased substance abuse, reduced self-esteem, and increased suicide attempts for girls (Kloos et al., 2009). More girls than boys (as young as the 6th grade) believe in self-medicating powers of alcohol to reduce depression, anger, or frustration, even before they begin to drink. Girls who believe that drinking alcohol reduces depression or helps them deal with negative thoughts and feelings report more alcohol use them those who do not (CASA, 2003). Other drugs such as ecstasy and marijuana are also used by girls to reduce depression (Kumpfer & Magalhães, in press).

Sexual abuse also appears to be a strong risk factor for girls and women, possibly due to the higher prevalence of victimization. On average, at least one in three women is beaten, coerced into sex, or otherwise abused by an intimate partner in the course of her lifetime (United Nations, 2008). Higher percentages

(55% to 95%) of women as compared to men in drug treatment facilities were sexually abused as a child (Kumpfer & Bays, 1995). In the USA, the prevalence of sexual abuse was reported to be 60% for incarcerated female and 20% for male adolescents (Dembo et al., 2000). Finally, youth who misuse alcohol, marijuana, or drugs are at increased risk of victimization, with female substance users at particularly elevated risk of sexual assault (Testa & Livingston, 2009).

For these reasons, more effective prevention and treatment programs for girls and women are needed. Unfortunately, the prevention field has not conducted much research to determine how to design more effective prevention programs and policies for adolescent females. Also, the etiological causal factors are complex and research on girls is lacking. A gender-attentive approach would implement gender-specific strategies for girls that address their specific risk factors for behavioral and health issues.

Effectiveness of Family-Based Programs for Boys and Girls

A survey of evidence-based prevention programs conducted for a UNODC gender guideline (Kumpfer & Magalhães, in press) revealed 13 family-based programs that worked for girls. Of the seven generic evidence-based family programs that had done a gender analysis, all reported equally effective results for girls and boys and one reported better results for girls (i.e., Multidimensional Treatment Foster Care). In addition, all six gender-specific family-based programs reported positive results for girls.

Gender-specific family-based programs

Very few of the evidence-based family programs have developed gender-specific versions for girls, partially because the need to do so was only recently discovered. Of the three gender-specific programs, randomized control trials of a mother–daughter substance use prevention program delivered through CDs or internet showed good results for reducing HIV risk and alcohol and drug use among inner city Hispanic, African American, and Asian American girls (Fang & Schinke, 2013; Schinke, Cole, & Fang, 2009; Schinke, Fang, Cole, & Cohen-Cutler, 2011; Schwinn, Schink, & Di Noia, 2010). Two gender and ethnic adaptations of *SFP 6–11 Years* targeting mothers and daughters also reported positive results for Hawaiians (Kameoke, 1996) and Hispanic mothers and daughters (Alvarado, 1996).

A recent gender analysis of a large SFP normative database of over 4,000 families from SFP groups worldwide found that SFP is equally effective for girls as for boys and in some cases even more effective for girls despite lower base rates of risk factors, possibly because girls are more influenced by family relationships (Magalhães, 2013). Finally, a recent gender analysis of *SFP 12–16*

Years with high-risk adolescents in Ireland found SFP to be equally effective for adolescent girls as for boys (Mahoney, Kumpfer, Xie, & Cofrin Allen, 2014).

The general positive results of family-based programs are consistent with both the brief discussion above regarding vulnerability and resilience factors that are particular to girls, as well as with other general reviews of the effectiveness of family-based programs (Kumpfer, 2014; Petrie, Bunn, & Byrne, 2007). In particular, family-based strategies are generally effective for both boys and girls (Kumpfer et al., 2003; Petrie et al., 2007), while school-based and community-based programs are often not as effective for girls.

Recommended Gender Adaptations

Enhancing existing EBPs to be even more effective for girls would require that program developers take into account girls' unique needs. Specific recommendations for making prevention programs more effective for girls include:

1. In general, topics to include in adolescent females programming should include dealing with stress, depression, and body image, and improving relations and communication with parents and significant others.
2. Girls need developmentally appropriate positive models and practice of skills such as conflict negotiation, drug refusal skills, and social assertiveness.
3. Program modules on dating, the meaning of love and sexual relationships, protection from date rape, unwanted pregnancy, and sexually transmitted diseases would be helpful for girls. Program design could include: a) separate activities for boys and girls, focusing on knowledge and skill development around open cross-gender communication; and b) opportunities for mixed-gender group discussions that could promote both skill development and greater shared understanding of these issues.
4. Given the importance of abuse, and particularly sexual abuse, as a significant risk factor in the development of substance abuse disorders, especially among girls and women, programs to prevent such abuse and, particularly, to support the victims and to address post-traumatic stress disorders appear to be essential (United Nations, 2008).
5. Gender-specific prevention programs should include opportunities for relationship building between girls and adult female role models and should incorporate the everyday realities of women's and girls' lives, including opportunities for girls to debunk societal and media pressures to engage in health compromising behaviors.
6. Effective gender-specific programs should be culturally tailored to address the unique needs of girls and women from varying races, ethnicities, and social classes. For example, two gender and ethnic adaptations of *SFP 6–11 Years* targeting mothers and daughters reported positive results for Hawaiians (Kameoke, 1996) and Hispanic mothers and daughters (Alvarado, 1996).

Recommendations for Future Research and Practice

The majority of substance abuse prevention programs that are not family-based are not as effective in reducing behavioral health problems in adolescent girls as in boys, possibly because these programs are not designed specifically to address the unique needs of girls. Most prevention programs are developed for universal school-based populations of both girls and boys, so they do not attend to important gender differences in the etiology of behavioral and health problems. In the prevention of substance abuse, this includes the differing pathways for girls' initiation and continued use of substances as well as the differences in the kinds of substance used and the effects of those substances. Therefore, it is important to encourage researchers with epidemiological or etiological data to conduct separate gender analyses to enhance our current understanding of the precursors of substance use among girls (Kumpfer, Smith et al., 2008). These models should be comprehensive and include family, peer, community, and school processes, and should consider both risk and protective factors (e.g., stress, depression and anxiety, social roles, assertiveness, social competencies). In addition, secondary data analyses should be conducted on prevention program data sets to determinate the factors that influence program effectiveness for girls as compared to boys (Kumpfer, 2014).

Because family-based programs appear to be the most effective in preventing behavioral health problems in both boys and girls (Foxcroft, Ireland, Lister-Sharp, Lowe, & Breen, 2003; Foxcroft & Tsertsvadze, 2012; Kumpfer, 2014; Kumpfer & Hansen, 2014; Miller & Hendrie, 2008), more funds should be allocated for dissemination of proven programs to high-risk populations of girls. More cost-effective ways of dissemination such as DVD, web, mail-out booklets, and smart phone apps should be developed, tested, and compared to the more costly group or individual family delivery. Professional training and continuing education programs for prevention specialists should include training in family-based programs as well as better specification of the practices associated with improved gender outcomes. Identifying and specifying which aspects of girls' development and girls' patterns of substance use/abuse must be incorporated into a program in order for it to be considered "gender-specific" is another critical element in addressing the growing problems with girls' substance use (Kumpfer, Smith et al., 2008).

Conclusion

To improve engagement and program efficacy, evidence-based family prevention programs should consider adaptations for both culture and gender. Culturally adapted prevention programs do increase enrollment and retention in family interventions, but it is not clear yet if they always improve outcomes. Cultural adaptation can be achieved for the least cost by hiring and training implementers from the same cultural group, who can make the language and cultural improvements even "on the spot" in interacting with families. Generic culturally sensitive family programs that have video clips or graphics that represent the major ethnic groups would be the next step in cultural adaptation.

At this point, there is insufficient research evidence or published articles to conclude whether most prevention programs are as effective for girls as for boys. A recent gender subgroup analysis of a large SFP normative database of over 4,000 families from agencies worldwide did find that the traditional 14-session SFP is equally effective for girls as for boys (Kumpfer, 2014; Magalhães & Kumpfer, 2014). In some cases, SFP was even more effective for girls despite lower base rates of risk factors, possibly because girls are more influenced by family relationships. Although this finding is laudable, the degree of effectiveness for girls as compared to boys for other evidence-based prevention programs should be investigated. In particular, parenting and family interventions with the potential to have greater protective impact on girls should publish their gender-by-program interaction analyses. Component or mediational analyses are also needed to determine which aspects of the interventions contribute to effectiveness for the two genders. Additionally, we do not know if making evidence-based programs more gender-specific would strengthen outcomes for girls. Cultural adaptation research does suggest that enrollment and retention can increase dramatically with adaptations (UNODC, 2009) and this might conceivably apply also in the case of gender.

References and Further Reading

Alvarado, R. (1996). Evaluation of the Strengthening Hispanic Mothers and Daughters Program. (Evaluation report submitted to SAMHSA Center for Substance Abuse Prevention). Unpublished manuscript.

Annenberg Institute of School Reform (2009). *Annual Report.* Providence, RI: Annenberg Institute of School Reform, Brown University.

Ary, D.V., Duncan, T. E., Biglan, A., Metzler, C. W., Noell, J.W., & Smolkowski, K. (1999). Developmental model of adolescent problem behavior. *Journal of Abnormal Child Psychology, 27*(2), 141–150.

Baker, J. H., Mitchell, K. S., Neale, M. C., & Kendler, K. S. (2010). Eating disorder symptomatology and substance use disorders: Prevalence and shared risk in a population based sample. *International Journal of Eating Disorders, 43*, 648–658.

Barber, J. G., Bolitho, F., & Bertrand, L. D. (1999). Intrapersonal versus peer group predictors of adolescent drug use. *Children and Youth Services Review, 21*(7), 565–579.

Bauman, K. E., Ennett, S. T., Foshee, V. A., Pemberton, M., King, T. S., & Koch, G. G. (2000). Influence of a family-directed program on adolescent cigarette and alcohol cessation. *Prevention Science, 1*(4), 227–237.

Beauvais, F., & Trimble, J. E. (2006). The effectiveness of alcohol and drug abuse prevention among American-Indian youth. *Handbook of Drug Abuse Prevention,* 393–410.

Berkel, C., Knight, G. P., Zeiders, K. H., Tein, J. Y., Roosa, M. W., Gonzales, N. A. et al. (2010). Discrimination and adjustment for Mexican American adolescents: A prospective examination of the benefits of culturally-related values. *Journal of Research on Adolescence, 20,* 893–915.

Bernal, G., Bonilla, J., & Bellido, C. (1995). Ecological validity and cultural sensitivity for outcome research: Issues for the cultural adaptation and development of psychosocial treatments with Hispanics. *Journal of Abnormal Child Psychology, 23*(1), 67–82.

Bernal, G. E., & Domenech Rodríguez, M. M. (2012). *Cultural adaptations: Tools for evidence based practice with diverse populations.* Washington, DC: American Psychological Association.

Biglan, A., & Metzler, C. (1999). A public health perspective for research on family-focused interventions. In R. Ashery, E. Robertson, & K. Kumpfer (Eds.), *Drug abuse prevention through family interventions* (National Institute of Drug Abuse Research Monograph on family-focused prevention research). Rockville, MD: National Institute on Drug Abuse.

Boyd-Franklin, N. (2001). Reaching out to larger systems. In interventions with multi-cultural families (Part 2). *The Family Psychologist, 17*(3), 1–4.

Brody, G. H., Chen, Y.-f., Kogan, S. M., Murry, V. M., & Brown, A. C. (2010). Long-term effects of the Strong African American Families program on youths' alcohol use. *Journal of Consulting and Clinical Psychology, 78*(2), 281–285.

Brody, G. H., Chen, Y.-f., Kogan, S. M., Yu, T., Molgaard, V. K., DiClemente, R. J., & Wingood, G. M. (2012). Family-centered program to prevent substance use, conduct problems, and depressive symptoms in Black adolescents. *Pediatrics, 129*(1), 108–115.

Burke, S., Cremeens, J., Vail-Smith, K., & Woolsey, C. (2010). Drunkorexia: Calorie restriction prior to alcohol consumption among college freshman. *Journal of Alcohol & Drug Education, 54*(2), 17–34.

Burkhart, G. (2013). *North American drug prevention programmes: Are they feasible in European cultures and contexts?* European Monitoring Center for Drugs and Drug Addiction (EMCDDA) http://www.emcdda.europa.eu/publications/thematicpapers/north-american-drug-prevention-programmes.

Cabassa, L., & Baumann, A. (2013). A two-way street: Bridging implementation science and cultural adaptations of mental health treatments. *Implementation Science, 8,* doi:10.1186/1748-5908-8-90.

Califano, J. A. (2001). Food for thought: Substance abuse and eating disorders. Paper presented at the National Center on Addiction and Drug Abuse (CASA) at Columbia University Conference, New York.

CASA. (2003). *The formative years: Pathways to substance abuse among girls and young women ages 8–22.* New York: CASA.

Caspi, A., Lynam, D., Moffitt, T. E., & Silva, P. A. (1993). Unraveling girls' delinquency: Biological, dispositional, and contextual contributions to adolescent misbehavior. *Developmental Psychology, 29,* 19–30.

Centers for Disease Control and Prevention (CDC). (2013). *Asian American populations.* Retrieved from http://www.cdc.gov/minorityhealth/populations/REMP/asian.html.

Center for Substance Abuse Prevention (2000). *Final report: The national cross-site evaluation of high-risk youth programs* (ORC MACO, 4.18-4.22). Local: EMT Associates.

Chamberlain, P., Price J. M., Reid, J. B., Landsverk, J., Fisher, P. A., & Stoolmiller, M. (2006). Who disrupts from placement in foster and kinship care? *Child Abuse and Neglect, 30,* 409–424.

Champagne, F. A. (2010). Epigenetic influence of social experiences across the lifespan. *Developmental Psychobiology, 52*(4), 299–311.

Coombes, L., Allen, D. M., & Foxcroft, D. H. (2012). An exploratory pilot study of the Strengthening Families Programme 10–14 (UK). *Drugs: Education, Prevention, and Policy, 19*(5), 387–396.

Cofsky, L. (2012). Drunkorexia: A prevalent disorder on college campuses. *The Daily Pennsylvanian.* Retrieved from http://www.thedp.com/r/17f289d6.

Dembo, R., Wothke, W., Shemwell, M., Pacheco, K., Seeberger, W., Rollie, M., & Schmeidler, J. (2000). A structural model of the influence of family problems and child abuse factors on serious delinquency among youths processed at a juvenile assessment center. *Journal of Child and Adolescence Substance Abuse, 10*(1), 17–31.

Domenech Rodríguez, M. M., & Bernal, G. (2012). Bridging the gap between research and practice in a multicultural world. In G. Bernal & M. M. Domenech Rodriguez (Eds.), *Cultural adaptations: Tools for evidence-based practice with diverse populations* (pp. 265–287). Washington, DC: American Psychological Association Press.

Donovan, J. E. (2002). Gender differences in alcohol involvement in children and adolescents: A review of the literature. In J. M. Howard, S. E. Martin, P. D. Mail, M. E. Hilton, & E. D. Taylor (Eds.). *Women and alcohol: Issues for prevention research: NIAAA research monograph no. 32* (NIH Pub. No. 96-3817, pp. 133–162). Bethesda, MD: US Department of Health and Human Services.

Dow, H. D. (2011). The acculturation processes: The strategies and factors affecting the degree of acculturation. *Home Health Care Management & Practice, 23*(3), 221–227.

Fang, L., & Schinke, S. P. (2013). Two-year outcomes of a randomized, family-based substance use prevention trial for Asian American adolescent girls. *Psychology of Addictive Behaviors, 27*(3), 788–798.

Farver, J. A. M., Bhadha, B. R., & Narang, S. K. (2002). Acculturation and psychological functioning in Asian Indian adolescents. *Social Development, 11*(1), 11–29.

Feldman, S. S., & Rosenthal, D. A. (1993). Culture makes a difference . . . or does it? A comparison of adolescents in Hong Kong, Australia, and the USA. In R. Silbereisen & E. Todt (Eds.), *Adolescence in context.* New York: Springer.

Ferrer-Wreder, L., Adamson, L., Kumpfer, K. L., & Eichas, K. (2012). Advancing intervention science through effectiveness research: A global perspective. *Child and Youth Care Forum, 41*, 109–117.

Ferrer-Wreder, L., Sundell, K., & Mansoory, S. (2012). Tinkering with perfection: Theory development in the intervention cultural adaptation field. *Child and Youth Care Forum, 41*, 149–171.

Fothergill, K. E., & Ensminger, M. E. (2006). Childhood and adolescent antecedents of drug and alcohol problems: A longitudinal study. *Drug and Alcohol Dependence, 82*, 61–76.

Foxcroft, D., Allen, D., & Coombes, L. (2005). Adaptation and Implementation of SFP 10–14 Years for U.K. Abstract submitted to Society for Prevention Research, San Antonio, May 2005. School of Health and Social Care, Oxford Brookes University, Oxford, UK.

Foxcroft, D. R., Ireland, D., Lister-Sharp, D. J., Lowe, G., & Breen, R. (2003). Longer-term primary prevention for alcohol misuse in young people: A systematic review. *Addiction, 98*, 397–411.

Foxcroft, D. R., & Tsertsvadze, A. (2012). Universal alcohol misuse prevention programmes for children and adolescents: Cochrane systematic reviews. *Perspectives in Public Health, 132*, 128–134.

Gonzalez-Guarda, R. M., Ortega, J.,Vasquez, E., & De Santis, J. (2010). La maneha negra: Substance abuse, violence and sexual risks among Hispanic males. *Western Journal of Nursing Research, 32*(1), 128–148.

Gottfredson, D., Kumpfer, K., Polizzi-Fox, D., Wilson, D., Puryear, V., Beatty, P., & Vilmenay, M. (2006). The Strengthening Washington D.C. Families Project: A randomized effectiveness trial of family-based prevention. *Prevention Science, 7,* 57–74.

Guilamo-Ramos, V. (2009). Maternal influence on adolescent self-esteem, ethnic pride and intentions to engage in risk behavior in Latino youth. *Prevention Science, 10,* 366–375.

Henggeler, S. W. (1997). The development of effective drug abuse services for youth. In J. A. Egertson, D. M. Fox, & A. I. Leshner (Eds.), *Treating drug abusers effectively* (pp. 253–279). New York: Blackwell.

Inman, A. G., Howard, E. E., Beaumont, R. L., & Walker, J. A. (2007). Cultural transmission: Influence of contextual factors in Asian Indian immigrant parents' experiences. *Journal of Counseling Psychology, 54*(1), 93.

Jirtle, R. (2010). Epigenetic mechanisms on gene expression. Plenary session I, Annual Conference of the Society for Prevention Research. Denver, Colorado (June 2, 2010).

Johnson, K., Strader, T., Berbaum, M., Bryant, D., Bucholtz, G., Collins, D. et al. (1996). Reducing alcohol and other drug use by strengthening community, family, and youth resiliency: An evaluation of the Creating Lasting Connections program. *Journal of Adolescent Research, 11*(1), 36–67.

Kameoke, V. A. (1996). *The effects of a family-focused intervention on reducing risk for substance abuse among Asian and Pacific-island youths and families: Evaluation of the Strengthening Hawaii's Families Project.* Honolulu: University of Hawaii, Social Welfare Evaluation and Research Unit.

Kerr, D., Leve, L. D., & Chamberlain, P. (2009). Pregnancy rates among juvenile justice girls in two RCTs of Multidimensional Treatment Foster Care. *Journal of Consulting and Clinical Psychology, 77,* 588–593.

Kimber, B. (2005). Cultural adaptation and preliminary results of the Strengthening Families Program 6–11 in Sweden. Paper presented at Society for Prevention Research, San Antonio, TX, full report at Department of Public Health Sciences, Karolinska Institutet, Stockholm, Sweden.

Kloos, A., Weller, R., Chan, R., & Weller, E. (2009). Gender differences in adolescent substance abuse. *Current Psychiatric Reports, 11*(2), 120–126.

Knowlton, J., Noe, T., Collins, D., Strader, T., & Bucholtz, G. (2000). Mobilizing church communities to prevent alcohol and other drug abuse: A model strategy and its evaluation. *Journal of Community Practice, 7*(2), 1–27.

Kumpfer, K. L. (2014). Family-based interventions for the prevention of substance abuse and other impulse control disorders in girls. *ISRN Addiction, 2014,* Article ID 308789.

Kumpfer, K. L., Alvarado, R., Smith, P., & Bellamy, N. (2002). Cultural sensitivity and adaptation in family-based prevention interventions. *Prevention Science, 3*(3), 241–246.

Kumpfer, K. L., Alvarado, R., & Whiteside, H. O. (2003). Family-based interventions for substance abuse prevention. *Substance Use and Misuse, 38*(11–13), 1759–1789.

Kumpfer, K. L., & Bays, J. (1995). Child abuse and alcohol and other drug abuse. In J. H. Jaffe (Eds.), *The encyclopedia of drugs and alcohol* (pp. 217–222). New York: Macmillan.

Kumpfer, K. L., & Hansen, W. (2014). Family-based prevention programs. In L. Scheier & W. Hansen, *Parenting and Teen Drug Use,* Ch. 8. Oxford: Oxford University Press.

Kumpfer, K. L., & Johnson, J. (2007). Strengthening family interventions for the prevention of substance abuse in children of addicted parents. *Adicciones, 11*(1), 1–13.

Kumpfer, K. L., & Johnson, J. L. (2009). Enhancing positive outcomes for children of substance-abusing parents, In B. Johnson (Ed.), *Addiction medicine: Science and practice.* New York: Springer.

Kumpfer, K., & Magalhães, C. (in press). *Gender guidelines on substance abuse prevention among adolescent females and males.* Vienna, Austria: United Nations Office on Drugs and Crime.

Kumpfer, K. L., Magalhães, C., & Kanse, S. (in press). Family structure, culture, and family-based interventions for health promotion. In M. Korin (Ed.), *The handbook of health promotion for children and adolescents.* New York: Springer.

Kumpfer, K. L., Magalhães, C., & Xie, J. (2012a). Cultural adaptations of evidence-based family interventions to strengthen families and improve children's outcomes. *European Journal of Developmental Psychology, 9*(1), 104–116.

Kumpfer, K. L., Pinyuchon, M., de Melo, A., & Whiteside, H. (2008). Cultural adaptation process for international dissemination of the Strengthening Families Program (SFP). *Evaluation and Health Professions, 31*(2), 226–239.

Kumpfer, K. L., Pinyuchon, M., Baharudin, R., Nolrajsuwat, K., & Xie, J. (in press). Evidence-based parenting education in the Asian and Pacific Region. In J. Ponzetti (Ed.), *Evidence-based parenting education: A global perspective*, Chapter 18. New York: Routledge.

Kumpfer, K. L., Smith, P., & Summerhays, J. (2008). A wake-up call to the prevention field: Are prevention programs for substance use effective for girls? *Substance Use and Misuse, 43*(8), 978–1001.

Kumpfer, K. L., Xie, J., & O'Driscoll, R. (2012b). Effectiveness of a culturally adapted Strengthening Families Program 12–16 Years for high risk Irish families. *Child and Youth Care Forum, 41*, 173–195.

Lanza, S. T., & Collins, L. M. (2002). Pubertal timing and the onset of substance use in females during early adolescence. *Prevention Science, 3*, 69–81.

Liddle, H. A., Dakof, G. A., Henderson, C. E., & Rowe, C. L. (2011). Implementation outcomes of Multidimensional Family Therapy-Detention to Community: A reintegration program for drug-using juvenile detainees. *International Journal of Offender Therapy and Comparative Criminology, 55*, 587–604.

Liddle, H. A., Dakof, G. A., Parker, K., Diamond, G. S., Barrett, K., & Tejeda, M. (2001). Multidimensional Family Therapy for adolescent drug abuse: Results of a randomized clinical trial. *Journal of Drug and Alcohol Abuse, 27*(4), 651–688.

Liddle, H. A., Rowe, C. L., Dakof, G. A., Henderson, C. E., & Greenbaum, P. E. (2009). Multidimensional family therapy for young adolescent substance abuse: Twelve-month outcomes of a randomized controlled trial. *Journal of Consulting and Clinical Psychology, 77*, 12–25.

Magalhães, C. (2013). *Effectiveness of the Strengthening Families Program 6–11 Years among US Portuguese immigrant families and families in Portugal compared to SFP norms* (PhD dissertation). University of Lisbon, Lisbon.

Magalhães, C., & Kumpfer, K. L. (2014). Effectiveness of the SFP 6–11 Years for Portuguese girls and boys. Paper presented at European Society of Prevention Research, Palma, Mallorca, Spain, 17 October.

Mahoney, C., Kumpfer, K., Xie, J., & Cofrin Allen, K. (2014). Effectivenesed of SFP 12–16 Years in high risk Irish youth. Paper presented at the European Society for Prevention Research annual conference, Palma, Mallorca, Spain, October, 2014.

Malouf, W. (2014). Implementing family skills pilots in South East Europe: Infrastructures needed, cost implications, value added and lessons learned. Paper presented at the 5th International Conference of the European Society for Prevention Research (EUSPR), Palma, Mallorca, Spain, October 2014.

Marek, L., Brock, D., & Sullivan, R. (2006). Cultural adaptations to a family life skills program: Implementation in rural Appalachia. *Journal of Primary Prevention*, *27*(2), 113–133.

Mazzucchelli, T. G., & Sanders, M. R. (2010). Facilitating practitioner flexibility within an empirically supported intervention: Lessons from a system of parenting support. *Clinical Psychology: Science and Practice*, *17*, 238–252.

McLean, C. A., & Campbell, C. M. (2003). Locating research informants in a multi-ethnic community: Ethnic identities, social networks and recruitment methods. *Ethnicity and Health*, *8*(1), 41–61.

Miller, T. A., & Hendrie, D. (2008). *Substance abuse prevention: Dollars and cents: A Cost-benefit analysis*. DHHS Pub. No. 07-4298. Rockville, MD: Center for Substance Abuse Prevention (CSAP), SAMHSA.

National Center on Addiction and Substance Abuse (NCASA). (2003). The formative years: Pathways to substance abuse among girls and young women ages 8–22, Report February 2003.

Ogden, T., & Halliday-Boykins, C. A. (2004). Multisystemic treatment of antisocial adolescents in Norway: Replication of clinical outcomes outside of the US. *Child & Adolescent Mental Health*, *9*(2), 77–83.

Onrust, S., & Bool, M. (2006). *Evaluatie van de Cursus Gezin aan Bod: Nederlandse versie van het Strengthening Families Program (SFP) [Evaluation of Cursus Gezin aan Bod: The distribution*. Dutch adaptation of the Strengthening Families Program (SFP)]. Utrecht, the Netherlands: Trimbos Institute.

Orte, C., March, M., Ballester, L., & Touza, C. (2007, May). Results of a family competence program adapted for Spanish drug abusing parents (2005–2006). Poster presented at the 15th Annual Conference of the Society for Prevention Research, Washington, DC.

Petrie, J., Bunn, F., & Byrne, G. (2007). Parenting programmes for preventing tobacco, alcohol or drugs misuse in children <18: A systematic review. *Health Education Research*, *22*, 177–191.

Phinney, J. (1996). When we talk about American ethnic groups, what do we mean? *American Psychologist*, *51*, 917–918.

Pickens, R. W., Svikis, D. S., Mcgue, M., Lykken, D. T., Heston, L. L., & Clayton, P. J. (1991). Heterogeneity in the inheritance of alcoholism: A study of male and female twins. *Archives of General Psychiatry*, *48*, 19–28.

Pinyuchon, M. (2010). *The effectiveness of father involvement in the Strengthening Thai Families Program*. Paper at NIDA International Forum, Scottsdale, AZ, June 12, 2010.

Reel, J. J., & Beal, K. (2009). *The hidden faces of eating disorders*. Reston, VA: AAPHERD.

Resnicow, K., Soler, R., Braithwaite, R. L., Ahluwalia, J. S., & Butler, J. (2000). Cultural sensitivity in substance use prevention. *Journal of Community Psychology*, *28*, 271–290.

Rodnium, J. (2007). Causes of delinquency: The Social Ecology Model for Thai Youth. Unpublished dissertation, Department of Health Promotion and Education, University of Utah, Salt Lake City.

Sales, E., Sambrano, S., Springer, F. J., & Turner, C. (2003). Risk, protection, and substance use in adolescents: A multi-site model. *Journal of Drug Education*, *33*(1), 91–105.

Sanders, M. R. (1999). Triple P positive parenting program: Towards an empirically validated multilevel parenting and family support strategy for the prevention of behaviour and emotional problems in children. *Clinical Child and Family Psychology Review, 2*, 71–90.

Sanders, M. R., & Kirby, J. N. (2012). Consumer engagement and the development, evaluation and dissemination of evidence-based parenting programs. *Behavior Therapy Journal, 10*, doi:10.1016/j.beth.2011.01.005.

Sanders, M., Calam, R., Durand, M., Liversidge, T., & Carmont, S. A. (2008). Does self-directed and web-based support for parents enhance the effects of viewing a reality television series based on the Triple P–Positive Parenting Programme? *Journal of Child Psychology and Psychiatry, 49*, 924–932.

Sanders, M. R., Turner, K. M. T., & Markie-Dadds, C. (2002). The development and dissemination of the Triple P—Positive Parenting Program: A multilevel, evidence-based system of parenting and family support. *Prevention Science, 3*, 173–189.

Schaeffer, C. M., & Borduin, C. M. (2005). Long-term follow-up to a randomized clinical trial of multisystemic therapy with serious and violent juvenile offenders. *Journal of Consulting and Clinical Psychology, 73*(3), 445–453.

Schinke, S. P., Cole, K. C., & Fang, L. (2009). Gender-specific intervention to reduce underage drinking in early adolescent girls: Test of a computer-mediated Mother-Daughter Program. *Journal of Studies on Alcohol Drugs, 70*, 70–77.

Schinke, S. P., Fang, L., Cole, K. C., & Cohen-Cutler, S. (2011). Preventing substance abuse among Black and Hispanic adolescent girls: Results from a computer-delivered, mother-daughter intervention approach. *Substance Use and Misuse, 46*(1), 35–45.

Schwinn, T. M., Schinke, S. P., & Di Noia, J. (2010). Preventing drug abuse among adolescent girls: Outcome data from an internet-based intervention. *Prevention Science, 11,* 24–32.

Skärstrand, E., Larsson, J., & Andreasson, S. (2008). Cultural adaptation of the Strengthening Families Programme to a Swedish Setting. *Health Education, 108*, 287–300.

Sypeck, M. F., Gray, J. J., & Ahrens, A. H. (2004). No longer just a pretty face: Fashion magazines' depictions of ideal female beauty from 1959 to 1999. *International Journal of Eating Disorders, 36*, 342–347.

Testa, M., & Livingston, J. (2009). Alcohol consumption and women's vulnerability to sexual victimization: Can reducing women's drinking prevent rape? *Substance Use and Misuse, 44*(9–10), 1349–1376.

United Nations (2008). *Depth study on violence against women, 2006.* Electronic document http://www.un.org/en/women/endviolence/pdf/VAW.pdf.

United Nations Office on Drugs and Crime (2009). *Guide to implementing family skills training programmes for drug abuse prevention.* Vienna, Austria: United Nations Office on Drugs and Crime. Electronic document https://www.unodc.org/documents/prevention/family-guidelines-E.pdf.

United Nations Office on Drugs and Crime (2010). *Compilation of evidence-based family skills training programmes.* Vienna, Austria: United Nations Office on Drugs and Crime. Retrieved from http://www.coe.int/t/dg3/children/corporalpunishment/positive%20parenting/UNODCFamilySkillsTrainingProgrammes.pdf.

US Census Bureau (2012). *America's families and living arrangements: 2012.* Retrieved from http://www.census.gov/hhes/families/data/cps2012.html.

Valentine, J. C., Biglan, A., Boruch, R. F., Castro, F. G., Collins, L. M., Flay, B. R. et al. (2011). Replication in prevention science. *Prevention Science, 12*, 103–117.

Watson, J. (2005). *Active engagement: Strategies to increase service participation by vulnerable families.* Ashfield: New South Wales: Centre for Parenting & Research.

Webster-Stratton, C. (1994). Advancing videotape parent training: A comparison study. *Journal of Consulting and Clinical Psychology, 62*(3), 583–593.

Webster-Stratton, C., Reid, M., & Stoolmiller, M. (2008). Preventing conduct problems and improving school readiness: Evaluation of the Incredible Years Teacher and Child Training Programs in high-risk schools. *Journal of Child Psychology and Psychiatry, 5,* 471–488.

Printed in the United States
by Baker & Taylor Publisher Services